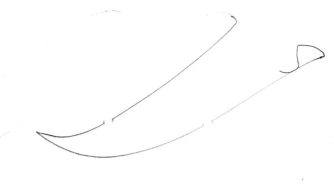

In memory of Harriette Miller,
who taught me the importance
of a wholistic approach to science and life

Contents

OPIATES

10 **Structure and Function of the Endogenous Opiate Systems: An Overview**
Henry Khachaturian and Michael E. Lewis **209**

11 **Behavioral Effects of Opiates During Development**
Gordon A. Barr **221**

12 **Development of Multiple Opioid Receptors**
Frances M. Leslie and Sandra E. Loughlin **255**

13 **Regulation of the Opioid System by Exogenous Drug Administration**
Ann Tempel **285**

14 **Consequences of Early Exposure to Opioids on Cell Proliferation and Neuronal Morphogenesis**
Ronald P. Hammer, Jr., and Kurt F. Hauser **319**

15 **Effects of Perinatal Opiate Addiction on Neurochemical Development of the Brain**
Cynthia M. Kuhn, Rolf T. Windh, and Patrick J. Little . . **341**

16 **Prenatal Ethanol Exposure: Endogenous Opioid Systems, Inappropriate Emotional Responsiveness, and Autism**
William J. Shoemaker, Priscilla Kehoe, and Ross A. Baker . **363**

Index **379**

Contributors

Ross A. Baker
Department of Psychiatry,
University of Connecticut Health
Center, Farmington, CT 06030 [**363**]

Gordon A. Barr
Hunter College, City University of
New York, and New York State
Psychiatric Institute, Columbia
University College of Physicians
and Surgeons, New York, NY 10032
[**221**]

Claire D. Coles
Human and Behavior Genetics
Laboratory, Department of
Psychiatry, Emory University
School of Medicine, and Georgia
Mental Health Institute, Atlanta,
GA 30306 [**9**]

Mary J. Druse
Department of Molecular and
Cellular Biochemistry, Loyola
University of Chicago, Stritch
School of Medicine, Maywood, IL
60153 [**139**]

Loretta Finnegan
Department of Pediatrics, Jefferson
Medical College, Thomas Jefferson
University, Philadelphia, PA
19107-5092 [**37**]

Ronald P. Hammer, Jr.
Department of Anatomy and
Reproductive Biology, University of
Hawaii School of Medicine,
Honolulu, HI 96822 [**319**]

Kurt F. Hauser
Department of Anatomy and
Neurobiology, University of
Kentucky Medical Center,
Lexington, KY 40536-0084 [**319**]

Karol A. Kaltenbach
Department of Pediatrics, Jefferson
Medical College, Thomas Jefferson
University, Philadelphia, PA
19107-5092 [**37**]

Priscilla Kehoe
Psychobiology Laboratory, Trinity
College, Hartford, CT 06106 [**363**]

Henry Khachaturian
Neuroimaging and Applied
Neuroscience Research Branch,
National Institute of Mental Health,
Rockville, MD 20857 [**209**]

Cynthia M. Kuhn
Department of Pharmacology, Duke
University Medical Center, Durham,
NC 27710 [**341**]

Frances M. Leslie
Department of Pharmacology,
University of California Irvine,
Irvine, CA 92717 [**255**]

Michael E. Lewis
Cephalon, Inc., West Chester, PA
19380 [**209**]

Patrick J. Little
Department of Pharmacology, Duke
University Medical Center, Durham,
NC 27710 [**341**]

The numbers in brackets are the opening page numbers of the contributors' articles.

Sandra E. Loughlin
Department of Anatomy and Neurobiology, University of California Irvine, Irvine, CA 92717 [255]

Michael W. Miller
Veterans Administration Medical Center and Department of Psychiatry, University of Iowa College of Medicine, Iowa City, IA 52242 [1, 47, 71]

Sam N. Pennington
Department of Biochemistry, East Carolina University, Greenville, NC 27834 [189]

Roberta J. Pentney
Department of Anatomical Sciences, School of Medicine and Biomedical Sciences, State University of New York at Buffalo, Buffalo, NY 14214 [71]

P. Kevin Rudeen
Department of Anatomy and Neurobiology, University of Missouri School of Medicine, Columbia, MO 65212 [169]

William J. Shoemaker
Department of Psychiatry, University of Connecticut Health Center, Farmington, CT 06030 [363]

Ann Tempel
Department of Psychiatry, Hillside Hospital, Long Island Jewish Medical Center, Glen Oaks, NY 11004 [285]

Glenn R. Ward
Alcohol and Brain Research Laboratory, Department of Anatomy, University of Iowa College of Medicine, Iowa City, IA 52242 [109]

James R. West
Alcohol and Brain Research Laboratory, Department of Anatomy, University of Iowa College of Medicine, Iowa City, IA 52242 [109]

Rolf T. Windh
Department of Pharmacology, Duke University Medical Center, Durham, NC 27710 [341]

Preface

During the past two decades, research on the effects of early exposure to substances of abuse has increased steadily. It was my goal to compile a book that summarizes the significant advances made in this research and that identifies gaps in our knowledge. The early literature on the toxicity of drugs in the developing nervous system was mostly phenomenological descriptions. More recent investigations have explored the mechanisms of drug action and toxicity in developing animals. These studies not only shed light on the etiology of fetal drug syndromes, but also provide insights into the mechanisms of normal development that otherwise would not be achieved from performing studies of normal development alone.

It has been my goal that this book be a multidisciplinary treatment of a single issue—the development of the central nervous system. As such, it is obviously a reflection of my conception of neuroscience, which in turn is a reflection of my training. In this regard, I would like to thank two science teachers who were crucial to my physical and intellectual development, my parents Walter and Harriette Miller. I remember fondly the times when my father and I discussed chemistry and physics over ice cream sodas. Although I have had many other teachers who deserve mention, I would like to acknowledge particularly Alan Peters. Dr. Peters was courageous enough to train a visual psychophysicist to be a developmental neuroscientist, and under his tutelage I learned classical and modern neuroanatomical techniques. I would also like to thank Richard Rieck and Brent Vogt for helping hone my craft, technically and philosophically.

This book evolved from a symposium presented at the annual meeting of the Research Society of Alcoholism in Wild Dunes, South Carolina on June 5, 1988. The symposium focused on the effects of prenatal exposure to ethanol on the development of cerebral cortex. I thank the participants of the symposium, Mary Druse, William Shoemaker, and James West, for their immediate and total support in organizing this volume. As this volume began to take shape, its scope broadened to probe more fully the mechanisms of normal and abnormal development. The chapters on opiate exposure were added to compare with those on the effects of ethanol. I appreciate greatly the diligence and the fine work of the authors in this book.

Various governmental agencies, especially the National Institute of Alcohol Abuse and Alcoholism, have supported the ongoing research in my laboratory and in neuroscience laboratories across the country. Without this support, the research described in this book would not have been done. Recently, we entered the "Decade of the Brain." It is my hope that this federal support will not flag, and that the biomedical community will be able to maintain the level of excellence upon which the citizens of the United States have come to rely and expect.

I thank the numerous scientists with whom I have spoken or whose writings I have read over the years. These interactions have stimulated my thoughts and continually replenished my batteries. I would be remiss if I do not thank Laurie Foudin, Carrie Randall, and Ed Riley, who have been particularly helpful in my growth as an alcohol researcher and have provided me with needed advice at crucial times in my career.

Finally, this book would not have taken shape were it not for the support of many people, only a few of whom I will mention. Robert Waters, an unsung hero in the award of my first grant, has sharpened my writing and editing skills. I thank the staff of Wiley-Liss for their patience and their belief that this book would be completed. My heartfelt appreciation goes to my wife Christine Waters and my daughters Hannah and Tovah. My interest in fetal alcohol syndrome began shortly before my wife became pregnant with our first child, a time when our sensitivities to the fragility of pregnancy and a subsequent new life were heightened. My family has supported and amused me when circumstances were less than ideal. They have served repeatedly as my fountain of vitality.

Michael W. Miller

Development of the Central Nervous System:
Effects of Alcohol and Opiates, pages 1–8
© 1992 Wiley-Liss, Inc.

1

The Necessity of Biomedical Research on Substance Abuse

MICHAEL W. MILLER
*Veterans Administration Medical Center and Department of Psychiatry,
University of Iowa College of Medicine, Iowa City, Iowa*

The adverse effects of substance abuse (notably ethanol) by a pregnant woman on her offspring have been discussed since biblical and medieval times (see Warner and Rosett, 1975; Randall and Nobel, 1980; Abel, 1984). The references in the old literature have been somewhat anecdotal and frequently contested. Nevertheless, until recently, alcohol and opiates were routinely used as analgesics during the birthing process. As much as 100 years ago, the scientific community was debating the existence and severity of ethanol teratogenicity (e.g., Nicloux, 1899, 1900; Sullivan, 1899; Stockard, 1910; Stockard and Craig, 1912; Stockard and Papanicolaou, 1916; Nice, 1917; Arlitt, 1919). Studies explored the effects of ethanol on the development of fish and rodents. Although these early studies were often poorly controlled, the consensus was that the exposure of developing animals to ethanol caused learning deficits, craniofacial malformations, and reductions in litter size and in the size of the surviving offspring.

The modern recognition that early exposure to ethanol affects the development of the immature organism has not been longstanding. The first report associating the consumption of ethanol during pregnancy with adverse outcomes was presented by a group of French physicians (Lemoine et al., 1968). It was not until 5 years after Jones and his colleagues published a pair of papers (Jones and Smith, 1973; Jones et al., 1973) that fetal alcohol syndrome (FAS) was given serious attention. Even so, acceptance of this syndrome by the medical community was slow. Over the past 17 years, however, interest and recognition in FAS have grown exponentially, as the original observations have been repeated and extended. Now, ethanol is among the most thoroughly studied and best understood teratogens.

The acceptance that ethanol disrupts development has come in part from biochemical studies using rats as models of FAS. The concentration of ethanol in the blood of (human and rat) fetuses is similar to that in the pregnant female (Ho et al., 1972; Kesaniemi and Sippel, 1975; Belinkoff and Hall, 1980; Guerri and Sanchis, 1985), and the placental transfer of nutrients is compromised by ethanol, not only in humans but in rats as well (e.g., Fisher et al., 1981; Henderson et al., 1981; Lin, 1985; Sanchis and Guerri, 1986). Furthermore, data from embryological and morphological studies identify some of the targets of ethanol toxicity and they show some of the permanent changes induced by early ethanol exposure (e.g., Papara-Nicholson and Telford, 1957; Clarren et al., 1978; Samson and Diaz, 1981; West et al., 1981; Phillips and Cragg, 1982; Miller, 1986; Miller and Potempa, 1990). Such changes include microencephaly, abnormal and exuberant connections, and inappropriate positioning of neurons. The function of this abnormally structured brain has been explored in physiological and behavioral investigations. These studies have shown that the functional alterations associated with ethanol exposure result from permanent effects on the developing central nervous system. Ethanol-induced defects include hyperactivity, losses in fine motor coordination, learning and memory deficits, and mental retardation (e.g., Vincent, 1958; Jones et al., 1973; Abel, 1979; Shaywitz et al., 1980; Cogan et al., 1983; Vingan et al., 1986; Miller et al., 1990; Riley and Barron, 1989). In fact, recent evidence indicates that ethanol is *the* primary cause of mental retardation for people living in the Western world (Abel and Sokol, 1986).

Interestingly, the history of research on the developmental effects of opiates somewhat parallels that on ethanol teratogenicity. As early as the late 19th century, a number of case reports were written which describe how neonates exposed to morphine in utero underwent withdrawal much like that observed in withdrawing adults (Fere, 1883; Preyer, 1885; Happel, 1892; Tate, 1899; Pettey, 1913; Menninger-Lerchenthal, 1934; Pohlisch, 1934). The bulk of this early evidence was that infants of addicted mothers often exhibited withdrawal symptoms (such as restlessness, breathing difficulties and distress, and an inconsolable shrill cry) which could be ameliorated by oral administration of paregoric. Clinical evidence indicated that as with ethanol, opiates in a pregnant woman's circulation readily cross the placental "barrier" into the fetal circulation (Preyer, 1885; Shute and Davis, 1933; Apgar et al., 1952). Early evidence demonstrated that in the rabbit, too, morphine crosses the placenta (Snyder, 1949). It was the general consensus of these early studies that after the infant had passed through withdrawal episodes, the child would not suffer any permanent damage. Thus, one of the major voids in this early literature was determining whether prenatal exposure to opiates has long-term effects on the function of the central nervous system. Recent data from human and animal studies show that early exposure to opiates has a great impact on the offspring. For example, the sizes of the body and brain of opiate-exposed offspring are reduced and the number and morphology of surviving neurons is altered (e.g., Crofford and Smith, 1973; Wilson, 1975; Zagon and McLaughlin, 1977, 1986; Ostrea and Chavez, 1979; Hauser et al., 1989; Seatriz and Hammer, 1991).

In summary, there are many similarities in the response of the developing nervous system to ethanol and to opiates. It should be noted, however, that the sequelae of early exposure to these substances are strikingly different in some respects; for example, their teratogenic effectiveness in causing craniofacial malformations. Ethanol is a potent teratogen that induces a reproducible array of craniofacial malformations, e.g., microcephaly, short palpebral fissures, hypoplastic philtrum, lowered pinnae, and thin vermillion border of the upper lip (e.g., Jones et al., 1973; Sulik et al., 1981; Clarren et al., 1988). Such dysmorphisms result from exposure to relatively low doses and/or for periods as short as 20 minutes (Kesaniemi and Sippel, 1975; Sulik et al., 1981). On the other hand, reports of craniofacial malformations resulting from early exposure to opiates are few (cf. Meyers, 1931; Ostrea and Chavez, 1979). The paucity of such reports may reflect the narrowness of the range between the dose effective in inducing facial dysmorphisms and the LD_{50} (Harpel and Gautieri, 1968).

Concurrent with the advances in our understanding of the phenomenology of early exposure to ethanol and opiates, there have been quantal leaps in our knowledge and approaches to the study of the development of the central nervous system. Investigators have made tremendous strides in attaining our current understanding of neural communication, be it at a systemic, cellular, or molecular level. One hypothesis for the etiology of various diseases that has emerged from recent research activity is that diseases recapitulate or unshield normal developmental processes. One example is the family of oncogenes. Originally, these proteins were identified as mitogens that promote the cell division of neuronal and glial precursors during the unabated growth of tumors (e.g., Aaronson et al., 1986; Klein, 1988). Evidently, however, these mitogens are of crucial importance in normal developmental processes. The chief difference in the two roles played by oncogenes is that during development, oncogenes function within the context of normal checks and balances, whereas during the progress of cancer such governances apparently are eliminated or dysfunctional. Thus, it appears that the growth of cancerous tissue results from the disinhibition of normal developmental processes. Another example is the protein identified by the antibody ALZ-50 (Wolozin et al., 1986). In immature animals, this protein is expressed in neurons which apparently degenerate as a natural consequence of normal development. The epitope identified by ALZ-50 is re-expressed in the brains of Alzheimer's patients (Wolozin et al., 1988; Al-Ghoul and Miller, 1989; Ueda et al., 1990).

Centuries-old questions basic to neuroscience have received large infusions of activity that have brought about new insights into how the nervous system develops and functions. For example, during the past 5 years, hypotheses on the molecular bases of learning and memory have been forwarded. Such hypotheses include the gating of the neurotransmitter glutamate at the N-methyl-d-aspartate receptor and the role of oncogene products such as FOS as signal transducers essential for mediating short-term memory (Morgan and Curran, 1989; Nicoll et al., 1988; Wickens, 1988). Whether right or wrong, these hypotheses provide useful frameworks for future research. This background of activity has provided incentives and tools with which to explore the toxic effects of ethanol and opiates on the central nervous system. Our challenge is to incorporate these new ideas and techniques in our efforts to unravel the mechanism of drug toxicity in the developing animal. Furthermore, it cannot be overemphasized that such inquiries are much more than simple examinations of pathological processes; they provide a unique opportunity to explore the intricacies of normal neuronal ontogeny.

This volume is divided into three segments. Chapters 2 and 3 describe the clinical ramifications of the prenatal exposure to ethanol or to opiates. These chapters broach issues related to the behavior and learning deficits of substance-exposed children.

The next two sets of chapters carefully examine the effects of ethanol and opiates on neural ontogeny at the molecular, cellular, and systemic levels. Chapters 4–9 focus on the effects of ethanol on the various stages of neuronal development, cell proliferation, migration, differentiation, and death, as well as examine the permanent defects in neuronal structure, synaptology, and plasticity. Particular interest is devoted to an examination of some of the possible mechanisms by which ethanol alters the development of various chemical systems (e.g., hormonal, neurotransmitter, and second messenger systems) that are crucial to the normal development and function of the nervous system.

Chapters 10–16 explore the effects of opiates on neuronal development. Unlike ethanol, a number of opioids are produced endogenously, hence three chapters examine the structure and function of opiate systems, the behaviors that are attributed to opiate systems, and the development of these systems. Three of the chapters examine the effects of early exposure to opiates on the development of the central nervous system in a manner which parallels the chapters on ethanol toxicity. That is, the effects of opiates on cell proliferation, neuronal morphogenesis, and neurochemical development are described. The last chapter serves as a bridge between the presentations on the effects of ethanol and opiates; it relates how early exposure to ethanol affects the endogenous opioid systems and the behaviors associated with these systems.

The authors in this book refer to many models that have been used to parallel the human situation of substance abuse. Accordingly, laboratory animals have been exposed acutely or chronically during the prenatal and/or postnatal period. In most cases, the laboratory animal of choice has been the rat; however, the specific choices are described in each chapter. Suffice it to say that the development occurring during the gestation period of the rat (usually 22 days) is equivalent to the maturation occurring during the first two trimesters of human pregnancy, and that the first 10 days in the rat's life is equivalent to the development that occurs during the third trimester of a human's pregnancy.

The history of research on the effects of early exposure to ethanol contrasts with that on opiate exposure. Simplified, basic science research on the effects of ethanol has preceded the clinical descriptions of FAS, whereas clinical descriptions of the problems caused by early exposure to opiates have preceded the biomedical investigations. While some steps have been made, the scientific community is now in a position to operate as one in addressing the important clinical, social, and biomedical issues of substance abuse.

During the past two decades, basic scientists and substance abuse researchers have experienced revolutions, but unfortunately, these gains have largely followed parallel tracks. The products of both lines of research can be synergistic, but we need more cross-pollination among researchers. It is my hope that after reading this volume, readers can begin to fathom the numbers of unformed, but essential questions that have yet to be addressed. More investigators (e.g., biochemists, cell and molecular biologists, pharmacologists, and physiologists) must be enlisted if we are to understand the mechanisms of how the exquisite balance of neural development is disrupted by drugs of abuse. Such research is important not only for the narrow goal of understanding the effects of such drugs on the developing nervous system, but also in providing a unique insight into the normal development and function of the brain. As Theognis wrote 2,500 years ago, "Wine is wont to show the mind of man." [*Sententiae. No. 500*]

REFERENCES

Aaronson SA, Bishop JM, Sugimura T, Terada M, Toyoshima K, Vogt PK (1986): "Oncogenes and Cancer." Utrecht: VNU Science Press BV.

Abel E (1979): Prenatal effects of alcohol on adult learning in rats. Pharmacol Biochem Behav 10:239–243.

Abel EL (1984): "Fetal Alcohol Syndrome and Fetal Alcohol Effects." New York: Plenum.

Abel EL, Sokol RJ (1986): Fetal alcohol syndrome is now a leading cause of mental retardation. Lancet 2:1222.

Al-Ghoul WM, Miller MW (1989): Transient expression of Alz-50-immunoreactivity in developing rat neocortex: A marker for naturally occurring neuronal death? Brain Res 481:361–367.

Apgar V, Burns JJ, Brodie BB, Papper EM (1952): Transmission of meperidine across human placenta. Am J Obstet Gynecol 64:1368–1370.

Arlitt AH (1919): The effect of alcohol on the intelligent behavior of the white rat. Psychol Monogr 26:1–50.

Belinkoff S, Hall OW (1980): Intravenous alcohol during labor. Am J Obstet Gynecol 59:429–432.

Clarren S, Ellsworth C, Sumi M, Streissguth A, Smith DW (1978): Brain malformations related to prenatal exposure to ethanol. J Pediatr 92:64–67.

Clarren SK, Astley SJ, Bowden DM (1988): Physical anomalies and developmental delays in nonhuman primate infants exposed to weekly doses of ethanol during gestation. Teratology 37:561–569.

Cogan DC, Cohen LE, Sparkman G (1983): Effects of gestational alcohol on the development of neonatal reflexes in the rat. Neurobehav Toxicol Teratol 5:517–522.

Crofford M, Smith AA (1973): Growth retardation in young mice treated with *dl*-methadone. Science 181:947.

Férè C (1883): De la morphomanie au point de vue de la grossees et de la née du foetus. Comm Soc Biol Sem Med p. 294.

Fisher SE, Barnicle, MA Steis B, Holzman I, Van Thiel DH (1981): Effects of acute ethanol exposure upon in vivo leucine uptake and protein synthesis in the fetal rat. Pediatr Res 15:335–339.

Guerri C, Sanchis R (1985): Acetaldehyde and alcohol levels in pregnant rats and their fetuses. Alcohol 2:267–270.

Happel JJ (1892): Morphinism in its relation to the sexual functions and appetite, and its effect on the off-spring of the users of the drug. Med Surg Rep 68:403–407.

Harpel HS, Jr, Gautieri RF (1968): Morphine-induced fetal malformations. I. Exencephaly and axial skeletal fusions. J Pharm Sci 57:1590–1597.

Hauser KF, McLaughlin PJ, Zagon IS (1989): Endogenous opioid systems and the regulation of dendritic growth and spine formation. J Comp Neurol 290:13–22.

Henderson GI, Turner D, Patwardhan RV, Lumeng L, Hoyumpa AM, Schenker S (1981): Inhibition of placental valine uptake after acute and chronic maternal ethanol consumption. J Pharmacol Exp Ther 216:465–472.

Ho BT, Fritchie GE, Idanpaan-Heikkila JE, McIssac WM (1972): Placental transfer and tissue distribution of ethanol-1-C^{14}. A radioautographic study in monkeys and hamsters. Q J Stud Alcohol 33:485–494.

Jones KL, Smith DW (1973): Recognition of the fetal alcohol syndrome in early infancy. Lancet 2:999–1001.

Jones KL, Smith, DW, Ulleland CN, Streissguth AP (1973): Pattern of malformation in offspring of alcoholic mothers. Lancet 1:1267–1271.

Kesaniemi YA, Sippel HW (1975): Placental and fetal metabolism of acetylaldehyde in rat. I. Contents of ethanol and acetylaldehyde in placenta and fetus of the pregnant rat during ethanol oxidation. Acta Pharmacol Toxicol 37:43–48.

Klein G (1988): "Cellular Oncogene Activation." New York: Marcel Dekker.

Lemoine PH, Harousseau H, Borteyru JP, Menuet JC (1968): Les enfants de parents alcooliques: Anomalies observées à propos de 127 cas. Ouest Med 21:476–482.

Lin GW-J (1985): Altered placental folate coenzyme distribution by ethanol consumption during pregnancy. Nutr Rep Int 31:1375–1383.

Menninger-Lerchenthal E (1934): Die Morphin Kronkheit der Neugeborenen Morphinstischer Mutter. Monastsschr Kinderheilkd 60:182–193.

Meyers HB (1931): The effect of chronic poisoning upon growth, the oestrus cycle and fertility of the white rat. J Pharmacol Exp Ther 41:317–323.

Miller MW (1986): Fetal alcohol effects on the generation and migration of cerebral cortical neurons. Science 233:1308–1311.

Miller MW, Chiaia NL, Rhoades RW (1990): Intracellular recording and labeling study of corticospinal neurons in the rat somatosensory cortex: Effect of prenatal exposure to ethanol. J Comp Neurol 296:1–15.

Miller MW, Potempa G (1990): Numbers of neurons and glia in mature rat somatosensory cortex: Effects of prenatal exposure to ethanol. J Comp Neurol 293:92–102.

Morgan JI, Curran T (1989): Stimulus-transcription coupling in neurons: Role of cellular immediate-early genes. Trends Neurosci 12:459–462.

Nice LB (1917): Comparative studies on the effects of alcohol, nicotine, tobacco smoke and caffeine on white mice. I. Effects on reproduction and growth. J Exp Zool 12:133–147.

Nicloux M (1899): Sur le passage de l'alcool ingeré de la mère au foetus, en particulier chez la femme. C Roy Soc Biol 51:980–982.

Nicloux M (1900): Passage de l'alcool ingeré de la mère au foetus et passage de l'alcool ingeré dans le lait, en particulier chez la femme. Obstétrique 5:97–132.

Nicoll RA, Kauer JA, Malenka RC (1988): The current excitement in long-term potentiation. Neuron 1:97–103.

Ostrea EM, Chavez CJ (1979): Perinatal problems (excluding neonatal withdrawal) in maternal drug addiction: A study of 830 cases. J Pediatr 94:292–295.

Papara-Nicholson D, Telford IR (1957): Effects of alcohol on reproduction and fetal development in the Guinea pig. Anat Rec 127:438–439.

Pettey GE (1913): "Narcotic Drug Diseases and Allied Ailments." Tennessee: J.A. Davis Co.

Phillips SC, Cragg BG (1982): Change in susceptibility of rat cerebellar Purkinje cells to damage by alcohol during fetal, neonatal, and adult life. Neuropathol Appl Neurobiol 8:441–454.

Pohlisch K (1934): Die Kinder mannlicher and weiblicher Morphinisten. Leipzig, George Thieme.

Preyer W (1885): Specialle Physiologie des Embryo. Leipzig, T. Grieben.

Randall CL, Nobel EP (1980): Alcohol abuse and fetal growth and development. Adv Subst Abuse 1:327–367.

Riley EP, Barron S (1989): The behavioral and neuroanatomical effects of prenatal alcohol exposure in animals. Ann NY Acad Med 562:173–177.

Samson HH, Diaz J (1981): Altered development of brain by neonatal ethanol exposure: Zinc levels during and after exposure. Alcohol Clin Exp Res 5:563–569.

Sanchis R, Guerri C (1986): Alcohol-metabolizing enzymes in placenta and fetal liver: Effect of chronic ethanol intake. Alcohol Clin Exp Res 10:39–44.

Seatriz JV, Hammer RP (1991) Effects of endogenous and exogenous opiates on neuronal development in rat cerebral cortex. Brain Res Bull (in press).

Shaywitz SE, Cohen DJ, Shaywitz BA (1980): Behavior and learning difficulties in children of normal intelligence born to alcoholic mothers. J Pediatr 96:978–982.

Shute E, Davis ME (1933): The effect on the infant of morphine administered in labor. Surg Gynecol Obstet 57:727–736.

Snyder FF (1949): "Obstetric Analgesia and Anesthesia. Their Effects Upon Labor and the Child." Philadelphia: W.B. Saunders.

Stockard CR (1910): The influence of alcohol and other anesthetics on embryonic development. Am J Anat 10:369–392.

Stockard CR, Craig DM (1912): An experimental study of the influence of alcohol on the germ cells and the developing embryos of mammals. Arch Entw Mech 35:569–597.

Stockard CR, Papanicolaou G (1916): A further analysis of the hereditary transmission of degeneracy and deformities by the descendants of alcoholized mammals. Am Nat 50:144–177.

Sulik KK, Johnston MC (1983): Sequence of developmental alterations following acute ethanol exposure in mice: Craniofacial features of the fetal alcohol syndrome. Am J Anat 166:257–269.

Sulik KK, Johnston MC, Webb MA (1981): Fetal alcohol syndrome: Embryogenesis in a mouse model. Science 214:936–938.

Sullivan WC (1899): A note on the influence of maternal inebriety on the offspring. J Ment Sci 45:489–503.

Tate MA (1899): The transmissibility of morphine. Cincinnati Lancet- Clinic 43:598–603.

Ueda K, Masliah E, Saitoh T, Bakalis SL, Scoble, H, Kosik KS (1990): Alz-50 recognizes a phosphorylated epitope of *tau* protein. J Neurosci 10:3295–3304.

Vincent NM (1958): The effects prenatal alcoholism upon motivation, emotionality, and learning in the rat. Am Psych 13:401.

Vingan RD, Dow-Edwards DL, Riley EP (1986): Cerebral metabolic alterations in rats following prenatal alcohol exposure: A deoxyglucose study. Alcohol Clin Exp Res 10:22–26.

Warner RH, Rosett HL (1975): The effects of drinking on offspring. An historical survey of the American and British literature. J Stud Alcohol 36:1395–1420.

West JR, Hodges CA, Black Jr AC (1981): Prenatal exposure to ethanol alters the organization of hippocampal mossy fibers in rats. Science 211:957–959.

Wickens J (1988): Electrically coupled but chemically isolated synapses: Dendritic spines and calcium in a rule for calcium modification. Prog Neurobiol 31:507–528.

Wilson GS (1975): Somatic growth effects of perinatal addiction. Addict Dis 2:333–345.

Wolozin BL, Pruchnicki A, Dickson DW, Davies P (1986): A neuronal antigen in the brain of Alzheimer's patients. Science 232:648–650.

Wolozin BL, Scicutella A, Davies P (1988): Re-expression of a developmentally regulated protein in Alzheimer's disease and Down's syndrome. Proc Natl Acad Sci USA 85:6202–6206.

Zagon IS, McLaughlin PJ (1977): Morphine and brain growth retardation in the rat. Pharmacology 15:276–282.

Zagon IS, McLaughlin PJ (1986): Opioid antagonist (naltrexone) modulation of cerebellar development: Histological and morphometric studies. J Neurosci 6:1424–1432.

Development of the Central Nervous System:
Effects of Alcohol and Opiates, pages 9–36
© 1992 Wiley-Liss, Inc.

2

Prenatal Alcohol Exposure and Human Development

CLAIRE D. COLES
Human and Behavior Genetics Laboratory, Department of Psychiatry, Emory University School of Medicine, and Georgia Mental Health Institute, Atlanta, Georgia

INTRODUCTION

The use of alcoholic beverages is apparently as widespread as human culture. In most cultures where alcohol is permitted, women, including women of childbearing age, drink alcohol regularly although they may do so somewhat less heavily than men (Blume, 1986) and may be more subject to social sanctions for abusive drinking (Sandmaier, 1980). A national survey (National Institute on Drug Abuse [NIDA], 1988) estimated that two-thirds of American women of childbearing age drank alcohol. These figures probably differ somewhat in different populations (Smith et al., 1986a; Holtzman, 1991).

Given the extent of alcohol use (and abuse), it seems extraordinary that it was not until 20 years ago that its potential for causing birth defects and damage to the central nervous system (CNS) as a result of prenatal exposure was described. At that time, several researchers (Lemoine et al., 1968; Ulleland, 1970) reported on the offspring of alcoholic women, and Jones and Smith (1973) named the fetal alcohol syndrome (FAS). Warner and Rosett (1975) found that there were a number of historical references to the effects of alcohol in pregnancy during the 18th and 19th centuries but that the existence of FAS and other alcohol-related birth defects (ARBD) was denied or ignored for most of the 20th century.

In the two decades since FAS was rediscovered, a great deal of research (Abel, 1982, 1984) has focused on describing the extent and nature of the effects of prenatal alcohol exposure on human development, on animal models of development, and on the search for a mechanism that will explain the means by which alcohol has its effects on the developing organism. The results suggest that the effects of prenatal alcohol exposure are significant in many ways—theoretically, socially, economically, and in terms of human suffering.

According to estimates compiled by the Centers for Disease Control (Holtzman, 1990), full FAS may occur one to three times in every 1,000 births, making alcohol exposure one of the most frequent causes of mental retardation (Abel and Sokol, 1987). In addition, a substantial number of individuals may show less severe but still observable effects of exposure. These have been termed ARBD or fetal alcohol effects (FAE). It has been estimated that three to four infants per 1,000 may show ARBD at birth. Finally, an unknown number of individuals may have more subtle effects on the CNS whose consequences for behavior and development are still under investigation.

Rosett and Weiner (1984) postulated that 5–10% of pregnant women drink at levels high enough to place their fetuses at risk for some of the effects described above. Abel and Sokol (1987) estimated that the cost of treatment of infants and children with fetal alcohol exposure may amount to $321 million a year in the United States alone. These costs include hospitalization in the neonatal period, treatment of organic and sensorineural disorders, and care and treatment of the mentally retarded. These authors also pointed out that, given these costs and the fact that FAS is preventable, the amount of money spent on research and treatment is very low relative to other handicapping disorders.

In addition, there are other, less well defined costs, both to the individual who is affected and to the rest of society. Exposed children, even those who do not show the full syndrome, are more likely to need medical, social, and educational services than are unexposed children. Their parents and caretakers may be less able to provide them with these services, as well as other kinds of positive parenting.

Given the real and potential problems associated with prenatal alcohol exposure, it is important to understand the nature and extent of the effects which have been documented at this time, as well as the gaps which still exist in the understanding of this area.

RANGE OF DEVELOPMENTAL EFFECTS OF PRENATAL ALCOHOL EXPOSURE

A teratogen is any agent which leads to physical defects in the developing offspring. As Streissguth (1986) has pointed out, alcohol is a classic teratogen capable of producing the whole range of outcomes identified with such agents. These can range from mortality through dysmorphia and growth retardation to behavioral deficits.

Fetal Wastage

For the individual fetus, the most serious possible consequence is nonviability. Pregnancies complicated by alcohol abuse are associated with a higher risk for a number of obstetrical and perinatal complications due both to the effects of the alcohol exposure and to associated factors like cigarette smoking and poor prenatal care (Kaminski et al., 1978; Russell and Skinner, 1988). Negative outcomes include reduced fertility (Russell, 1985), a higher frequency of spontaneous abortions and fetal deaths (Anokute, 1986; Harlap and Shlon, 1980), and preterm birth (Abel, 1982). Research has demonstrated (Kline et al., 1980) a higher incidence of pregnancy loss when reported drinking reaches 2 ozs of alcohol per week, although usually much larger amounts are reported.

Fetal Alcohol Syndrome

The most serious consequence of prenatal alcohol exposure in surviving offspring is FAS, which is usually defined by the presence of three kinds of signs (Sokel and Clarren, 1989).

Dysmorphia

The most obvious and, therefore, the usually documented consequences of teratogenic exposure are the physical defects. These dysmorphic effects, or congenital anomalies, occur as a result of exposure during the embryonic or early fetal period of development. A number of physical deficits have been observed to be the results of prenatal alcohol exposure. Most well known is the facial dysmorphia (craniofacial anomalies) associated with FAS. These include an underdevelopment of the midline of the face (hypoplastic midface) which is often associated with an absence of the philtrum, the groove in the upper lip between the base of the nose and the vermillion or colored portion of the lip. The upper vermillion is often thinned and the opening of the eye (palpebral fissure) is shortened (Jones et al., 1973). Ears may be low set and rotated and this may be associated with abnormalities of the inner ear. In addition, children may have cardiac problems, defects of the urogenital region, skeletal abnormalities (Streissguth et al., 1985), vision (Stromland, 1981), hearing problems (Church and Gerkin, 1988), and dental abnormalities (Barnett and Shusterman, 1985). Immunological problems (Johnson et al., 1981) have also been reported in one study. Physical therapy examination may reveal abnormalities of gait, persistence of primative reflexes, and other motor deficits (Kyllerman et al., 1985).

There has been some suggestion that the dysmorphic facial features that distinguish children with FAS or FAE are less apparent in middle and later childhood (Spohr et al., 1989). However, other researchers, following samples of FAS and alcohol-affected children, have found that the dysmorphia is persistent and easily identified even after many years, and that its extent can be predicted reliably during the neonatal period (Smith et al., 1990; Streissguth et al., 1985).

Growth retardation

Growth retardation is another defining characteristic of FAS and is said to occur when the individual is in the lowest 10th percentile for that age. In infants who are exposed to alcohol, growth retardation occurs in utero and encompasses several measures of growth—birthweight, length, and head circumference—resulting in full-term infants who are small for gestational age. Among FAS children, this deficit is persistent over childhood, although the mechanism for their lack of growth is not clear (Streissguth, 1986; Kyllerman et al., 1985). In fact, Ulleland (1970) first noticed that alcohol might be an etiological factor in a sample of children hospitalized for failure to thrive. The growth deficit associated with alcohol is evidently different from that seen as result of cigarette smoking, which often accompanies alcohol abuse, because although infants of women who smoke cigarettes are smaller at birth (Pirani, 1978), they usually gain weight and grow normally after birth. Streissguth, who has been following a number of children with a diagnosis of FAS, has found that growth, particularly for head circumference and height, is persistently about two standard deviations below normal, although weight may be less affected (Streissguth et al., 1985).

Among children who are not FAS or FAE and who receive adequate nutrition, the relatively milder growth deficit seen at birth may not be persistent, although Barr et al. (1984) reported that it was still measurable among 8-month-olds in their middle-class sample of social and moderate drinkers. In addition, these growth variables may interact with other factors. In prospective studies of exposed children who were not necessarily FAS or FAE, Coles et al. (1991) found persistent differences in height and head circumference but not weight among 6-year-olds from a low-income black population, while Stresssiguth et al. (1989a) reported no such effects in 7-year-old white middle-class children.

CNS damage

Evidence of damage to the CNS is the third defining feature of FAS. In addition to the large animal literature (Abel, 1982), there is evidence of direct and extensive neurological damage in autopsy studies of FAS children (Clarren, 1986).

Among surviving offspring, neurological damage can be inferred from the increased incidence among alcoholized children of mental retardation, (Streissguth, 1986), motor problems (Kyllerman et al., 1985), and neonatal evidence of CNS effects (Coles et al., 1985). More difficult to demonstrate is that alcohol is specifically a behavioral teratogen that even in the absence of dysmorphia and growth deficits can affect behavior in more subtle ways through its effect on the CNS.

A behavioral teratogen can be expressed through deficits in cognition, arousal and attention, fine and gross motor control, and social and emotional development (Vorhees, 1986), presumably as the consequence of damage to the CNS. Because of these possible consequences, the behavioral effects of prenatal alcohol exposure have been an area of growing concern (Meyers and Riley, 1986).

Fetal Alcohol Effects or Alcohol-Related Birth Defects

Less seriously affected children who cannot be classified as showing full FAS may be classified as having FAE or ARBD if they demonstrate signs in two of the three defining categories or if they have some other deficit which is probably the result of their prenatal exposure (Sokol and Clarren, 1989). In many ways, this distinction is arbitrary since it relies on a categorical classification of a continuous phenomenon. However, it can be useful in indicating that individuals are less seriously affected by their exposure or have some effects which do not usually appear as part of the classic definition of FAS. Thus, a child who is not growth retarded but shows some dysmorphia, cardiac anomalies, and evidence of mild neurological problems would be said to be showing fetal alcohol effects. This class of individuals is probably larger, but less noticeable, than those with FAS. The outcome for such children may be problematic. Although they are less frankly affected than those with FAS, such children were found by Streissguth and Randels (1988) to have equal academic and greater social problems. The authors attributed this finding to social factors but also cautioned that prediction of intelligence and adaptive skills from physical status was unreliable.

Nondysmorphic Children and Offspring of Moderate Drinkers

A final group of affected individuals is also hypothesized. These are the offspring of moderate drinkers or children with no evident physical effects of their prenatal exposure who may have some behavioral effects. Given the distribution of alcohol use among women of childbearing age (NIDA, 1988) as well as the variable effects of exposure, this mildly affected group may be much larger than those who are obviously affected at birth. However, for many reasons, it is difficult to demonstrate that problems in such individuals are the result of their prenatal alcohol exposure. Effects of mild damage to the CNS would be primarily behavioral and it is difficult to demonstrate that these are specifically the result of alcohol exposure and not associated factors. The evidence for these effects has been provided by prospective studies of children with known prenatal exposure.

BEHAVIORAL EFFECTS OF PRENATAL ALCOHOL EXPOSURE

In some ways, the behavioral outcomes of alcohol exposure are of greatest long-term significance for the affected individuals and for society which must provide educational, medical, and social services. However, these outcomes are the most difficult to study. Complex human behavioral phenomena require a variety of methods, each of which may contribute its own portion of the "truth." In the examination of human development, experimental studies are not possible for ethical reasons, and animal studies cannot answer questions about more complex human behaviors although they are invaluable in confirmation of hypotheses about structural and biological effects. As a result, our understanding of the behavioral consequences of prenatal alcohol exposure in humans is dependent on limited evidence from retrospective and prospective studies of children whose mothers drank in pregnancy. As is usually the case, the individuals who are investigated through these two kinds of research protocols tend to be quite different. Retrospective studies of children identified as affected or as offspring of alcoholic mothers have described a number of behavioral features associated with FAS and FAE. Prospective studies, on the other hand, have followed infants born to mothers with various drinking behaviors and charted their development as a function of that exposure. The majority of the children in prospective studies are not FAS, FAE, or children of alcoholics. Therefore, prospective studies allow examination of the more subtle effects of a wide range of prenatal alcohol exposure.

Studies of Dysmorphic Children

Because their appearance identifies them and because of the association of dysmorphia with the other negative consequences of alcohol exposure, dysmorphic children are more likely than other alcohol-affected children to be identified and referred for evaluation and treatment. If it is indeed true that such children are the most seriously affected, they should be expected to manifest the most extreme kinds of behavioral and intellectual problems associated with alcohol exposure. Therefore, study of these children may outline the areas of behavioral concern.

In a number of studies, these children have been found to show mental retardation, usually with intelligence quotients (IQs) in the mild (50–70) range. However, the range of outcomes is quite broad. Individuals are seen who are severely and profoundly affected (IQ <50) while higher intelligence is possible with borderline (IQ = 70–85) and low normal scores (IQ = 86–100) not uncommon. Intelligence appears to be correlated in a general way with degree of dysmorphia and growth retardation but the relationship is far from linear (Streissguth, 1986).

Iosub et al. (1981) reported on a sample of 63 patients diagnosed as FAS whose mothers were chronic alcoholics. Some children had been reared in foster homes and some with their biological mothers. Although abnormal facies (57%), mental retardation (46%), developmental delays (41%), and growth retardation (39–57%) were often noted, the most common deficits cited for this group were "hyperactivity" (74%) and speech problems (80%). School problems were common. Speech problems and hyperactivity were found even in individuals who lacked dysmorphic features. While the last two findings are interesting, verification of their relationship to prenatal alcohol exposure requires evaluation of a similarly disadvantaged control group to assure that they are not the result of environmental factors.

Steinhausen et al. (1982) examined children with FAS in relation to control groups of nonaffected children. Although mental retardation was the most frequent outcome found in the alcohol group, other deficits noted included speech and language problems, hyperactivity, sleep disturbances, stereotypic behavior, and an increased incidence of behavior problems.

Horowitz (1985), comparing FAE children aged 7–12 years with children with learning disabilities and with normal children of the same age, educational experience, and social class, found that alcohol-exposed children had poorer test scores than both other groups and were more often referred for special educational services.

Platzman et al. (1986) found that dysmorphic infants were smaller and had more problematic medical histories than children of nondrinkers and a matched group of children of drinkers who were not dysmorphic. In addition, dysmorphic children were consistently lowest on tests of mental and motor development at 6, 12, and 24 months, while the scores of the nondysmorphic infants and the nonexposed infants did not differ significantly. Also noted in these children were poor weight gain (sometimes to the extent that failure to thrive was a concern), distractibility, delayed language development, particularly expressive language development, and frequent illnesses. There were also differences in the medical and social histories of substance abusing mothers who had dysmorphic children that may have been related to children's outcome.

In general, when clinically referred dysmorphic children are examined, they show not only the abnormal physical features associated with alcohol exposure but often are smaller physically and intellectually impaired. In addition, they appear to have behavioral impairments as well, including speech deficits, hyperactivity, and an increased incidence of school failure and psychiatric disorders. However, understanding of these outcomes is confounded by other factors associated with maternal substance abuse.

Studies of Exposed Children of Alcoholic Mothers

A second (and probably overlapping) group of children who have been studied retrospectively are children who were not identified primarily as FAS but whose mothers have been diagnosed as alcoholics who were drinking during the child's gestation.

Aronsson et al. (1985) paired 21 children born to alcoholic mothers with controls matched for sex, age, birthweight, gestational age, and living area. Children of alcoholics were found to have significantly lower mean cognitive scores (X = 95, s.d. = 12) than did controls (X = 112, s.d. = 10) and to have more perceptual problems. No differences in development were found as a result of biological versus foster home placement. In a further report (Aronsson and Olegard, 1987), 60% of 8- and 9-year-old children were found to have significant intellectual deficits and to require special educational services.

Shaywitz et al. (1980) reported behavior and learning problems as well as fine and gross motor difficulties among 15 children of normal intelligence born to alcoholic mothers. School failure and referral for special educational services were common with hyperactivity noted in all but one child. Larsson and Bohlin (1987) reported that 80% of the children of alcohol abusing mothers whom they studied had either behavioral or psychomotor problems.

In summary, among children who have alcoholic mothers, many of the same behavioral deficits were noted as were seen among dysmorphic children, although in somewhat attenuated form. This difference may be related to the wider range of outcomes in this group since not all were FAS.

These retrospective studies, while they cannot discriminate postnatal environmental from prenatal influences, do indicate areas for further study. Based on these reports, investigation of various aspects of development is indicated. These aspects are intellectual levels, language development, motor performance, perceptual/motor development, emotional and social status, attention and hyperactivity, and academic performance.

Developmental Risk and Alcohol Exposure: Prospective Studies

Another approach to the study of the effects of prenatal alcohol exposure on development is to study prospectively a broader range of exposure among women who drink at various levels. If alcohol has particular behavioral effects, these should be evident in statistical differences between groups of infants with different exposure.

There have been several such studies (Holtzman, 1990) and these have differed somewhat in methodology so that, despite a general similarity, there are some discrepancies in outcome. Important differences include: type of population studied (middle versus lower class; predominantly white, predominantly black, mixed); methods for ascertaining drinking (e.g., number of assessment points); point in pregnancy at which drinking was assessed (first, second, third trimester, postpartum); types of dependent measures used; and length of follow-up. Some studies have focused on outcome in the neonatal period (e.g., Rosett et al., 1980) and others have followed children for longer periods.

At the present time, there is a good deal of published information about the effects of prenatal exposure in the neonatal period and very little about development beyond that period. The information about neonatal effects is suggestive but not adequate to predict what the long-term effects will be. This difficulty arises from the nature of the developmental process in infancy which makes prediction from neonatal status very difficult, particularly when effects are relatively mild. Because of the discontinuities in development (McCall, 1979), discovery of the relationship between prenatal factors and neonatal status with later cognitive, emotional, and social consequences requires following large samples of exposed infants and appropriate control groups from the prenatal period through adolescence. While this process is not yet complete, the studies which have been done have documented effects after infancy and into the early school age period.

To date the following patterns have been found by prospective studies of alcohol-exposed children.

Neonatal period: alterations in growth and behavior

The studies of prenatal alcohol exposure in samples of women followed prospectively have produced results that are similar to those found in the studies of children of heavier drinkers but in attenuated form. A reduction in birthweight is the most obvious and consistently found consequence in alcohol-exposed children who are somewhat smaller than nonexposed children even when no other signs of FAS are present (Little, 1977). This effect is found consistently and also appears to be related to the duration of exposure (Olegard et al., 1979; Rosett et al., 1980).

In the low socioeconomic status (SES) Atlanta sample, 293 full-term black infants were placed in three birthweight categories (eliminating those who weighed less than 1,500 g who were all dysmorphic and obviously alcohol affected). This was done in order to establish the relative risk (RR) for lower birthweight as the result of duration of maternal drinking (Coles et al., 1987a). The weight categories were: low birthweight (< 2,500 g), "questionable" (2,500–< 3,000 g), and full weight (> 3,000 g). Drinking categories concerned the length of time during pregnancy that exposure occurred. These were: 1) never drank in pregnancy; 2) stopped in the second trimester; 3) continued throughout gestation. It was found that alcohol use throughout pregnancy was associated with a higher incidence of low (< 2,500 g) and questionable (< 3,000 g) birthweights. In this population, the RR of low birthweight (< 2,500 g) was 3.08 for those who stopped drinking and 5.45 for those who continued compared with the control group. For the questionable category, the RR was 1.04 and 1.15, and for the normal weight category, drinking and stopping in the second trimester reduced the probability of this weight range to 0.87 versus the nonexposed infants; for those who continued to drink, the probability of having a normal weight infant was only 0.69 compared with the controls.

Because low birthweight, resulting either from preterm birth or from being small for gestational age, is associated with poor developmental outcome, there has been a good deal of concern regarding this aspect of alcohol's effects. Although it can be argued that the usual 400–500 g mean effect (in comparison to children of nondrinkers) is the direct result of alcohol and other drug exposure (e.g., cigarettes), it is not necessarily the case that any negative developmental deficits are the result of the low birthweight per se. Rather, low birthweight may be a marker variable indicating that the infant's prenatal development has not been optimal; the child has been born preterm, has suffered malnutrition in utero, or has been exposed to some other factor, like cigarette smoking, which has interfered with growth.

Because lower birthweight may indicate that an alcohol-exposed child has been vulnerable to the drug, like dysmorphic features, it may be able to serve as a screening device to identify children at high risk for behavioral effects. In this pilot study of the relationship of birthweight to developmental outcome (Coles et al., 1987a), it was hypothesized that alcohol-exposed children of the normal birthweight (> 3,000 g) were probably unaffected by their exposure, while those who weighed less might show cognitive deficits as well. To examine this idea, a subsample (N = 60) of the 293 children was given developmental testing with the Bayley Scales at 12 months (Bayley, 1969). For infants of nondrinkers, the mean mental development index (MDI) for all three weight groups was within the normal range (MDI = 98–114) suggesting that birthweight was not very predictive of outcome in this group. However, for those children whose mothers continued to drink throughout pregnancy and who had birthweights less than 2,500 g, the mean MDI was 77. In the < 3,000 g category the mean score was 81, and if the child was of full weight, the MDI average was 110. These results are of concern particularly because 52.1% of those who continued to drink in the larger sample of 293 had children in the low birthweight and questionable categories. There are two possible explanations for these data which should be explored further. First, is the possibility that growth effects may be related to a genetic or biological vulnerability to alcohol and, therefore, can be used as an early marker for cognitive deficits, at least on a group basis. A second explanation is that these children are at higher risk, like other low(er) birthweight infants (Zeskind and Ramey, 1981), and because they are exposed to a less positive rearing environment, have poorer outcomes than the full weight infants whose mothers also drink alcohol. Of course, it is certain that other factors, many of which were related to maternal substance use, also influenced these results. However, the intention was to demonstrate that birthweight could be useful in defining risk categories associated with substance abuse.

There are also alterations in *neonatal behavior* associated with alcohol exposure and these have occurred across samples in different populations using various measures. Children of drinkers may show behavioral alterations (Landsman-Dwyer et al., 1978), problems with habituation and suck (Streissguth et al., 1983), and changes in electroencephalogram (EEG) associated with sleep disturbances (Havlicek et al., 1977; Scher et al., 1988). Similarly, Coles et al. (1985) reported alterations in activity levels, motor tone, and orientation among infants whose mothers continued to drink throughout pregnancy. These effects were persistent over the first month (Coles et al., 1987b) and predicted developmental outcome at 6 months in a low SES primarily black sample (Coles et al., 1987c). Such findings are not universal. Ernhart et al. (1985) and Richardson et al. (1989), who were also using the Brazelton neonatal examination (Brazelton, 1984), found no behavioral effects in their samples, which they attributed to the much lower drinking levels in their populations.

Thus, in many neonatal studies, growth and behavioral effects of alcohol exposure have been noted. However, the meaning of these neonatal effects for long-term development is not clear. It is quite possible that these behaviors are associated with prenatal tolerance to alcohol leading to neonatal withdrawal (Coles et al., 1984) which will gradually resolve. Equally, some of these effects may represent alterations in the CNS which will be compensated for over time as is so frequently the case for other sorts of prenatal and perinatal insults (Sameroff and Chandler, 1975). Finally, early effects may be indicators of more permanent damage which will be associated with real alterations in developmental outcome.

Development in infancy

The data which have been published concerning this age period are as yet limited; however, when prospectively studied alcohol-exposed children are examined in later infancy and in the preschool period, there are group differences. These differences suggest that those who were exposed most (either most heavily or for the longest period) show the poorest cognitive and motor development and the least weight gain. In the middle-class Seattle sample, children of heavy drinkers had lower mental and motor development scores on the Bayley Scale at 8 months than other children (Streissguth et al., 1980). In a middle-class Canadian sample, prenatal alcohol, marijuana, and cigarette use contributed to depressed mental development scores at 12 and 24 months with the effect being stronger at 2 years (Fried and Watkinson, 1988). In the low SES Atlanta sample, there were significant differences at 6 and 12 months in the Bayley cognitive and motor development scores of offspring of women who continued to drink versus those who stopped in the second trimester and those who never drank (Smith et al., 1987a).

Larssen et al. (1985) also reported that drinking which persisted through the third trimester was associated with poorer outcome in off-spring on physical, behavioral, and psychiatric measures in the second and third years of life. These outcomes did not appear to be associated with environment because they were also seen in children who were placed in nonalcoholic foster homes. Hyperactivity, language problems, and fine and gross motor deficits were most often observed in the continued-to-drink group.

Preschool period: behavior and intellectual development

During the preschool period, behavioral effects may be more apparent than are cognitive deficits. Morrow-Tlucuk and Ernhart (1987) reported on evaluation of the Cleveland sample of low SES mothers and their 3-year-old children who were rated on nine different behaviors as well as intellectual development. No differences were noted in intellectual or language development, but using multivariate procedures, they noted that as maternal substance abuse increased, there were changes in behavior patterns with heavier alcohol use associated with a reduction in the amount of activity, emotional reactivity, irritability and dependence, and an increase in rigidity and task absorption.

In contrast, at 4 years old, 128 middle-class subjects from a Seattle sample were observed for behavioral effects (Landesman-Dwyer et al., 1981). None of the mothers of these children were alcoholics or alcohol abusers during pregnancy although a group of "moderate" drinkers was included. The study focused on home environment, children's temperament, and the child's spontaneous behavior. Although there were no alcohol-related differences in home environment, children's activity levels were found to be related to prenatal alcohol and nicotine use in a manner suggesting that use of these substances might be associated with later hyperactivity and attentional deficit disorder. The authors stressed that the positive home environments of these middle-class families should have reduced the potency of the prenatal effects.

In the follow-up of the Seattle sample, intelligence was measured at 4 years among 421 children (Streissguth et al., 1989b). The size of the sample allowed many major confounding factors (e.g., sex, parental education, other drug use) to be statistically controlled. These authors reported that use during pregnancy of more than 1.5 oz of alcohol daily (about three drinks) was associated with an IQ decrement of about five (5) points on the Wechsler Preschool and Primary Scales of Intelligence (WPPSI), a standardized measure of intelligence.

Cognition at school age

By school age, relative deficits in cognitive performance are noted to be associated with greater exposure to alcohol. Russell et al. (1987) examined 6-year-olds whose mothers had been identified as heavy drinkers prenatally. They found no significant differences related to drinking in intellectual development or in auditory processing in the children of "social" and moderate drinkers. However, in a subsample of "problem" drinkers (N = 14), children were found to have lower verbal IQ scores than the other children in the sample (X = 99.1, s.d. = 11.7, versus X = 107.4, s.d. = 14.2) as well as lower scores on the Token test, a measure of receptive language, and a higher error rate on a dichotic listening test.

Streissguth et al. (1989 a,c) reported that heavier drinking and particularly drinking in a "binge" pattern (more than five drinks per occasion) was associated with a variety of deficits in cognitive functioning at 7 years. Although exposed children were not clinically impaired, the children of drinkers had lower scores on standardized tests of intelligence, memory, problem solving and flexibility, visual/motor performance, and academic skills, particularly arithmetic. Despite the evidence from retrospective studies, verbal behavior and language skills were not as affected. The authors reported that this relationship with language development had been consistent throughout the repeated assessments, suggesting that poor language was not a characteristic of this group of children. The authors also reported that the latent effects of prenatal alcohol were more strongly evident when environmental stresses were present (e.g., single mother; large family) but appeared to be ameliorated when conditions were relatively positive.

In a very dissimilar sample, similar effects were apparent. In a follow-up of some of the Atlanta sample (Coles et al., 1991) with children having a mean age of 5 years, 10 months, specific cognitive deficits were noted in alcohol-exposed children with those having the great duration of exposure (e.g., throughout the third trimester) showing the most obvious effects. In addition to total cognitive score (equivalent to IQ) on the Kaufman Achievement Battery (Kaufman and Kaufman, 1983), children exposed through the third trimester showed significant decrements in sequential processing of information and in academic achievement. Problems were noted in short-term memory, math skills, and decoding of letters and words. Language as measured by verbal fluency, word finding, and vocabulary was less affected.

These studies suggest that alcohol effects may become more apparent over time or as different cognitive functions develop; however, the only data available at the time this report was prepared came from studies which have consistently found behavioral and cognitive effects while the Cleveland (Ernhart et al., 1985) and Pittsburgh (Richardson et al., 1989) studies, which have found fewer behavioral effects in infancy, have not yet published results of their studies of older children.

Hyperactivity and attention

In retrospective studies, attention deficit hyperactivity disorder (ADHD) has been widely reported among dysmorphic children and children of alcoholic mothers. Gold and Sherry (1984) have suggested that there may be a relationship between prenatal alcohol exposure and later hyperactivity, learning disabilities, and attentional problems. As a result, this aspect of cognition and behavior has been a focus of interest in prospective studies.

Some of the human studies of prenatally exposed children are supportive of this view while others are not (Morrow-Tlucuk and Ernhart, 1987). At 4 years, 452 children in the Seattle sample were tested using a vigilance task to examine reaction time and sustained attention (Streissguth et al., 1984), and both maternal alcohol use and cigarette smoking were found to be related to poorer attention even in the absence of evidence of parental alcohol abuse. In this same cohort, Streissguth et al. (1986) measured attention at 7 years using a computerized continuous performance test. Greater alcohol exposure was associated with poorer test performance, distractibility, and impulsivity.

In the Atlanta sample at 6 years, a similar procedure was used to measure a variety of attention-related tasks, including sustained attention, distractibility, and impulsivity (Brown et al., 1991). When mothers continued to drink throughout pregnancy, children showed an inability to sustain attention but no difficulties with impulsivity. Hyperactivity and impulsivity also were assessed through standardized checklists as well as videotaped observations, and results suggested that these children could not be classified as showing ADHD although they did have problems with attention that were probably neurologically based.

These outcomes support the suggestion that alcohol exposure affects attentional processes, although the data are not strong enough to maintain that the outcomes seen in the prospective studies are actually ADHD. It may be that these effects are milder than those seen in more seriously affected children. However, there may also be environmental factors which affect children's behavior in homes where substance abuse is a problem. Obviously, this is an issue that will require further study.

Summary of Effects of Prenatal Alcohol Exposure in Prospective Studies

In summary, when prospective studies examine the outcomes of a wide range of prenatal alcohol exposure, behavioral effects can be noted in the neonatal period, in later infancy, and at early school age. To some extent, these outcomes confirm, between groups, in a statistical manner, the effects noted in the more obviously affected offspring of alcoholics. In the majority of studies, however, most of the infants and children are only mildly affected behaviorally and do not have obviously dysmorphic features or significant growth retardation. Had these individuals not been participating in research studies, their behavioral differences would usually not have been noted or, if noted, would not have been associated with exposure to alcohol.

In addition, a number of areas which are important to the understanding of the long-term development of children with prenatal alcohol exposure have not been examined adequately. These areas include emotional and social development and attitudes about and response to substance abuse.

FACTORS THAT APPEAR TO AFFECT OUTCOMES

Not all children exposed to alcohol have negative developmental consequences. Even among alcoholics, only 35–40% of those women who were drinking during pregnancy had children with FAS. In the 20 years that these issues have been under study, some of the variables that are associated with the presence or absence of certain effects of alcohol have been examined, and there appear to be certain factors which are related to the probability of poor outcomes. However, it is important to understand that methods of collection, social trends, and similar factors may have influenced some of these results. In addition, many questions about the reasons for alcohol's effects are not yet answered.

Genetic Vulnerability

Vorhees (1986) suggested that there are several principles of teratogenetics that are applicable to the study of alcohol's effects. The first of these suggests that an organism is susceptible to the effects of a teratogenic substance if it has a genetic vulnerability and if it is exposed to the substance. Such a genetic vulnerability would explain why not all alcoholic women who drink during pregnancy have affected children. However, in relation to the actual occurrence of fetal alcohol effects, evidence for genetic effects is quite limited. Support for this hypothesis comes from the suggestion that fetal alcohol effects are seen more frequently among blacks (Sokol et al., 1986a) and certain groups of American Indians (May et al., 1982). However, these studies are open to criticism that social factors such as differences in drinking patterns or availability of research subjects may have influenced ascertainment rates in different racial and ethnic groups (Bray and Anderson, 1988). In addition, it is difficult to support the contention that American blacks can be considered a genetically homogenous group such that incidence rates should be so significantly different from the majority population. Finally, reports of incidence data from indisputably white European populations (Olegard et al., 1979) have similar rates to those reported in the United States among minority groups.

Twin studies are often used to discriminate the effects of heredity and environmental factors. Unfortunately, there are only a few published reports of twins who show FAS (Chasnoff, 1985; Christoffel and Salafsky, 1975; Palmer et al., 1974; Santolaya et al., 1978), and the majority of these case studies are of dizygotic twins. Examination of these studies suggests that while there may be some differences in vulnerability, the effect of prenatal exposure itself is substantial.

Even though at the present time the evidence for a genetic vulnerability in FAS is quite limited, this remains an attractive hypothesis that may be explored when the mechanisms underlying alcohol's effects are better known.

Maternal Factors

All mothers are not equal when the probability of having an alcohol-affected child is calculated. The "typical" mother of an FAS child is older (in her thirties), has had several children, has a history of reproductive problems as well as a history of alcohol abuse (Abel, 1984). Sokol et al. (1986a) reported that four factors—proportion of drinking days, positive status on the Michigan Alcohol Screening Test, black race, and high parity—predicted those women who had a 50 fold greater chance of producing an FAS offspring than did other women in the Cleveland sample.

Women who are able to stop drinking in pregnancy have children with substantially better outcomes than those who continue to drink. Smith et al. (1987b) found that there were differences in social and health-related factors between women who did and did not stop drinking after an educational intervention. Women who continued to drink reported beginning to drink at an earlier age, had more family members who were drinkers, and had more physical problems associated with alcohol use despite drinking a similar amount at the time of intervention.

Other factors that probably influence outcome include access to and use of prenatal care, access to alcohol treatment, adequate nutrition, social support and other, similar factors which may be affected by maternal lifestyle. A common problem in alcohol using women is the concomitant use of other drugs. The polydrug abuse usually includes cigarette and marijuana use while cocaine abuse is increasingly common.

Health problems in alcohol abusing women may include disorders specifically related to alcohol abuse, like liver damage and gastritis, but may also include an increased incidence of sexually transmitted and other infectious diseases. Recently, Frezza et al. (1990) reported that prolonged alcohol abuse led to an inability of the body to produce alcohol dehydrogenase, which helps in the metabolization of alcohol. They reported that this was a particular problem in women who were, therefore, at greater risk from alcohol. For the pregnant woman who is a heavy drinker, such a deficiency may allow a greater concentration of alcohol to pass the placental barrier and reach the developing fetus (Schenker and Speeg, 1990). It is important, therefore, that maternal factors, particularly physical factors, be considered in examination of alcohol effects on the fetus.

Dose/Drinking Patterns

Another area in which alcohol's teratogenic effects have been investigated is in the *type of exposure*. To some extent, the expression of outcome depends on the amount (dose) and the pattern of exposure experienced by the fetus.

Dose/response

A classic and very intellectually satisfying phenomenon usually occurs with exposure to a toxin. This is the dose/response curve in which, with increasing exposure (dose), there is increasing effect (response). In the study of the prenatal effects of alcohol exposure, the usual dose/response curve has not been completely evident, probably because of the interaction of alcohol exposure with other factors. However, while most effects observed have not shown a simple dose/response curve, there is strong evidence from prospective studies that drinking greater amounts of alcohol leads to more negative results. In fact, the full syndrome does not occur among nonalcoholic women. Streissguth et al. (1981) reported that increased maternal alcohol use was associated with a number of negative outcomes including smaller infant size, a higher frequency of minor dysmorphic features, and the occurrence of a number of behavioral effects.

In a number of studies, birthweight has been found to be particularly sensitive to dose levels even when potential confounding variables such as smoking, maternal age, hypertension, marital status, and prenatal care were statistically controlled (Kuzma and Sokol, 1982; Mills et al., 1984). Smith et al. (1986b) reported that both dose and duration of exposure affected birthweight and behavior even in nondysmorphic infants. Birthweight is probably more easy to examine in this way than dysmorphic features or behavioral effects because it is a single, unambiguous trait whose measurement employs a metric scale.

Ernhart et al. (1987b) quantified craniofacial and other congenital anomalies and used multivariate techniques to control confounding variables. They also used a mean substitution method to account for missing data and estimated drinking levels during the period of embryonic development based on findings from a later study. When these procedures were used, estimated maternal drinking was related to incidence of craniofacial anomalies in a dose/response manner.

Behavioral effects of alcohol exposure have not been reported to be related to dose in the same kind of dose/response pattern, although it is clear that higher doses produced more negative results (Streissguth et al., 1989a,c).

Binge versus continuous exposure

Drinking levels are usually reported in terms of the average amount of absolute alcohol (AA) per day or per week. In determining use, drinkers are often asked to report number of drinking occasions per specific time period and usual number of drinks per occasion (Cahalan et al., 1969). These figures can be multiplied to determine risk level. For instance, if a woman drinks two times a week and has a six pack of beer each time, she has consumed 6 oz of absolute alcohol in a single week or 0.857 oz AA per day—slightly less than 1 oz per day. Similarly, a woman who has a glass of wine preceding dinner and another glass with the meal 6 days a week would also have a mean of 0.857 per day. However, it is possible that the exposure both of the mother and the fetus is different in each case, since when greater quantities are consumed in a shorter period of time, the alcohol is not metabolized as effectively and a greater blood alcohol concentration (BAC) is achieved. Animal studies (Bonthius and West, 1988; Clarren et al., 1988) indicated that such higher BACs, which are usually the result of a "binge" pattern of drinking, may be much more damaging for the developing offspring's CNS than is a similar dose which is given over a longer period of time. In prospective research on humans, Streissguth et al. (1989c) reported that the negative neurobehavioral effects observed in the 7-year-old Seattle sample were related to the probability of a "binge" pattern of alcohol consumption (which was defined as more than five drinks per occasion). These studies suggest that the BAC may be more important in understanding the effects of dose than is the usual method of reporting as a daily average.

Critical period/duration

Another significant factor in the effects on offspring is the timing and duration of the exposure. Exposure during different developmental periods will have different effects because there are critical periods during gestation when introduction of toxic substances will disrupt specific aspects of development. This issue is examined most easily in animal models in which timing of exposure can be controlled. In this volume, Pentney and Miller (Chapter 5) and Miller (Chapter 4) review this work and suggest that there are specific and significant effects of exposure during different periods of development.

However, such rigor is not possible in clinical research with a human sample. As a result, our understanding of effects of exposure during particular periods of gestation is still limited. It is probable that heavy, very early exposure leads to nonviability although this is difficult to measure since pregnancy may not have been identified. However, the effects of different periods of exposure on other factors like dysmorphia and birthweight have been examined more fully. Study of the effect of exposure during different periods on behavior is more difficult since understanding of the neural structures supporting various aspects of behavior is less fully developed. However, it has been possible to examine some aspects of behavior.

Since facial dysmorphia occurs during the period of organogenesis in the embryonic period, craniofacial anomalies could be expected to be associated with drinking during the first trimester of pregnancy. Animal studies have demonstrated that exposure on specific days of gestation, which are analogous to the third week of gestation in humans, produce animals with the same kinds of anomalies seen in human infants (Sulik et al., 1981)

In statistical studies of craniofacial anomalies in non-FAS children, Sokol et al. (1986b) reported that such a pattern was evident also and was related to later intellectual development (Ernhart et al., 1987a). Similarly, the level of alcohol-related congenital anomalies is the same in children of women who stop drinking during the second trimester and those who continue to drink even when other outcomes are very different (Coles et al., 1985; Smith et al., 1990), indicating that such defects are the result of early exposure. Graham et al. (1988) also reported that anomalies at birth and at 4 years were related to heavier drinking in the very early "prior to pregnancy recognition" period rather than at midpregnancy.

In contrast, birthweight is reduced in prenatally exposed infants particularly if the exposure continues throughout the third trimester. When drinking is discontinued by the second trimester, children of drinkers may not differ in growth from children of nondrinkers (Coles et al., 1985; Olegard et al., 1979; Rosett et al., 1980). This finding may indicate either that the growth effect associated with alcohol exposure occurs in the third trimester or that being alcohol-free during that time allows the fetus to "catch up" in growth.

For several reasons, behavioral effects have not been examined as closely in relation to critical periods of exposure. First, the neurological substrate of many behaviors is not well known and similar behaviors may have more than one "cause." Second, it is evident, given the range of possible outcomes resulting from fetal alcohol exposure, that a wide variety of behavioral outcomes can be expected. Severe CNS damage associated with microcephaly in FAS children probably results from different drinking patterns than do mild effects which are evident in otherwise normal children only as a result of experimental procedures. Therefore, it is probably true that behavioral effects result from exposure during all of gestation. However, it is possible to tease out some relationships between exposure during different periods and particular behaviors. This process is clearer when the behavioral outcomes are relatively specific and are quantifiable.

In order to measure behavioral effects of fetal alcohol exposure during particular periods of gestation, it is necessary to have measured maternal drinking during these periods. Although this has been done in some cases (e.g., Richardson et al., 1989), in most prospective studies only one estimate was taken at the point of recruitment. This limitation makes investigation of this issue difficult although some researchers have been very ingenuous in overcoming this limitation (e.g., Ernhart et al., 1987b).

A second way to examine this phenomenon is to take advantage of the effects of intervention and recruitment on drinking levels. Coles et al. (1985) and Larsson et al. (1985) have done this by comparing behavioral differences in offspring of those who did and did not stop drinking in the second trimester. These studies have found differences in intellectual abilities as well as other behaviors in those who where exposed throughout pregnancy. However, it is necessary to interpret these results cautiously because it is possible that women who continue to drink despite an educational intervention also differ in other ways from those who are able to stop. Still, support for the idea that there are specific effects of third trimester exposure has been found in animal research where confounding factors are not present (West and Pierce, 1986).

Postnatal Effects/Interaction With a Negative Environment

In discussing behavior teratogens, Vorhees (1986) also stressed the importance of the interaction of the environment with the effects of the teratogen. As is the case with other kinds of risk factors evident in infancy (Sameroff and Chandler, 1975), the expression of the effects of the teratogen will depend on the organism's pre and postnatal environment. This factor has been extensively researched in the study of children born preterm (Hunt, 1986) and to a lesser degree, among methadone maintained mothers and their offspring (Hutchings and Fifer, 1986). From this viewpoint, development is an interactive and reciprocal process carried on between the individual child and the environment. Factors that affect the individual child can include health, temperament, physical attractiveness, cognitive competence, and interactive capacity. Social/environmental factors include social class, competence of the parent/caretaker, social and emotional support provided to the caretaker, as well as substance abuse. The relationship among these factors will shape the process of development. Unless the individual is badly damaged, a supportive and nurturing environment may mitigate the effects of the earlier teratogenic insult (Zeskind and Ramey, 1981). Similarly, a negative, neglectful, or abusive environment may potentiate those deficits.

It is evident that there are profoundly important environmental and social factors which influence individuals whose parents are substance abusers. A child who has been exposed to alcohol prenatally, particularly if the mother has been *abusing* alcohol, is likely to grow up in a less than optimal environment. The relatively recent literature on children of alcoholics (Adler and Raphael, 1983; Woodside, 1983) provides strong support for the prominent role in the child's development played by environmental factors. To study how much additional risk occurs when the child has been prenatally exposed is difficult. Clinically identified children who remain with their natural mothers may be exposed to a number of other risk factors which can affect cognitive and emotional outcome. Problems that have been noted in research studies or anecdotally include early maternal death (Streissguth et al., 1985), failure to thrive (Ulleland, 1970), neglect and abuse (Burgess and Conger, 1978), lack of adequate medical care, and lack of environmental stimulation (Wilson et al., 1984).

It is hard to discriminate the effect of these factors from the effect of the teratogen. To examine the issue of environment, development of exposed children who have remained with their natural mother has been compared with that of children placed in foster care. Streissguth (1986) and Aronsson et al. (1985) found that children placed in nonalcoholic foster homes did not show significantly higher IQ scores than did those who remained in their own homes; however, these were not controlled studies. It is possible that children were only removed from the worst environments. In addition, the poor quality of care provided in many foster placements is well known.

The follow-up prospective studies which assessed children in the preschool period (Landesman-Dwyer et al., 1981; Morrow-Tlucuk & Ernhart, 1987) have examined environment without finding significant differences related to alcohol use. Because of the complexity of the problem of environmental effects, studies will have to focus more sharply on specific issues and on the interaction of the caretaking environment with alcohol-specific traits of the affected children. Recent theoretical trends in the study of infant development suggest that it may be important to examine what the child brings to its interaction with its environment. The traditional unidirectional model of development which viewed the child as the product of its environment and its geneotype has been replaced by a transactional model (Sameroff and Chandler, 1975) which stresses the active participation of the infant with its environment.

SUGGESTIONS FOR FUTURE RESEARCH

Although a great deal has been learned about the effects of prenatal alcohol exposure, it is evident that there are many more questions. As our knowledge is refined and technologies improve, some of these may be answered.

Is There a Threshold for Alcohol Effects?

Some authors have suggested that there is a *threshold* effect in the exposure to alcohol with amounts less than 1–2 oz per day showing few effects (Richardson et al., 1989; Roman et al., 1988). Florey (1988) contends that, at moderate drinking levels, the variance associated with alcohol exposure is negligible and suggests that unless drinking is abusive, it is inappropriate to recommend abstinence in pregnancy. Others believe that a more conservative approach is appropriate and recommend that pregnant women avoid any substance use. Longitudinal studies which demonstrate effects in children with moderate exposure support this viewpoint. Obviously, there are many variables involved including both those associated with maternal drinking as well as experimental variables which affect understanding of exposure. Equally, the outcomes measured will be related to the putative safety of various levels of exposure. As a result, this is a question which will require more study.

Role of Genetic Factors in Alcoholism and in Fetal Alcohol Effects

At the present time, there is a tremendous interest in the extent to which genetic factors influence health, development, and pathology. This is due to the recent incredible advances in molecular genetics that have allowed the identification of the genes which underlie a number of disorders (e.g., Duchenne's muscular dystrophy). For this reason, the search is on to find the gene(s) that are responsible for many physical and behavioral conditions which appear to be familial in nature. Alcoholism and alcohol abuse have long been identified as occurring more frequently in certain families and cultures (Devor and Cloninger, 1989; Tabakoff and Hoffman, 1988) and are, therefore, a focus of interest as well (Hill et al., 1988; Tanna et al., 1988). Blum et al. (1990) reported an association between the dopamine D_2 receptor and a history of alcoholism, finding that presence of the A1 allele of this receptor gene was sufficient to correctly classify more than 70% of samples taken postmortem from brain tissue of alcoholics and controls. The authors suggested that there may be an association between this receptor and the brain reward system which contributes to the addiction process. However, these authors and others (Gordis et al., 1990) caution that alcoholism, which has a very high incidence in the population, is not a genetically "simple" phenomenon. Rather, it is evidently the end product of several different processes and, if genetically influenced, is polygenetic in nature with several, and perhaps many, genes contributing to the outcome.

Alcoholism, however, is a necessary but not a sufficient condition for the occurrence of FAS. Even if a genetic basis for alcoholism is identified, it may be still another step to the understanding of vulnerability to FAS. The resulting investigation will be complex and, if a genetic component is found, may involve intervening factors between the genetic and behavioral levels.

Imaging Studies of Affected Children and Animals

Anatomical studies of brain structures in alcohol-affected offspring (Clarren, 1986) indicate that prenatal exposure has significant effects. Unfortunately, such studies are done necessarily when the organism is no longer able to exhibit behavior. Therefore, it is difficult to establish, except by inference, the relationship between specific damage and particular behaviors. Technological advances now allow investigation of the living brain through various imaging methods and this seems an obvious direction for future study of the effects of fetal alcohol exposure on the CNS. Through such studies in affected individuals, the relationship between specific neurological deficits and particular behaviors can be explored. In addition, experimental work with animals, particularly primates, could establish effects of different amounts and periods of exposure.

Pentney and Miller (Chapter 5) review studies of metabolic effects of prenatal exposure in the rat, which suggest that such techniques may be fruitful. Miller and Dow-Edwards (1988) found alterations in motor cortex as well as a significant decrease in glucose utilization specific to certain areas using a 2-deoxyglucose autoradiographic technique. Vingan et al. (1986) found a relationship between behavioral deficits and chronic changes in brain metabolism (glucose utilization) in rats with prenatal alcohol exposure. These studies suggest that similar patterns could be identified in a human sample through association of specific behavioral assessments with appropriate imaging techniques.

Long-term Development in Exposed Children

Although a few children with FAS have been followed into adulthood, the short period of time during which alcohol effects have been of interest limits our understanding of the long-term effects of this disorder. The many unknowns include the relationship between prenatal exposure and later alcohol and other drug use, and the effect of prenatal exposure on reproduction, the aging process, and the life span. In addition, understanding of the outcomes for more mildly exposed children is still very limited. Although there have been a few studies of some aspects of attention and cognition, most areas of development have not been examined and the period of development studied is short. Prospective data exist only up to the early school age period so that there is no knowledge about the rest of the life span.

Specific Versus Global Effects

At the present time, it appears that the kind of serious damage that occurs in FAS affects most behaviors through its damage to the CNS. However, when exposure is more moderate, brain damage or alterations and, therefore, behavioral effects, may be more specific. This is an area which may be very rewarding to examine. Theoretically based studies of development in specific areas should be carried out using more limited measures of outcome. For instance, if alcohol exposure is hypothesized to affect attention specifically, such deficits should be identified early in infancy, using experimental techniques, and the effects of that factor followed over time. Studies of this kind would not only provide information about the effects of alcohol but would illuminate aspects of the process of development itself.

Polydrug Effects

In human studies, it is difficult to avoid studying polydrug abuse since the majority of women who abuse alcohol also use marijuana and cigarettes (Fried and Watkinson, 1988; Russell and Skinner, 1988). Increasingly, cocaine and other drugs of abuse are becoming very common, particularly in the inner city populations that are often the focus of systematic research. This historical effect may necessitate the investigation of interactions between alcohol and other drugs, as well as focus attention on the extent to which "lifestyle" related factors contribute to the negative outcomes associated with fetal alcohol effects.

Relationship Among "Levels" of Understanding

While there has been a great deal of research on the effects of prenatal alcohol exposure, the majority of it has been confined to a particular "level" of study. Epidemiologists have studied exposure and outcome in terms of mortality and birthweight within large samples. Developmental psychologists have examined mental and motor development, intelligence, and similar factors. Anatomists have focused on animal models of ethanol-induced abnormalities in craniofacial and brain structures. Cell biologists have examined the effects on the cell and the cell membrane. Molecular biologists are beginning to examine the DNA. Each level of this effort has been valuable in bringing meaning to the whole. However, at this time there is a great need to begin the integration of these levels in a meaningful way. For instance, what does a "weak" statistical effect, or a statistically nonsignificant trend, mean for the individual? Factors which may have meaning statistically or be predictive in terms of populations may not be clinically important for a single individual who may not have any of the many other risk factors associated with negative outcomes. Therefore, it is important to identify not only the effects of the teratogen itself but the conditions associated with it in making statements which will be applied practically.

The relationship between structural and functional effects of prenatal alcohol exposure is also of great importance. We have been able to establish many structural effects but do not yet understand how these are related to behavior. We have established that alcohol produces effects at the receptor site but cannot yet explain how changes in the cell membrane affect response to environmental stressors (for instance).

There are many questions which would reward further study. Choice depends on the interests and understanding of the investigator as well as the state of knowledge. Nevertheless, it is clear that, although the last 20 years of research into the effects of prenatal alcohol exposure have provided many answers, there is much more work to be done in this area.

ACKNOWLEDGMENTS

Support for some of the work discussed in this chapter was received from the Georgia Department of Human Resources, Alcohol and Drug Abuse Section, and from the March of Dimes Social and Behavioral Research grants 12-140 and 12-190.

REFERENCES

Abel EL (1982): "Fetal Alcohol Syndrome, Vol III." Boca Raton, FL: CRC Press, Inc.

Abel EL (1984): "Fetal Alcohol Syndrome and Fetal Alcohol Effects." New York: Plenum Press.

Abel EL, Sokol RJ (1987): Incidence of fetal alcohol syndrome and economic impact of FAS-related anomalies. Drug Alcohol Depend 19:51–70.

Adler R, Raphael B (1983): Review: Children of alcoholics. Aust N Z J Psychiatry 17:3–8.

Anokute CC (1986): Epidemiology of spontaneous abortions: The effects of alcohol consumption and cigarette smoking. J Natl Med Assoc 78: 771–775.

Aronsson M, Kyllerman M, Sabel K-G, Sandin B, Olegard R (1985): Children of alcoholic mothers: Developmental, perceptual, and behavioural characteristics as compared to matched controls. Acta Paediatr Scand 74:27–35.

Aronsson M, Olegard R (1987): Children of alcoholic mothers. Pediatrician 14:57–61.

Barnett R, Shusterman S (1985): Fetal alcohol syndrome: Review of literature and report of cases. JADA 111:591–593.

Barr HM, Streissguth AP, Martin DC, Herman CS (1984): Infant size at 8 months of age: Relationship to maternal use of alcohol, nicotine, and caffeine during pregnancy. Pediatrics 74:336–341.

Bayley N (1969): "Bayley Scales of Infant Development." New York: Psychological Corp.

Blum K, Noble EP, Sheridan PJ, Montgomery A, Ritchie T, Jagadeeswaran P, Nogami H, Briggs AH, Cohn JB (1990): Allelic association of human dopamine D_2 receptor gene in alcoholism. JAMA 263:2055–2060.

Blume SB (1986): Women and alcohol: A review. JAMA 256:1467–1470.

Bonthius DJ, West JR (1988): Blood alcohol concentration and microencephaly: A dose-response study in the neonatal rat. Teratology 37:223–231.

Bray DH, Anderson PD (1988): Appraisal of the epidemiology of fetal alcohol syndrome among Canadian native peoples. Can J Public Health 80:42–45.

Brazelton TB (1984): "Neonatal Behavioral Assessment Scale, 2nd Ed." Philadelphia: Lippincott.

Brown RT, Coles CD, Smith IE, Platzman KA, Silverstein J, Erickson S, Falek A (1991): Effects of prenatal alcohol exposure at 6-years postpartum: II Attention and Behavior. Neurotoxicol Teratol 13:12.

Burgess RL, Conger CD (1978): Family interaction in abusive, neglectful, and normal families. Child Dev 49:1163–1173.

Cahalan D, Cisin I, Crossley HM (1969): "American Drinking Practices." New Haven, CT: College and University Press.

Chasnoff IJ (1985): Fetal alcohol effect in twin pregnancy. Acta Genet Med Gemellol (Roma) 34:229–232.

Christoffel KK, Salafsky I (1975): Fetal alcohol syndrome in dizygotic twins. J Pediatr 87:963.

Church MW, Gerkin KP (1988): Hearing disorders in children with fetal alcohol syndrome: Findings from case reports. Pediatrics 82:147–154.

Clarren SK (1986): Neuropathology in fetal alcohol syndrome. In West JR (ed): "Alcohol and Brain Development." New York: Oxford University Press, pp 158–166.

Clarren SK, Astley SJ, Bowden DM (1988): Physical anomalies and developmental delays in nonhuman primate infants exposed to weekly doses of ethanol during gestation. Teratology 37:561–569.

Coles CD, Brown RT, Smith IE, Platzman KA, Erickson S, Falek A (1991): Effects of prenatal alcohol exposure at 6 years: I. Physical and cognitive development. Neurotoxicol Teratol 13:1–11.

Coles CD, Smith IE, Falek A (1987a): A neonatal marker for cognitive vulnerability to alcohol's teratogenic effects. Alcoholism 11:197 (Abstract).

Coles CD, Smith IE, Falek A (1987c): Prenatal alcohol exposure and infant behavior: Immediate effects and implications for later development. Adv Alcohol Subst Abuse 4:85–103.

Coles CD, Smith IE, Fernhoff PM, Falek A (1985): Neonatal neurobehavioral characteristics as correlates of maternal alcohol use during gestation. Alcoholism 9:1–7.

Coles CD, Smith IE, Fernhoff PM, Falek A (1984): Neonatal ethanol withdrawal: Characteristics in clinical normal, nondysmorphic, neonates. J Pediatr 105:445–451.

Coles CD, Smith IE, Lancaster JS, Falek A (1987b): Persistence over the first month of neurobehavioral alterations in infants exposed to alcohol prenatally. Infant Behav Dev 10:23–37.

Devor EJ, Cloninger CR (1989): Genetics of alcoholism. Annu Rev Genet 23:19–36.

Ernhart CB, Morrow-Tlucak M, Sokol R (1987a): Anatomic alcohol-related birth defects (ARBD); The relationship to early child development. Alcoholism 11:198 (Abstract).

Ernhart CB, Sokol RJ, Martier S, Moron P, Nadler D, Ager JW, Wolf A (1987b): Alcohol teratogenicity in the human: A detailed assessment of specificity, critical period, and threshold. Am J Obstet Gynecol 156:33–39.

Ernhart CB, Wolf AW, Linn PL, Sokol RJ, Kennard MJ, Filipovich HF (1985): Alcohol-related birth defects: Syndrome anomalies, intrauterine growth retardation and neonatal assessment. Alcoholism 9:447–453.

Frezza M, di Padova C, Pozzato G, Maddalena T, Baraona E, Lieber CS (1990): High blood alcohol levels in women: The role of decreased gastric alcohol dehydrogenase activity and first-pass metabolism. N Engl J Med 322:95–99.

Florey C du V (1988): Weak associations in epidemiological research: Some examples and their interpretation. Int J Epidemiol 17:950–954.

Fried PA, Watkinson B (1988): 12- and 24-Month neurobehavioural follow-up of children prenatally exposed to marijuana, cigarettes, and alcohol. Neurotoxicol Teratol 10:305–313.

Gold S, Sherry L (1984): Hyperactivity, learning disabilities, and alcohol. J Learn Dis 17:3–6.

Gordis E, Tabakoff B, Goldman D, Berg K (1990): Editorial: Finding the gene(s) for alcoholism. JAMA 263:2094–2095.

Graham JM, Hanson JW, Darby BL, Barr HM, Streissguth AP (1988): Independent dysmorphology evaluations at birth and 4 years of age for children exposed to varying amounts of alcohol in utero. Pediatrics 81:772–778.

Harlap S, Shlon PH (1980): Alcohol, smoking, and incidence of spontaneous abortion in the first and second trimesters. Lancet 2:173–176.

Havlicek V, Childiaeva R, Chernick V (1977): EEG frequency spectrum characteristics of sleep states in infants of alcoholic mothers. Neuropaediarie 8:360.

Hill SY, Aston C, Rabin B (1988): Suggestive evidence of genetic linkage between alcoholism and the MNS blood group. Alcohol Clin Exp Res 12:811–814.

Holtzman NA (1990) The prevention of developmental disabilities associated with the consumption of alcohol during pregnancy. Centers for Disease Control, Atlanta, GA, unpublished manuscript.

Horowitz SH (1985): Fetal alcohol effects in children: Cognitive, educational, and behavioral considerations. Diss Abstr Int 45, No 8, 2482-A.

Hunt JV (1986): Developmental risk in infants. Adv Special Ed 5:25–59.

Hutchings DE, Fifer WP (1986): Neurobehavioral effects in human and animal offspring following prenatal exposure to methadone. In Riley EP, Vorhees CV (eds): "Handbook of Behavioral Teratology." New York: Plenum Press, pp 141–160.

Iosub S, Fuchs M, Bingol N, and Gromisch DS (1981): Fetal alcohol syndrome revisited. Pediatrics 68:475–479.

Johnson S, Knight R, Marmer DJ, Steele RW (1981): Immune deficiencies in fetal alcohol syndrome. Pediatr Res 15:908–911.

Jones KL, Smith DW (1973): Recognition of the fetal alcohol syndrome in early infancy. Lancet 2:989.

Jones KL, Smith DW, Ulleland CN, Streissguth AP (1973): Pattern of malformation in offspring of chronic alcoholic mothers. Lancet 1:1267–1271.

Kaminski M, Rumeau C, Schwartz D (1978): Alcohol consumption in pregnant women and the outcome of pregnancy. Alcoholism 2:155–163.

Kaufman AS, Kaufman NL (1983): "Kaufman Assessment Battery for Children: Interpretive manual." Circle Pines, MI: American Guidance Service.

Kline J, Stein Z, Shrout P, Susser M, Warburton D (1980): Drinking during pregnancy and spontaneous abortion. Lancet 2:176–180.

Kuzma JW, Sokol RJ (1982): Maternal drinking behavior and decreased intrauterine growth. Alcoholism 6:396–402.

Kyllerman M, Aronsson M, Sabel K-G, Karlberg E, Sandin B, Olegard R (1985): Children of alcoholic mothers: Growth and motor performance compared to matched controls. Acta Paediatr Scand 74:20–26.

Landesman-Dwyer S, Keller S, Streissguth AP (1978): Naturalistic observation of the newborn: Effects of maternal alcohol intake. Alcoholism 2:171–177.

Landesman-Dwyer S, Ragozin AS, Little R (1981): Behavioral correlates of prenatal alcohol exposure: A four-year follow-up study. Neurotoxicol Teratol 3:187–193.

Larsson G, Bohlin A-B (1987): Fetal alcohol syndrome and preventive strategies. Pediatrician 14:51–56.

Larsson G, Bohlin A-B, Tunell R (1985): Prospective study of children exposed to variable amounts of alcohol in utero. Arch Dis Child 60:315–321.

Lemoine P, Haronsseau H, Borteyru J-P, Menuet J-C (1968): Les enfants de parents alcooliques: Anomalies observees a oriois de 127 cas. Ouest Med 25:477–482.

Little RE (1977): Moderate alcohol use during pregnancy and decreases in infant birthweight. Am J Public Health 67:1154–1156.

May PA, Hymbaugh KJ, Aase JM, Somet JM (1982): Epidemiology of fetal alcohol syndrome among American Indians in the Southwest. Soc Biol 30:374–387.

McCall RB (1979): The development of intellectual functioning in infancy and the prediction of later I.Q. In Osofsky JD (ed): "Handbook of Infant Development." New York: Wiley, pp 707–741.

Meyers LS, Riley EP (1986): Behavioral teratology of alcohol. In Riley EL, Vorhees CV (eds): "Handbook of Behavioral Teratology." New York: Plenum Press, pp 101–140.

Miller MW, Dow-Edwards DL (1988): Structural and metabolic alterations in rat cerebral cortex induced by prenatal exposure to ethanol. Brain Res 474:316–326.

Mills JL, Graubard BI, Harley EE, Rhoads GG, Berendes HW (1984): Maternal alcohol consumption and birthweight: How much drinking during pregnancy is safe? JAMA 252:1875–1879.

Morrow-Tlucuk M, Ernhart CB (1987): Maternal prenatal substance use and behavior at age 3 years. Alcoholism 11:213 (Abstract).

National Institute on Drug Abuse (1988): National household survey on drug abuse: Main findings (1985). USDHHS Pub No. Adm 88-1586.

Olegard R, Sobel KG, Aronsson M, Sander B, Johansson RR, Carlsson C, Kyllerman M, Iverson K, Hrbek A (1979): Effects on the child of alcohol abuse during pregnancy. Acta Paediatr Scand Suppl 275:112–121.

Palmer RH, Ouellette EM, Warner L, Leichtman SR (1974): Congenital malformations in offspring of a chronic alcoholic mother. Pediatrics 53:490.

Pirani BBK (1978): Smoking during pregnancy. Obstet Gynecol Surv 33:1–13.

Platzman KA, Coles CD, Rubin CP, Smith IE (1986): Developmental profiles of infants with fetal alcohol syndrome and fetal alcohol effect. Paper presented at the Southeastern Psychological Association Annual Meeting, Orlando, FL.

Richardson GA, Day NL, Taylor PM (1989): The effect of prenatal alcohol, marijuana and tobacco exposure on neonatal behavior. Infant Beh Dev 12:199–209.

Roman E, Beral V, Zuckerman B (1988): The relationship between alcohol consumption and pregnancy outcome in humans: A critique. Issues Rev Teratol 4:205–236.

Rosett HL, Weiner L (1984): "Alcohol and the Fetus: A Clinical Perspective." New York: Oxford University Press.

Rosett HL, Weiner L, Zuckerman B, McKinlay S, Edelin KC (1980): Reduction of alcohol consumption during pregnancy with benefits to the newborn. Alcoholism 4:178–184.

Russell M (1985): Alcohol abuse and alcoholism in the pregnant woman: Identification and intervention. Alcohol Health Res World 10:28–31.

Russell M, Cowan R, Czarnecki D (1987): Prenatal alcohol exposure and early childhood development. Alcoholism 225:11.

Russell M, Skinner JB (1988): Early measures of maternal alcohol misuse as predictors of adverse pregnancy outcomes. Alcoholism 12:824–830.

Sameroff AJ, Chandler JJ (1975): Reproductive risk and the continuum of caretaking casualty. In Horowitz FD, Heatherington M, Scarr-Salapatek S, Seigel G (eds): "Review of Child Development Research," Vol 4. Chicago: University of Chicago Press, pp 187–244.

Sandmaier M (1980): "The Invisible Alcoholics: Women and Alcohol Abuse in America." New York: McGraw-Hill.

Santolaya JM, Martinez G, Gorostiza E, Aizpiri J, Hernandez M (1978): Alcoholismo fetal. Drogalchol 3:183.

Schenker S, Speeg KV (1990): The risk of alcohol intake in men and women: All may not be equal. N Engl J Med 322:127–129 (Letter).

Scher MS, Richardson GA, Coble PA, Day NL, Stoffer DS (1988): The effects of prenatal alcohol and marijuana exposure: Disturbances in neonatal sleep cycling and arousal. Pediatr Res 24:101–105.

Shaywitz SE, Cohen DJ, Shaywitz BA (1980): Behavioral and learning difficulties in children with normal intelligence born to alcoholic mothers. J Pediatr 96:978–982.

Smith IE, Coles CD, Falek A, Fernhoff PM, Rubin C, Lancaster J (1987a): Prenatal alcohol exposure, cognitive and motor development in the first year. Paper presented at the Joint Meeting of the Research Society on Alcoholism and the Committee on Problems of Drug Dependence, Philadelphia, PA, June 16, 1987.

Smith IE, Coles CD, Fernhoff PM, Sloan K, Pollard J, Falek A (1990): Reliability and validity of dysmorphia assessment in children prenatally exposed to alcohol. Unpublished manuscript, Emory University School of Medicine.

Smith IE, Coles CD, Lancaster JS, Fernhoff PM, Falek A (1986b): The effect of volume and duration of prenatal ethanol exposure on neonatal physical and behavioral development. Neurotoxicol Teratol 8:375–381.

Smith IE, Lancaster JS, Falek A (1986a): A five year survey of patterns of drinking behavior in an inner-city prenatal population. Alcoholism 10:100 (Abstract).

Smith IE, Lancaster JS, Moss-Wells S, Coles CD, Falek A (1987b): Identifying high-risk pregnant drinkers: Biological and behavioral correlates of continuous heavy drinking during pregnancy. J Stud Alcohol 48:304–309.

Sokol RJ, Alger J, Martier S, Debanne S, Ernhart C, Kuzma J, Miller SI (1986a): Significant determinants of susceptibility to alcohol teratogenicity. Ann NY Acad Sci 477:87–102.

Sokol RJ, Clarren SK (1989): Guidelines for use of terminology describing the impact of prenatal alcohol on the offspring. Alcoholism 13:597–598.

Sokol RJ, Ernhart CN, Martier S (1986b): Critical period, specificity, and threshold for alcohol teratogenicity. Alcoholism 10:101 (Abstract).

Spohr HL, Willms-Bing J, Steinhausen HC (1989): A preliminary 10-year follow-up of 50 children diagnosed with fetal alcohol syndrome in infancy. Alcoholism 13:343 (Abstract).

Steinhausen HD, Nestler V, Spohr HL (1982): Development and psychopathology of children with the fetal alcohol syndrome. J Dev Behav Pediatr 3:49–54.

Streissguth AP (1986): The behavioral teratology of alcohol. Performance, behavioral and intellectual deficits in prenatally exposed children. In West J (ed): "Alcohol and Brain Development." New York: Oxford University Press, pp 3–44.

Streissguth AP, Barr HM, Martin DC (1983): Maternal alcohol use and neonatal habituation assessed with the Brazelton Scale. Child Dev 54:1109–1118.

Streissguth AP, Barr HM, Martin DC, Herman CS (1980): Effects of maternal alcohol, nicotine, and caffeine use during pregnancy on infant mental and motor development at eight months. Alcoholism 4:152–164.

Streissguth AP, Barr HM, Sampson PD, Bookstein FL, Darby BL (1989a): Neurobehavioral effects of prenatal alcohol: Part I. Research strategy. Neurotoxicol Teratol 11:461–476.

Streissguth AP, Barr HM, Sampson PD, Darby BL, Martin DC (1989b): IQ at age 4 in relation to maternal alcohol use and smoking during pregnancy. Dev Psych 25:3–11.

Streissguth AP, Barr HM, Sampson PD, Parrish-Johnson JC, Kirchner GJ, Martin DC (1986): Attention, distraction and reaction time at age 7 years and prenatal alcohol exposure. Neurotoxicol Teratol 8:717–725.

Streissguth AP, Bookstein FL, Sampson PD, Barr HM (1989c): Neurobehavioral effects of prenatal alcohol: Part III. PLS analyses of neuropsychologic tests. Neurotoxicol Teratol 11:493–507.

Streissguth AP, Clarren SK, Jones KL (1985): Natural history of the fetal alcohol syndrome: A 10-year follow-up of 11 patients. Lancet 2:85–91.

Streissguth AP, Martin DC, Martin JC, Barr HM, Sandman B (1984): Intrauterine alcohol and nicotine exposure: Attention and reaction time in 4-year old children. Dev Psych 20:533–541.

Streissguth AP, Martin DC, Martin JC, Barr HM (1981): The Seattle longitudinal prospective study on alcohol and pregnancy. Neurotoxicol Teratol 3:223–233.

Streissguth AP, Randels SP (1988): Long term effects of fetal alcohol syndrome. In Robinson G (ed): "Alcohol and Child/Family Health." Vancouver: University of British Columbia Press, pp 135–151.

Stromland K (1981): Eyeground malformations in the fetal alcohol syndrome. Neuropediatrics 12:97–98.

Sulik KK, Johnston MC, Webb MA (1981): Fetal alcohol syndrome: Embryogenesis in a mouse model. Science 214:936–938.

Tabakoff B, Hoffman PL (1988): Genetics and biological markers of risk for alcoholism. Public Health Rep 103:690–696.

Tanna VL, Wilson AF, Winokur G, Elston RC (1988): Possible linkage between alcoholism and esterase-D. J Stud Alcohol 49:472–476.

Ulleland CN (1970): The offspring of alcoholic mothers. Ann NY Acad Sci 197:167–169.

Vingan RD, Dow-Edwards DL, Riley EP (1986): Cerebral metabolic alterations in rats following prenatal alcohol exposure: A deoxyglucose study. Alcoholism: Clin Exp Res 10:22–26.

Vorhees CV (1986): Principles of behavioral teratology. In Riley EP, Vorhees CV (eds): "Handbook of Behavioral Teratology." New York: Plenum Press, pp 23–48.

Warner RH, Rosett HL (1975): The effects of drinking on offspring: An historical survey of the American and British literature. J Stud Alcohol 36:1395–1420.

West JR, Pierce R (1986): Perinatal alcohol exposure and neuronal damage. In West JR (ed): "Alcohol and Brain Damage." New York: Oxford University Press, pp 120–157.

Wilson PJ, Scott RV, Briggs FH, Ince SE, Quinton BA, Headings VE (1984): Characteristics of parental response to fetal alcohol syndrome. In Fine BA, Paul NW (eds): "Strategies in Genetic Counseling: Clinical Investigation Studies." White Plains, NY: March of Dimes Birth Defects Foundation.

Woodside M (1983): Children of alcoholic parents: Inherited and psychosocial influences. J Psychiatr Treatment Eval 5:531–537.

Zeskind PS, Ramey CT (1981): Preventing intellectual and interactional sequelae of fetal malnutrition. A longitudinal, transactional and synergistic approach to development. Child Dev 52:213–218.

Development of the Central Nervous System:
Effects of Alcohol and Opiates, pages 37–46
© 1992 Wiley-Liss, Inc.

3

Prenatal Opiate Exposure: Physical, Neurobehavioral, and Developmental Effects

KAROL A. KALTENBACH AND LORETTA FINNEGAN

Department of Pediatrics, Jefferson Medical College, Thomas Jefferson University, Philadelphia, Pennsylvania

INTRODUCTION

Although neonatal abstinence syndrome is a contemporary terminology, newborn drug withdrawal has been a known consequence of opiate dependency in pregnant women for more than a century. With the reemergence of heroin use among women of childbearing age in the late 1950s and early 1960s, clinical reports began to identify effects of opiates on the developing fetus as manifested in neonatal narcotic withdrawal. These early reports focused on the recognition and pharmacological management of neonatal abstinence syndrome and was further refined by work in the early 1970s with the development of a neonatal abstinence scoring system to assess the onset, progression, and delineation of symptoms.

The early 1970s was also distinguished by the onset of methadone maintenance for opiate dependence in pregnancy. With the advent of methadone maintenance, attention focused on the need to identify potential risks to the progeny of pregnant opiate-dependent women. Studies began to address both short- and long-term neurobehavioral effects in infants whose mothers were maintained on methadone during pregnancy.

The majority of data on the effects of prenatal opiate exposure in infancy and early childhood are based on methadone exposure, since populations accessible for study were primarily children of women in treatment. Methadone exposure, however, does not preclude exposure to other psychoactive agents. As will be discussed repeatedly throughout this chapter, research investigating prenatal opiate exposure usually includes exposure to both heroin and methadone, and does not necessarily exclude exposure to amphetamines and/or barbiturates, benzodiazepines, cocaine, alcohol, nicotine, and propoxyphenes.

METHADONE MAINTENANCE DURING PREGNANCY

Opioids are comprised both of natural and synthetic analgesic compounds that have morphine-like activity, with heroin and methadone the most frequently used opiates among women of childbearing age. Opiate drugs affect the neurons involved in respiration, pain perception, and affective behavior. Heroin is derived from morphine; methadone is a synthetic opioid that has been used for over 20 years as a treatment for heroin abuse (Levy and Koren, 1990). Methadone maintenance involves the oral administration of daily medical doses of methadone as a substitute for heroin. Since the early 1970s, methadone maintenance has been recommended for narcotic dependence in pregnancy (Blinick et al., 1973). A primary reason for the use of methadone as a maintenance therapy for pregnant women is to stabilize drug use so that the fetus is not subjected to repeated episodes of withdrawal.

The pharmacology of methadone in the pregnant woman has been well evaluated. It is widely distributed throughout the body after oral ingestion with extensive nonspecific tissue bonding creating reservoirs that release unchanged methadone back into the blood, thus contributing to its long duration of action (Dole and Kreek, 1973). After ingestion of a maintenance dose of methadone, peak plasma levels occur between 2 and 6 hours with 6% of the ingested dose in the total blood volume at this time. Lower sustained plasma concentration are present during the remainder of the 24-hour period (Inturrisi and Verebely, 1972; Kreek, 1973; Sullivan and Blake, 1972). Studies of methadone in pregnant women show marked intra- and inter-individual variations in the plasma levels, somewhat lower after a given dose during pregnancy than following delivery. This decrease in available methadone can be accounted for by the increased extracellular space and increased tissue and fluid reservoirs associated with pregnancy, as well as enhanced metabolism by placental and fetal units (Kreek et al., 1974).

Although infants born to heroin- or methadone-dependent mothers have a high incidence of neonatal abstinence, the relationship between maternal methadone dose and the severity of withdrawal symptoms has been difficult to establish. Wilson et al. (1981) reported that although the incidence in severity of neonatal abstinence was similar for heroin- and methadone-exposed infants, neonatal abstinence was of longer duration with the methadone-exposed infants. Ostrea et al. (1976) and Madden et al. (1977) both reported a significant relationship between severity of withdrawal and methadone dose during pregnancy. However, other investigators (Blinick et al., 1973; Rosen and Pippenger, 1976; Stimmel et al., 1982) found no relationship between severity of withdrawal and maternal methadone dose. Kaltenbach et al. (1990) examined maternal methadone dose during pregnancy and infant outcome and found no significant association for polydrug abuse, opiate use, use of drugs other than opiates, average methadone dose, total months on methadone, or sex of the infant. Again, it must be reiterated that in most studies, identifying methadone or heroin as an independent variable does not exclude prenatal exposure to other opiates and/or amphetamines, barbiturates, benzodiazepines, cocaine, alcohol, nicotine, and propoxyphenes.

NEONATAL ABSTINENCE

Neonatal abstinence is described as a generalized disorder characterized by problems of central nervous system (CNS) irritability and autonomous system dysfunction. Symptoms include gastrointestinal dysfunction, respiratory distress, yawning, sneezing, mottling, and fever. Neonates often suck frantically on their fists or thumbs, yet they may have extreme difficulty feeding because they have an uncoordinated and ineffectual sucking reflex. Infants who undergo abstinence generally develop tremors which are initially mild and occur only when the infant is disturbed but which progress to the point where they occur spontaneously without any stimulation. High pitched crying, increased muscle tone, and irritability develop.

The abrupt removal of the drug at delivery precipitates the onset of symptoms. The newborn infant continues to metabolize and excrete the drug, and withdrawal or abstinence signs occur when critically low tissue levels have been reached (Finnegan and Kaltenbach, 1991). Onset of withdrawal symptoms varies from minutes or hours after birth to 2 weeks of age, but the majority of symptoms appear within 72 hours. Many factors influence the onset of abstinence in individual infants, including the type of multi-drug exposure in utero, both the timing and the dose before delivery, the character of labor, type and amount of anaesthesia analgesic given during labor, the maturity, and the presence of intrinsic disease in the infant. The withdrawal syndrome may be mild and transient, may be delayed in onset, or may have a stepwise increase in severity, may be intermittently present, or may have a biphasic course that includes acute neonatal withdrawal signs, followed by improvement and then the onset of a sub-acute withdrawal reaction (Desmond and Wilson, 1975).

With appropriate pharmacotherapy, neonatal abstinence can be satisfactorily treated without any untoward neonatal effects. It has been recommended that an abstinence scoring system be used to monitor the passively addicted neonate in a comprehensive and objective way in order to assess the onset, progression, and diminution of symptoms of abstinence (Finnegan, 1990).

NEUROBEHAVIORAL CHARACTERISTICS

The neurobehavioral characteristics of newborns undergoing abstinence uniformly have been investigated using the Brazelton Neonatal Behavioral Assessment Scale (Brazelton, 1973). A number of researchers (Chasnoff et al., 1984; Jeremy and Hans, 1985; Kaplan et al., 1976; Strauss et al., 1975, 1976) have consistently found that the behavior of infants born to narcotic-dependent women differ from infants born to nondrug dependent women. Narcotic-exposed infants have been found to be more irritable, less cuddly, exhibit more tremors, and have increased tone. Several studies also report narcotic-exposed infants are less responsive to visual stimulation; moreover, it has been found that infants undergoing abstinence are less likely to maintain an alert state, so the orientation tasks used in the Brazelton assessment often are not able to be completed.

Strauss et al. (1975) report that when elicited, the orientation behavior of infants exposed to narcotics was comparable to those of nondrug-exposed infants.

The important aspects of these neonatal behavioral characteristics are their implications on mother-infant interaction. These infants are frequently difficult to nurture because of the behavioral changes resulting in poor mother-infant bonding. It is suggested by Hoegerman et al. (1990) that the behavioral consequences on maternal-child bonding may be the most pervasive and devastating legacy of perinatal addiction. A study by Kaltenbach and Finnegan (1988), investigating the effect of neonatal abstinence on the infant's ability to interact with the environment, found that infants born to women maintained on methadone were deficient in their capacity for attention and social responsiveness during the first few days of life. These deficiencies were present regardless of whether or not neonatal abstinence was severe enough to require treatment. The interactive behavior appeared to be affected until the infant was free of abstinence symptomatology and detoxification was complete. Fitzgerald et al. (1990) studied patterns of interaction between drug-dependent women and their infants and nondrug exposed dyads. Mothers and infants were videotaped at birth and at 4 months of age. Interaction behavior was evaluated by the Greenspan-Lieberman Observational System (GLOS), Newborn GLOS, and Clinical Global rating systems. At 4 months of age, infants were assessed by the Bayley Scales of Infant Development, including the Infant Behavior Record. Mother's life stress and social support were evaluated by the Social Readjustment Rating Scale and structured interviews, respectively. Drug-dependent mothers and their newborn infants had significantly lower global ratings of dyadic interaction quality than comparison dyads. Both drug-dependent mothers and their newborns performed poorer on a measure of social engagement. Drug-dependent mothers demonstrated significantly less positive affect and greater detachment, while drug-exposed newborns presented fewer behaviors promoting social involvement. At 4 months of age, dyadic interaction quality, social engagement, detachment, and negative affect among drug-exposed infants and their mothers no longer differed from comparisons. Drug-dependent mothers, however, reported significantly higher levels of stressful events in the past year, which were strongly correlated with their negative affect and detachment scores during interaction. Drug-exposed 4-month-old infants showed significantly greater body tension and poorer coordination on the Infant Behavior Record.

PERINATAL OUTCOME

Perinatal outcome in relation to intrauterine growth has also been an area of concern. A number of prospective studies have yielded somewhat inconsistent findings. Studies that have compared infants born to heroin-dependent women not maintained on methadone versus infants born to heroin-dependent mothers receiving methadone have found differential effects with greater birth weights for infants born to methadone-maintained women (Zelson, 1973; Connaughton et al., 1975, 1977; Kandall et al., 1976; 1977). Kandall et al. (1976) reported a significant relationship between the first trimester maternal methadone dose and birth weight. This study indicated that methadone promotes fetal growth in a dose-related fashion even after maternal heroin use, whereas heroin itself causes fetal growth retardation that persists beyond the period of addiction. Stimmel et al. (1982) analyzed the birth records of 239 infants born to narcotic-dependent women on supervised methadone maintenance, women on unsupervised methadone maintenance, women on street heroin, and women who were multiple drug users. They found that although the presence of withdrawal symptoms did not differ with respect to type of drug abused, perinatal outcome was significantly improved in those infants born to women on supervised methadone maintenance, as compared to all other groups. Some studies that compared methadone-exposed infants with non-drug-exposed infants found that methadone-exposed infants have lower birth weights than comparison infants (Chasnoff et al., 1982; Lifshitz et al., 1983). On the other hand, other investigators found no differences in birth weights (Rosen and Johnson, 1982; Strauss et al., 1976). A more recent study by Kaltenbach and Finnegan (1987) with a large sample of full-term infants found that although methadone-exposed infants have smaller birth weights and head circumference than comparison infants, the methadone-exposed infants were not small for their gestational age and there was a positive correlation between head circumference and birth weight for both the methadone-exposed infants and comparison infants.

A longitudinal study by Pasto et al. (1989) evaluated the cerebral sonographic characteristics of methadone-exposed infants and comparison infants at birth, 1 month, and 6 months of age. Sonographic characteristics of the cerebral ventricles (slit-like, i.e., no visible fluid, versus normal) were recorded, as well as transverse measurements of the intracranial hemidiameter (ICHD), right and left lateral ventricles (RLV, LLV), temporal lobe (TL), and thalamic area measurements (traced in a transaxial view). Methadone-exposed infants had significantly more slit-like ventricles at all three examinations. Although the number of infants with slit-like ventricles decreased with age, slit-like ventricles were slower to resolve in lower birth-weight infants irrespective of drug exposure. Lateral ventricle measures and ICHDs were smaller in the narcotic-exposed infants but thalamic areas and temporal lobe measurements did not differ at any time. The smaller ICHD and LV measurements suggest possible slower cortical growth.

The incidence of strabismus has been found to be greater in infants exposed to narcotics in utero than the general population. A study by Nelson et al. (1987) found a 24% incidence of strabismus among narcotic-exposed infants in contrast to 5–8% incidence in the general population. Birth weights were lower for the infants with strabismus but average maternal methadone dose during pregnancy was higher. Thus, it is unclear whether the strabismus was related to lower birth weight, to narcotic exposure, or a to combination of factors.

DEVELOPMENTAL OUTCOME

Developmental sequelae associated with in utero methadone exposure have been investigated in a number of longitudinal studies. The assessment procedures used in these follow-up studies are quite similar. Children are evaluated throughout infancy, typically at 6-month intervals, with the Bayley Scales of Infant Development. Children born to nondrug-dependent women from comparable socioeconomic and racial backgrounds are used as control groups. A review of infant data are presented in Table I.

A study by Strauss et al. (1976) found that both methadone-exposed infants and comparison infants scored well within the normal range of development on the Bayley Mental Development Index (MDI) and the Motor Development Index (PDI) at 3, 6, and 12 months of age. PDI scores for the methadone-exposed infants, however, declined with age and differed from comparison infants by 12 months of age. Wilson et al. (1981) also found no difference in MDI scores among the infants they studied at 9 months of age, but found lower PDI scores for the methadone-exposed infants. While Rosen and Johnson (1982) found no difference between groups on MDI and PDI scores at 6 months of age, they found methadone-exposed infants to have both lower MDI and PDI scores at 12 and 18 months of age. In comparison, Hans and Marcus (1983) reported no difference at 4 and 12 months of age; Chasnoff et al. (1984) reported no difference at 3, 6, 12, and 24 months of age; and Kaltenbach and Finnegan (1986) found no difference at 6, 12, and 24 months of age.

Unfortunately, too few studies have followed these children longitudinally past infancy. Wilson et al. (1979) reported differences between narcotic-exposed children and three different comparison groups comprised of a drug environment group, a high risk group, and a socioeconomic comparison group. Children in this study ranged from approximately 3–6 ½ years of age. Narcotic-exposed children performed poorer than comparison groups on the General Cognitive Index (GCI) of the McCarthy Scales of Children's Abilities and on the perceptual, quantitative, and memory subscales. In this study, heroin was the predominant drug used; only a few of the mothers were maintained on methadone so there is some difficulty in comparing the data. Strauss et al. (1979) evaluated children from the original Strauss et al. (1976) sample when the children were 5 years of age. They found no differences between groups on the McCarthy Scales of Children's Abilities or any of the McCarthy subscales. Lifshitz et al. (1985) evaluated 93 children between the ages 3 and 6 from their original longitudinal sample. Performance on the McCarthy GCI was comparable for heroin-exposed, methadone-exposed, and comparison children. Kaltenbach and Finnegan (1991) also found no differences between groups on the McCarthy or any of the subscales in their sample of children at 4-½ years of age. Although all of these studies found no difference between groups, there are marked differences in the data of Kaltenbach and Finnegan and the other two studies The McCarthy scores from the Kaltenbach and Finnegan study are higher than one would expect, considering that children from low

TABLE I. Results of Longitudinal Studies Investigating Developmental Outcome of Infants Born to Women Maintained on Methadone

		Bayley Scales of Infant Development							
		MDI				PDI			
		Methadone		Comparison		Methadone		Comparison	
Studies	Ages (months)	M	SD	M	SD	M	SD	M	SD
Strauss et al. (1976)	3	112.5	1.5	115.3	13.5	119.4	9.1	117.1	14.5
	6	115.7	16.8	114.3	20.9	109.4	12.2	111.7	14.5
	12	113.4	10.2	114.8	11.3	102.8	11.0	110.4**	9.8*
Wilson et al. (1981)	9	99.3	15.5	105.5	15.6	89.9	12.6	99.0**	14.5*
Rosen and Johnson (1982)	6	95.0	2.52	100.7	4.20	101.0	2.84	105.0	2.97
	12	98.4	2.68	107.0*	2.81	94.9	2.53	102.8*	2.30
	18	96.0	2.31	106.4*	3.56	92.6	2.38	105.3*	2.21
Hans and Marcus (1983)	4	110		115		117		117	
	12	108		108		107		107	
Chasnoff et al. (1984)	3	104.2	11.1	99.2	9.0	104.3	11.8	102.8	7.0
	6	103.6	13.5	111.0	12.3	102.2	11.9	107.6	15.1
	12	99.6	10.6	105.8	8.1	104.4	11.9	103.8	12.5
	24	98.7	16.0	96.2	15.9	100.3	14.2	98.2	8.9
Kaltenbach and Finnega (1986)	6	104.7	13.2	106.9	8.2				
	12	103.5	12.9	109.3	7.7				
	24	98.7	16.7	103.9	14.5				

*P = 0.05.
**P = 0.01

socioeconomic backgrounds usually score lower on cognitive tests than average (Ramey et al., 1985). It may well have been that this was a self-select sample of mothers, especially interested in their children's development and, thus, may have been more willing to participate in a 5-year longitudinal study.

Diverse findings between studies reflect the myriad of confounding variables that are present within human populations. The women differ on amounts of daily methadone dose, the length of methadone maintenance during pregnancy, and the amount of prenatal care. A large percentage of pregnant women maintained on methadone continue to use a number of other drugs such as heroin, diazepam, cocaine, barbiturates, nicotine, and alcohol (Wilson et al., 1981; Rosen and Johnson, 1982). Thus, the lack of consistency in the data may be related to the absence of uniformity in patient management and patient compliance.

SUMMARY

The delineation of the effects of prenatal opiate exposure is a complex task. Perinatal and developmental outcomes associated with prenatal opiate exposure must be viewed within a multifactorial perspective, i.e., the primary pharmacological/toxicological effects produced by the drug(s); postnatal environmental interactive effects; and possible genetic effects (Hutchings, 1985).

While the existing data for the effects of prenatal opiate exposure on development in infancy indicate that infants through 2 years of age function well within the normal range of development, and, although quite limited, the data on these children between the ages of 2–5 years of age also suggest that they do not differ in overall cognitive function from a high-risk population, several caveats must be offered. Foremost is the fact that the data generated are dependent upon the measures that are used. These studies are based on a linear model that focuses only on general developmental and cognitive function and as such cannot detect subtle cognitive, behavioral, or process deficits. Furthermore, the subtle protracted effects of opiate exposure may be either exacerbated or ameliorated by variables in the maternal drug population. It is important that future research identify not only the biological and socioenvironmental risk factors concomitant within this population, but the conjunct function of these factors, so that the risk of prenatal opiate exposure may be more adequately determined.

REFERENCES

Blinick G, Jerez E, Wallach RC (1973): Methadone maintenance, pregnancy, and progeny. JAMA 225:477.

Brazelton TB (1973): "Neonatal Behavior Assessment Scale." Philadelphia: Lippincott.

Chasnoff IJ, Hatcher R, Burns W (1982): Polydrug and methadone addicted newborns: A continuum of impairment? Pediatrics 70:210–213.

Chasnoff IJ, Schnoll SH, Burns WJ, Burns K (1984): Maternal non-narcotic substance abuse during pregnancy: Effects on infant development. Neurobehav Toxicol Teratol 6(4):277–280.

Connaughton JF, Finnegan LP, Schut J, Emich JP (1975): Current concepts in the management of the pregnant opiate addict. Addict Dis 2:21–35.

Connaughton JF, Reeser D, Finnegan LP (1977): Pregnancy complicated by drug addiction. In Perinatal Mine Bolognese R, Schwartz R (eds): "Perinatal Medicine." Baltimore: Williams & Wilkins.

Desmond MM, Wilson GS (1975): Neonatal abstinence syndrome, recognition and diagnosis. Addict Dis 2:113–121.

Dole VP, Kreek MJ (1973): Methadone plasma level: Sustained by a reservoir of drug in tissue. Proc Natl Acad Sci 70:10.

Finnegan LP, Kaltenbach K (1991): The assessment and management of neonatal abstinence syndrome. In Hoekelman, Friedman, Nelson, Seidel (eds): "Primary Pediatric Care. 3rd Ed." St. Louis: C.V. Mosby Company (in press).

Fitzgerald E, Kaltenbach K, Finnegan LP (1990.): Patterns of interaction among drug dependent women and their infants. Pediatr Res Abst.

Hoegerman G, Wilson C, Thurmond E, Schnoll S (1990): Drug-exposed neonates. West J Med 152:559–564.

Inturrisi CE, Verebely K (1972): A gas liquid chromatographic method for the quantitative determination of methadone in human plasma and urine. J Chromatogr 65:361.

Jeremy RJ, Hans SL (1985): Behavior of neonates exposed in utero to methadone as assessed on the Brazelton Scale. Inf Behav Dev 8:323–336.

Kaltenbach K, Finnegan LP (1986): Developmental outcome of infants exposed to methadone in utero: A longitudinal study. Pediatr Res 20:57.

Kaltenbach K, Finnegan LP (1987): Perinatal and developmental outcome of infants exposed to methadone in utero. Neurotoxicol Teratol 9:311–313.

Kaltenbach K, Finnegan LP (1988): The influence of the neonatal abstinence syndrome on mother-infant interaction. In Anthony EJ, Chilard C (eds): "The Child in His Family: Perilous Development: Child Raising and Identity Formation Under Stress." New York: John Wiley, pp 223–230.

Kaltenbach K, Finnegan LP (1991): Children exposed to methadone in utero: Assessment of developmental and cognitive ability. In Ann NY Acad Sci (in press).

Kaltenbach K Thakur N, Weiner S, Finnegan LP (1990.): The relationship between maternal methadone dose during pregnancy and infant outcome. Pediat Res Abstr.

Kandall SR, Albin RS, Gartner LM, Lee KS, Eidelman A, Lowinson J (1977): The narcotic dependent mother: Fetal and neonatal consequences. Early Hum Dev 1:159–169.

Kandall SR, Albin S, Lowinson J, Berle B, Eidelman AJ, Gartner LM (1976): Differential effects of maternal heroin and methadone use on birth weight. Pediatrics 58:681–685.

Kaplan SL, Kron RE, Phoenix MD, Finnegan LP (1976): Brazelton neonatal assessment at three and twenty-eight days of age: A study of passively addicted infants, high risk infants, and normal infants. In Alksne H, Kaufman E (eds): "Critical Concerns in the Field of Drug Abuse." New York: Marcel Dekker, Inc. pp 726–730.

Kreek MJ (1973): Plasma and urine levels of methadone. NY State J Med 23:2773.

Kreek MJ, Schecter A, Gutjahr CL, Bowen D, Field F, Queenan J, Merkatz I (1974): Analyses of methadone and other drugs in maternal and neonatal body fluids:

Use in evaluation of symptoms in a neonate of mother maintained on methadone. Am J Drug Alcohol Abuse 1:409.

Levy M, Koren G (1990): Obstetric and neonatal effects of drugs of abuse. Emerg Med Clin North Am·

Lifshitz MH, Wilson GS, Smith E, Desmond M (1983): Fetal and postnatal growth of children born to narcotic-dependent women. J Pediatr 102:686–691.

Madden JD, Chappel JM, Zuspan F, Gumpel H, Mejia A, Davis R (1977): Observations and treatment of neonatal narcotic withdrawal. Am J Obstet Gynecol 127:199.

Nelson LB, Ehrlich S, Calhoun JH, Matteucci T, Finnegan LP (1987.): Occurrence of strabismus in infants born to drug dependent women. Am J Dis Child 141:175–178.

Ostrea EM, Chavez CJ, Strauss ME (1976): A study of factors that influence the severity of neonatal narcotic withdrawal. J Pediatr 88:642.

Pasto ME, Ehrlich S, Kaltenbach K, Graziani L, Kurtz A, Goldberg B, Finnegan LP (1989): Cerebral sonographic characteristics and maternal and neonatal risk factors in infants of opiate dependent mothers. Ann NY Acad Sci·

Ramey CT, Bryant DM, Swarez TM (1985): Preschool compensatory education and the modifiability of intelligence: A critical review. In D. Detterman (ed): "Current Topics in Human Intelligence." Norwood, NJ: Ablex, pp 247–296.

Rosen RS, Pippenger CE (1976): Pharmacologic observation on the neonatal withdrawal syndrome. J Pediatr 88:1044.

Rosen RS, Johnson HL (1982): Children of methadone maintained mothers: Follow-up to 18 month of age. J Pediatr 101:192–196.

Stimmel B, Goldberg J, Reisman A, Murphy R, Teets K (1982): Fetal outcome in narcotic dependent women: The importance of the type of maternal narcotic used. Am. J. Drug Alcohol Abuse 9(4):383–395.

Strauss ME, Lessen-Firestone JK, Chavez CJ, Stryker JC (1979.): Children of methadone treated women at five years of age. Pharmacol Biochem Behav Suppl 11:3–6.

Strauss ME, Lessen-Firestone JK, Starr RH, Ostrea EM (1975): Behavior of narcotic-addicted newborns. Child Dev 46:887–893.

Strauss ME, Starr RH, Ostrea EM, Chavez CJ, Stryker JC (1976): Behavioral concomitants of prenatal addiction to narcotics. J Pediatr 89:842–846.

Sullivan HR, Blake DA (1972.): Quantitative determination of methadone concentration in human blood, plasma, and urine by gas chromatography. Res Commun Chem Pathol Pharmacol 3:467.

Wilson GS, Desmond MM, Wait RB (1981): Follow-up of methadone treated women and their infants: Health developmental and social implications. J Pediatr 98:716–722.

Wilson GS, McCreary R, Kean J, Baxter C (1979): The development of preschool children of heroin-addicted mothers: A controlled study. Pediatrics 63:135–141.

Zelson C (1973): Infant of the addicted mother. N Engl J Med 288:1391–1395.

Development of the Central Nervous System:
Effects of Alcohol and Opiates, pages 47–69
© 1992 Wiley-Liss, Inc.

4

Effects of Prenatal Exposure to Ethanol on Cell Proliferation and Neuronal Migration

MICHAEL W. MILLER

Veterans Administration Medical Center and Department of Psychiatry, University of Iowa College of Medicine, Iowa City, Iowa

INTRODUCTION

The development of the mammalian central nervous system takes place over an extended period of time. One of the early stages in the development of the immature nervous system is the formation of the neural plate which in the rat takes place about gestational day (G) 5 (Hebel and Stromberg, 1986). Neuronal development continues well into the third postnatal month when most neurons have achieved their mature morphology (e.g., Jacobson, 1978; Nowakowski, 1988; Stanfield and Cowan, 1988; Miller, 1988a).

As the central nervous system develops normally, cells pass through four ontogenetic phases—cell proliferation, migration, differentiation, and death. The proliferation (mitotic division) of neuronal precursors occurs in zones that line the neural tube (or ventricles) or in auxiliary germinal zones that are derived from these ventricular zones (e.g., Schaper, 1897; His, 1904; Schaper and Cohen, 1905; Sauer, 1935; Sidman et al., 1959; Miale and Sidman, 1961; Angevine and Sidman, 1961; Angevine, 1965; Altman and Das, 1966; 1972; Altman et al., 1969; Bayer, 1980; Stanfield and Cowan, 1988). Post-mitotic neurons leave the germinal zones and migrate through a topographically complex field using radial glial fibers as guides (e.g., Rakic, 1972, 1978, Nowakowski and Rakic, 1979; Pinto-Lord et al., 1982). These fibers extend from the germinal zones to the pial surface. After reaching their final position in the cortical plate, the post-migratory neurons begin to differentiate into their mature phenotypes. A significant portion of the neurons die (Hamburger and Oppenheim, 1982; Clarke, 1985; Finlay et al., 1987).

The number of neurons in a particular structure in the central nervous system represents the summation of the individual ontogenetic processes. In this sense, cell proliferation and neuronal migration are generative processes, i.e., these processes underlie the addition of new cells to the structure. Various extrinsic factors can affect these processes. For example, exposure to factors such as X-rays, bromodeoxyuridine, and methylazoxymethanol acetate reduces the number of proliferating cells, and can even cause the death of proliferating cells (e.g., Hicks et al., 1959; Altman et al., 1969; Altman and Anderson, 1972; Druckney and Lange, 1972; Matsumoto et al., 1972; Bannigan, 1987). Genetic and environmental factors can also affect neuronal migration so that many neurons do not complete their migration or migrate to an inappropriate position (Pearlman, 1988; Caviness et al., 1988; Nowakowski, 1988). On the other hand, neuronal death is a "regressive" or degenerative ontogenetic process which reduces the number of neurons in a structure. The death of neurons can result from factors that are inherent to the nervous system, naturally occurring neuronal death (Hamburger and Oppenheim, 1982; Clarke, 1985; Finlay et al., 1987). This death affects post-migratory neurons that may be competing for synaptic sites or trophic factors which are in limited supply. On the other hand, neuronal death can result from exposure to extrinsic factors including environmental changes or exposure to a toxin or drug. These factors may affect cells in any stage of their development. The effects of ethanol on neuronal death are examined by Ward and West in Chapter 6.

This chapter explores the mechanisms by which ethanol alters the generative processes of cell proliferation and neuronal migration. In this regard, the effects of pre- and postnatal exposure to ethanol on the number of neurons in various structures of the central nervous system are discussed. Attention is paid to the timing of the exposure to ethanol, particularly in relation to the ontogenetic phase through which the neurons are passing. References generally allude to experiments in which (a) rodents (usually rats) exposed to ethanol had peak blood ethanol concentrations of 100–200 mg/dl and (b) control rats were pair-fed a nutritionally balanced control diet.

NEUROGENESIS AND CELL PROLIFERATION
Neocortex

The brains of juvenile and mature rats exposed to ethanol pre- and/or postnatally are significantly smaller than the brains of pair-fed controls (e.g., Diaz and Samson, 1980; Lancaster et al., 1982; Burns et al., 1984; West et al., 1986; Nathaniel et al., 1986a; Miller, 1987). After prenatal exposure to ethanol, the brain weight is reduced 9–20%, whereas for postnatal exposure to ethanol produces a 17–19% smaller brain. Prenatal exposure to ethanol causes a 32% decrease in the DNA content of whole brain (Woodson and Ritchley, 1979). One of the structures which is particularly susceptible to the effects of prenatal exposure to ethanol is the cerebral cortex. The cortices of ethanol-treated rats are 13% smaller than for pair-fed controls (Miller, 1987). This translates into a significant decrease in the number of cortical cells (Miller and Potempa, 1990). There are 33.0% fewer neurons and 36.2% fewer glia in primary somatosensory cortex of ethanol-treated rats than in controls. All cortical layers are affected relatively equally.

In normal rats, neocortical neurons are generated during the second half of gestation (Miller, 1988a). Neurons in all layers of cortex are neither generated simultaneously nor haphazardly; cortical neuronogenesis is a highly ordered process. Cortical neuronogenesis can be described by the sum of three orthogonal spatiotemporal gradients, a lateral-to-medial, a rostral-to-caudal, and an inside-to-outside gradient (e.g., Angevine and Sidman, 1961; Gardette et al., 1982; Smart, 1983; Miller, 1985, 1987, 1988b). Accordingly, neurons in the deep laminae of rostromedial cortex are among the first generated and those in the superficial laminae of caudolateral cortex are among the last generated.

The timing and the pattern of neuronal generation is profoundly altered by ethanol (Fig. 1). Neuronogenesis is delayed 1–2 days by prenatal expo-

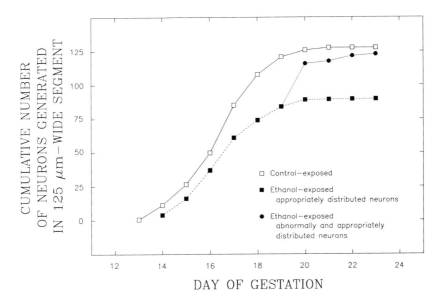

Fig. 1. Effect of prenatal exposure to ethanol on the density of cortical neurons generated daily. The cumulative density of neurons heavily labeled by single injections of [³H]thymidine placed during the period from G12–G23 is plotted against time. All values are based upon counts of neurons made on segments of tissue 125 μm wide. The data for the offspring of pair-fed controls can be described as a sigmoidal function. In contrast, the data for the rats prenatally exposed to ethanol is a complex curve which is the sum of two sigmoidal functions (open squares). One of these functions describes the density of neurons which is appropriately distributed in cortex based upon neuronal birthdate (solid squares). This curve lags behind the control values in steadily increasing amounts. The second, and smaller sigmoidal function represents the data on the density of neurons which are abnormally distributed in the "wrong" layer upon neuronal birthdates (solid circles). The delayed surge in the density of these abnormally distributed neurons compensates for the early reduction in neuronal generation. Thus, the total density of neurons in the ethanol-treated rats approximates that in the control rats. (Data taken from Miller, 1986.)

sure to ethanol (Miller, 1986, 1987, 1988b). The number of neurons born daily is altered by ethanol in a complex manner. Between G12 and G19, 30% fewer neurons are generated in ethanol-treated rats than in controls. After G19, however, there is a compensatory surge in neuronal generation; between G20–G23, 490% more neurons are born in ethanol-exposed rats than in controls. Interestingly, the abnormal, ethanol-induced surge in neuronal generation occurs coincidentally throughout neocortex. That is, there is no evidence of the lateral-to-medial or rostral-to-caudal gradient in the late surge in neuronal generation. The absence of these pan-cortical gradients suggests that cell proliferation in the cortical germinal zones is affected by a synchronizing factor(s), a factor(s) that is susceptible to the effects of ethanol.

Ethanol exposure has no effect upon the lateral-to-medial and rostral-to-caudal gradients of neuronogenesis, however, the inside-to-outside pattern of generation is disturbed (Miller, 1986, 1987, 1988b). Although early-generated neurons are distributed in the deep layers and some late-generated neurons are in superficial cortex, many late-generated neurons are distributed in the deep laminae. These data reflect changes in neuronal migration (see below).

Neocortical neurons are derived from a ventricular zone. The ventricular zone is a pseudostratified columnar epithelium, i.e., all cells contact the basement membrane and many extend to its apical limit (e.g., Schaper, 1897; His, 1904; Schaper and Cohen, 1905; Sauer, 1935; Boulder Committee, 1970; Hinds and Ruffett, 1971). This zone is most prominent during the first half of cortical neuronogenesis and wanes during the latter half (Miller, 1989).

Proliferative activity in the ventricular zone appears to be depressed by ethanol (Miller, 1989). It appears that the number of cells in the ventricular zone is decreased by ethanol exposure for despite no ethanol-induced changes in the size of the lateral ventricles, the ventricular zone is significantly thinner in ethanol-treated rats than in controls throughout much of the period of cortical neuronogenesis. Moreover, the fraction of ventricular cells labeled by a single dose of [³H]thymidine is reduced by ethanol exposure. From these data, it can be implied that ethanol exposure causes either a decrease in the number of proliferating cells or an increase in the length of the cell cycle.

As in other proliferating cell populations, mitotically active cells in the ventricular zone pass sequentially through four phases of the cell cycle. This cycle begins as a cell divides into two cells during the mitotic (M) phase. Subsequently, daughter cells enter a dynamic "gap" phase (G1), followed by a DNA synthetic phase (S). These transiently tetraploid cells pass through a second "gap" phase (G2) when the cells prepare for a mitotic division. During the period of cortical neuronogenesis in rodents, the cell cycle of telencephalic ventricular cells takes 11–21 hours, the amount of time increases with age (Atlas and Bond, 1965; Shimada and Langman, 1970; Waechter and Jaensch, 1972; Miller and Nowakowski, 1991). The most variable phase is G1; the durations of G1, S, and the summed duration of G2 and M are 4–11 hours, 7–9 hours, and 2–3 hours, respectively. As each cell in the ventricular zone moves through the phases of the cell cycle, the position of its nucleus and perikaryon changes. Mitotic cells are distributed along the ventricular surface whereas the cell bodies of cells in S are in the outer third of the ventricular zone (F. Sauer, 1935, 1936; M. Sauer, 1959; Leblond et al., 1959; Hinds and Ruffett, 1971; Seymour and Berry, 1975). This cyclic to-and-fro movement of the nucleus is known as "interkinetic nuclear migration."

Ethanol alters the duration of the cell cycle and the proportion of cells that are cycling. The cell cycle for ventricular cells is 29% longer in 21-day-old ethanol-treated fetuses than in age-matched controls (Miller and Nowakowski, 1991). In lieu of no changes in the proportion of mitotically active cells (Kennedy and Elliott, 1985; Miller, 1989) or in the duration of S (Miller and Nowakowski, 1991), it appears that the duration of G1 is most altered by ethanol. Additional support that ethanol affects the cell cycle comes from the effects of ethanol on the size of proliferating cells. In normal rats, the size of cells in different phases of the cell cycle is correlated with their DNA content (Sauer, 1935, 1936). The size of the nuclei of ventricular cells in S and G2, and the size of mitotic cells are markedly greater than the size of cells in G1. That is, nuclei of cells with DNA contents of greater than 2n are larger than those of diploid cells. Morphological evidence suggests that in rats prenatally exposed to ethanol, the size of the cells that have DNA contents greater than 2n is significantly greater than for diploid cells (Miller, 1989). Conceivably, this results from the effect of the ethanol on the packaging or synthesis of the DNA. It should be noted, however, that ethanol does not alter the spatial distribution of cells in S and in M. Therefore, it appears that interkinetic nuclear migration per se is not affected by ethanol.

Neocortical cells are also generated from a secondary proliferative zone, the cortical subventricular zone. This zone is located immediately suprajacent to the ventricular zone, i.e., toward the pial surface (Schaper and Cohen, 1905; Kershman, 1938; Smart, 1961; Lewis, 1968; Boulder Committee, 1970; Nowakowski and Rakic, 1981). The subventricular zone differs from the ventricular zone in several ways. The subventricular zone is not a pseudostratified columnar epithelium; there is no basement membrane and not all cells in this zone typically contact its basal limit, i.e., subventricular cells are stratified (Rakic et al., 1974). The cells of the subventricular zone do not participate in interkinetic nuclear migration. Instead, cells involved in mitosis and DNA synthesis are distributed in an apparently haphazard manner throughout the depth of the subventricular zone (Schaper and Cohen, 1905; Smart, 1961).

In contrast to the ventricular zone, proliferative activity in the subventricular zone is increased by ethanol exposure, particularly during the latter segment of the neuronogenetic period. Chronic exposure to ethanol during gestation using a standard liquid diet paradigm produces a thickening of the subventricular zone (Miller, 1989). Apparently the increased thickness of the subventricular zone compensates for the decreased thickness of the ventricular zone so that the overall thickness of the neocortical proliferative zones is unaffected by ethanol exposure (Kennedy and Elliott, 1985). Other indices of an ethanol-induced increase in cell proliferation within the subventricular zone are that the proportion of cells which take up [³H]thymidine (Miller, 1989) and the fraction of subventricular cells that are cycling is significantly greater in ethanol-treated rats than in pair-fed controls (Miller and Nowakowski, 1991). On the other hand, the total duration of the cell cycle, and apparently of each phase of the cell cycle, and the size of the cells in the subventricular cells, regardless of the phase of the cell cycle which they are in, is unaltered by ethanol.

Kennedy and colleagues administered ethanol by gavage in order to compare the effects of acute and chronic ethanol exposure on cell proliferation in the two neocortical germinal zones of the mouse (Kennedy et al., 1984; Kennedy and Elliott, 1985). Acute exposure to ethanol on G13–G15 has no effect upon the total thickness of the germinal zones or the cortical plate or on the distribution or density of mitotic cells. In contrast, chronic exposure to ethanol from G11–G18 leads to a reduction in the density of mitotic figures in the ventricular zone and an increase in the density of mitotic figures in the subventricular zone. The results of the chronic exposure experiment are akin to those described above. Thus, despite achieving a higher peak blood ethanol concentration in the study of acute exposure, the effects of chronic exposure are greater. It appears that the proliferating population can offset the damage resulting from an exposure to ethanol limited to the early part of the period of cortical neuronogenesis. On the other hand, the proliferating population is unable to accommodate to the trauma when the exposure to ethanol extends throughout the period of neuronogenesis.

The differential effects of ethanol on the ventricular and subventricular zones may underlie the ethanol-induced changes in neuronal generation (Miller, 1986, 1987, 1988b, 1989). Proliferative activity in the ventricular zone is depressed by ethanol. This zone is most prominent during the early period of neuronal generation. Ethanol depresses proliferative activity in this zone and it also reduces the number of early-generated neurons. In contrast, the subventricular zone is most prominent late in the period of neuronogenesis. Ethanol stimulates proliferative activity in this zone and the number of late-generated neurons is abnormally high in ethanol-treated rats.

Although it is known that the ventricular zone is a mosaic of glioblasts and neuroblasts (Levitt et al., 1981, 1983), the phenotypic expression of the derivatives of the subventricular zone is unknown. Based upon timing, it has been argued that the ventricular zone gives rise to neurons and the subventricular zone to glia or that derivatives of the ventricular zone become neurons and glia in deep cortex and subventricular zone decendants develop into cells in the superficial cortex (e.g., Berry, 1974; Nowakowski and Rakic, 1981; Miller, 1988b). The spatiotemporal correlation between the effects of ethanol on cell proliferation and neuronal generation supports the concept that the subventricular zone does give rise to neurons and likely neurons in the superficial laminal.

The differential expression of various factors may underlie the opposite effects of ethanol on the two neocortical proliferative zones. Such factors include α-fetoprotein and albumin which are present in the ventricular zone (Benno and Williams, 1978; Trojan and Uriel, 1979; Toran-Allerand, 1980). Moreover, opiate receptors are expressed in the subventricular zone (Kent et al., 1982) suggesting that opiates may have differential effects on the two zones. In the adult, ethanol alters the opiate system directly (Charness et al., 1983; Lucchi et al., 1985; Khatami et al., 1987) and indirectly (Lucchi et al., 1985). Ethanol has marked effects upon the opiate system and opiate-related behavior (Chapters 13 and 15) and current evidence shows that the opiates are intimately involved in the regulation of cell proliferation (Chapter 14).

Principal Sensory Nucleus

Examination of the effects of ethanol on the development of other structures in the central nervous system supports the concept that ethanol can affect proliferating populations in differential manners. Structures which have been examined are the principal sensory nucleus of the trigeminal nerve (PSN), the hippocampal formation, and the cerebellar cortex. The PSN is of interest because it receives somatosensory input from the face and prenatal exposure to ethanol causes craniofacial malformations in children and rodents alike (e.g., Jones et al., 1973; Clarren et al., 1978; Sulik et al., 1981; Sulik and Johnston, 1983; Edwards and Dow-Edwards, submitted). Moreover, the PSN is another structure which is derived solely from ventricular cells.

The generation of cells in the PSN occurs during the period from G12 through G22 (Nornes and Morita, 1979; Miller and Muller, 1989). Most neurons were born on G12–G14; these are the small neurons in the PSN. On G15, the few large neurons found in the PSN are born. Gliogenesis largely occurs after G16. Ethanol reduces the number of small neurons generated on G12–G14 by 40% and the generation of the large neurons is delayed by 1 day (Miller and Muller, 1989). A study of cell proliferation in the rhombencephalic ventricular zone of mice shows that high levels of ethanol cause no effect on the fraction of cells labeled by an injection of [^{3}H]thymidine (Bannigan and Burke, 1982). Acute high doses of ethanol, however, do cause many of the cycling cells to degenerate via pyknosis. The net result is that ethanol reduces the output from the ventricular zone. In addition, since pyknotic cells are not evident in other parts of the fetal neural tube, these data strongly indicate that the cycling cell is the target of ethanol.

Hippocampal Formation

The hippocampal formation is composed of two structures, the hippocampus and the dentate gyrus. Both structures are composed of three fundamental layers; in the hippocampus these strata are the molecular, pyramidal, and polymorphic layers and in the dentate gyrus they are the molecular, granular, and polymorphic layers.

Two studies have examined the effects of ethanol on the population of hippocampal neurons in mature and immature rats (Barnes and Walker,

1981; West et al., 1986). Following pre- or postnatal exposure to ethanol, the density of cells in the pyramidal layer reportedly decreases. These effects were time limited. Exposure to ethanol during the second half of gestation produced a 20% decrease in the density of cells in the pyramidal layer in the CA1 region (Barnes and Walker, 1981), whereas exposure between postnatal day (P) 4 and P10 had no effect on cell density in CA1, or for that matter in CA3 (West et al., 1986).

These data are difficult to interpret for rigorous stereological analyses were not applied. The cell bodies of hippocampal pyramidal neurons are significantly smaller in rats prenatally exposed to ethanol than in pair-fed controls (Davies and Smith, 1981). This change in size can lead to a stereological artifact such that the calculated cell packing density is overestimated (Floderus, 1944; Abercrombie, 1946; Smolen et al., 1983). Furthermore, there was no attempt to determine the effect of ethanol on the total volume of the pyramidal layer in CA1. If the volume of the hippocampal formation is altered by ethanol exposure, then the neuronal densities cannot be directly translated into numbers of neurons. Few pertinent data are available. Neither prenatal nor postnatal exposure to ethanol affects the area of the pyramidal layer in sections at the same level of the brain; however, these data do not take into account 3-dimensional changes in hippocampal size. A crude index of the 3-dimensional changes in hippocampal volume is the effect of pre- and postnatal exposure to ethanol on the size of the brain (cf. Barnes and Walker, 1981; West et al., 1986). In the model used by Barnes and Walker (1981), prenatal exposure to ethanol did not affect the overall weight of the brain, however, West et al. (1986) described that postnatal exposure to ethanol produced a significant reduction in the size of the brain (-20%).

Hippocampal neurons are generated prenatally and all of these neurons are derived from the ventricular zone (Angevine, 1965; Schlessinger et al., 1975; Bayer, 1980; Nowakowski and Rakic, 1981). Thus, since the number of neurons in the CA1 region are decreased only when the exposure to ethanol occurs during the period of neuronogenesis, it appears that as with neocortex, ethanol depresses cell proliferation in the ventricular zone.

The effect of ethanol on the developing dentate gyrus is paradoxical in comparison with that on the hippocampus. Prenatal exposure to ethanol has no effect or produces a slight, but not significant, decrease in the density of neurons in the granular layer (Barnes and Walker, 1981). In contrast, postnatal exposure to ethanol increases the density of granule neurons (West et al., 1986). As with the data on the hippocampal pyramidal neurons, caution must be used in interpreting these data because stereological methods were not used.

Granule cells in the dentate gyrus are generated over a long period of time. Neuronogenesis begins in the third week of gestation and continues until the rat is at least 1 year old (Schlessinger et al., 1975; Kaplan and Hinds, 1977; Bayer, 1980; Bayer et al., 1982). Only a small number of the granule cells (10–15%) in 21- or 60-day-old rats are generated prenatally; the remainder (85–90%) are generated after birth. The granule cells that are generated prenatally are derived from the ventricular zone, whereas those born postnatally are derived from an auxiliary proliferative zone, the intrahilar proliferative zone (also known as the CA4 region of the hippocampal formation). Thus, the data from the dentate gyrus are in concert with the data from the neocortex. That is, the differential effects of pre- and postnatal exposure to ethanol on the density of granule neurons appear to result from the depressive effects of ethanol on the ventricular zone and the stimulation of proliferation in the postnatally active intrahilar zone. The lack of a decrease in granule cell density after prenatal exposure to ethanol may merely be the reflection of the small number of granule neurons generated prenatally.

Cerebellum

The cerebellar cortex has been the focus of many studies on ethanol toxicity in the developing nervous system. Part of the attractiveness is 1) the role of the cerebellum in motor coordination, a function which is impaired by early exposure to ethanol, and 2) the anatomical simplicity of the cortex. The cerebellar cortex is composed of three layers. From the white matter to the pial surface, they are the granule cell layer, the Purkinje cell layer, and the molecular layer. These laminae are populated by three classes of neurons, granule cells (granule cell layer), Purkinje cells (Purkinje cell layer), and variety of inhibitory local circuit neurons (all three layers). Due to this apparent simplicity, the complex effects of environmental agents such as ethanol are more readily discerned in the cerebellum than other central nervous system structures.

One index of the complexity of the effects of ethanol on cerebellum development is the size of the cerebellum. The cerebellum of a 21-day-old rat exposed to ethanol during gestation and the first 3 postnatal weeks (blood ethanol concentrations were below 125 mg/dl) is 10% smaller than pair-fed controls (Borges and Lewis, 1982, 1983b). Comparable reductions in cerebellar size have been recorded following exposure to ethanol during the last 2 weeks of gestation (Kornguth et al., 1979; Nathaniel et al., 1986a,b) and following exposure to ethanol during the first postnatal weeks (Diaz and Samson, 1980). Unfortunately, it is difficult to equate the effects of pre- and postnatal exposure because the manner, timing, and amount of ethanol administered varied among the studies. For example, Borges and Lewis (1982, 1983b) fed the alcohol ad libitum and the peak blood ethanol concentration was 118m/dl. Nathaniel et al. (1986a,b) administered the ethanol via a liquid diet and the mean peak blood ethanol concentration in their rats was 150 mg/dl. On the other hand, Diaz and Samson (1980) administered the ethanol postnatally by gavage. The resulting mean blood ethanol concentration in these pups was 279 mg/dl.

An alternative approach has been to expose pregnant rats or neonates to ethanol by placing the subjects in an ethanol vapor-saturated atmosphere (Bauer-Moffett and Altman, 1975, 1977; Phillips and Cragg, 1982; Phillips, 1985). Five-day-old rats reared in this manner have blood ethanol concentrations in the range of 200–539 mg/dl. Prenatal exposure to ethanol leads to a 34% reduction in cerebellar size (Phillips and Cragg, 1982), whereas postnatal exposure to ethanol results in smaller reductions (4–12%; Bauer-Moffett and Altman, 1977; Phillips and Cragg, 1982).

A recent, carefully controlled study (Bonthius and West, 1990) in which the ethanol was delivered by gavage shows that the blood ethanol concentrations in pups postnatally exposed to ethanol is directly related to the reductions in cerebellar size. Peak blood ethanol concentrations of 45, 190, and 365 mg/dl result in 4.6, 18.8, and 36.5% reductions in the size of the cerebellum, respectively. Moreover, the total brain size was consistently less severely affected by these postnatal exposures. Thus, it appears that the cerebellum may be more susceptible to the effects of ethanol than many other parts of the brain. Taken together, all of the above data show that pre- and postnatal exposure to ethanol affect cerebellar size.

The data on cerebellar size provide crude indices that ethanol produces changes in the proliferation of cerebellar cells. Further insight can be gained by examining the effects of ethanol on the number of Purkinje and granule cells. Exposure to moderate amounts of ethanol during gestation and the first 3 postnatal weeks (which produce blood ethanol concentrations below 125 mg/dl) does not affect the density of Purkinje cells in 21-day-old rats (Volk et al., 1981; Borges and Lewis, 1983b). On the other hand, higher mean peak blood ethanol concentrations (between 200 mg/dl and above) result in significant decreases in Purkinje cell density. In vapor inhalation paradigms in which the blood ethanol cooncentrations are 200 mg/dl or more, prenatal exposure to ethanol leads to significant reductions (1–47%) in Purkinje cell density in a particular cerebellar lobe (Phillips and Cragg, 1982; Phillips, 1985). Postnatal exposure to ethanol produces a 1–51% reduction in Purkinje cell density (Bauer-Moffett and Altman, 1977; Phillips and Cragg, 1982; Phillips, 1985; Yanai and Waknin, 1985). It should be noted that ethanol-induced pyknosis of Purkinje cells has been described in experiments in which the mean peak blood ethanol concentration in neonates is 400–500 mg/dl (Cragg and Phillips, 1985). Unfortunately, it is difficult to compare the results of these studies since they did not employ rigorous morphometric analyses which account for changes in cell size and cerebellar volume. Nevertheless, since the size of the cerebellum is decreased and the density of Purkinje cells is not affected by prenatal exposure to ethanol, the number of Purkinje cells must be decreased. The lack of a change in cell density after exposure to the lower doses ethanol suggests that ethanol solely decreases cell proliferation. On the other hand, the finding of decreases in Purkinje cell density only in experiments in which the amount of ethanol administered and/or the blood ethanol concentrations are particularly high suggests that only with high doses does ethanol cause neuronal death.

The density of granule cells also has been examined extensively. In contrast to the Purkinje cells, pre- and postnatal exposure to ethanol decreases the density of granule cells (Bauer-Moffett and Altman, 1977; Anderson and Sides, 1978; Borges and Lewis, 1983b; Yanai and Waknin, 1985). The thesis that ethanol is primarily affecting proliferating populations is supported by finding of pyknotic cells in the external granule cell layer, a secondary proliferative zone (Anderson and Sides, 1978), and by the conspicuous lack of pyknosis and phagocytosis in the internal granule cell layer after postnatal exposure to ethanol (Bauer-Moffett and Altman, 1975, 1977; Phillips and Cragg, 1982; Phillips, 1985).

From the data on the numbers of Purkinje and granule cell numbers, various investigators have concluded that the deleterious effects of ethanol on the developing cerebellum, and particularly on maturing Purkinje cells, are greatest when the exposure to ethanol occurs during the period of synaptogenesis (e.g., Bauer-Moffett and Altman, 1975, 1977; Phillips and Cragg, 1982; Phillips, 1985). Alternatively, it has been proposed than the reductions in Purkinje and granule cell numbers result primarily from decreases in the stem cell populations (Bauer-Moffett and Altman, 1975; Borges and Lewis, 1982, 1983a). The development of cerebellar neurons occurs over a protracted period, however, the timing and site of generation of both Purkinje and granule cells do not overlap (e.g., Miale and Sidman, 1961; Altman and Das, 1966; Altman et al., 1969). Purkinje neurons arise prenatally from cells in the ventricular zone and granule cells are derived postnatally from the external granule cell layer. Thus, prenatal ethanol exposure causes the decrease in Purkinje cell number by directly affecting the pool of proliferating Purkinje cell precursors. On the other hand, postnatal exposure to ethanol cannot directly affect the Purkinje cell precursors, but it does influence the number of dividing cells in the external granule cell layer which ultimately alters the number of granule cells. Hence, the decreases in Purkinje cell number due to the postnatal exposure to ethanol may be secondary; secondary in that they result from a transneuronal degeneration caused by the ethanol-induced reduction in the number of granule cells.

Few data are available which can resolve the controversy as to whether the target of ethanol toxicity is the proliferating cerebellar cells or neurons which are forming synapses. It is expected that if the proliferating population is the target, then the number of Purkinje cells would be most affected by an exposure to ethanol prenatally, and that the number of granule cells would be most affected by an exposure to ethanol postnatally. Unfortunately, there has been only one study of cerebellar neuronogenesis (Bauer-Moffett and Altman, 1977). It that study, high doses of ethanol were delivered postnatally. The spatiotemporal pattern of granule cell generation was not affected by ethanol exposure. Thus, in light of the findings of a smaller cerebellum, it was concluded that the pool of granule cell precursors was decreased by ethanol. The reductions in granule cell generation may be more complex than simply a loss in the stem cell population. The decrease in granule cell generation may result from two other changes. 1) Ethanol exposure increases the duration of the cell cycle by 21%, particularly the durations of the G1 and S phases (Borges and Lewis, 1983a). 2) Ethanol may retard the migration of postmitotic neurons from the external granule cell layer (Kornguth et al., 1979; see below). The final resolution of the controversy will require a battery of carefully controlled longitudinal studies of the changes in neuronal numbers or an examination of the effects of ethanol on chimeras with cerebellar defects.

NEURONAL MIGRATION

After a proliferating cell divides, a daughter cell either remains in the proliferating zone to divide again or it begins its migration. As a neuron migrates from its proliferating zone, it passes through a zone composed of processes and other migrating neurons before it reaches its final residence in the developing structure.

The concept that ethanol affects neuronal migration originated in the studies on autopsy material from human children with fetal alcohol syndrome (e.g., Clarren et al., 1978). Following prenatal exposure to ethanol, sheets or clusters of ectopic neurons were identified. Such abnormalities were identified throughout the central nervous system, notably in neocortex, in cerebellar cortex, and in the floor of the fourth ventricle. Often ectopic clusters are located near the pial surface so that in addition to neurons, they are composed of glia, undifferentiated cells, and pial cells. Such features suggest that ethanol affects the mechanism for stopping the migration of the young neurons. But the defects are not restricted to the surface. For example, deep to the sheets of leptomengial heterotopias in neocortex, cortex is thinned and the lamination is disorganized. These findings indicate that ethanol has broad effects on neuronal migration and that the orderly spatiotemporal sequence of neuronal migration is profoundly altered by exposure to ethanol.

Consumption of moderate amounts of ethanol by pregnant rats does not produce severe disruptions in the lamination of neocortex (Jacobson et al., 1979; Miller and Dow-Edwards, 1988; Norton et al., 1988; Miller and Potempa, 1990), hippocampus (e.g., Davies and Smith, 1981; West et al., 1981), or cerebellar cortex (e.g., Bauer-Moffett and Altman, 1977; Kornguth et al., 1979; Phillips and Cragg, 1982; Borges and Lewis, 1983b) of the mature offspring. Nevertheless, there is evidence in each of these structures that neuronal migration is altered by ethanol exposure.

In neocortex, the emergence of the laminae is delayed by prenatal exposure to ethanol (Jacobson et al., 1979) and projection neurons with discrete laminar distributions (e.g., corticospinal and callosal neurons) are abnormally distributed (Miller, 1987; Kotkoskie and Miller, 1989). Moreover, acute administration of high doses of ethanol on G14 and G15 leads to the formation of ectopic clusters of neurons in 21-day-old fetuses (Kotkoskie and Norton, 1988). Although adequate control for defects induced by malnutrition were not used in this study, it should be noted that apparently there is no evidence that protein malnutrition produces abnormalities in neuronal migration (Morgane et al., 1978).

In the hippocampal formation, ectopic granule cells (which presumably were generated prenatally in the ventricular zone) can be observed at any of various places along the migratory path (Miller and Nowakowski, unpublished results).

Evidence in the rat cerebellum also suggests that neuronal migration is altered by pre- and/or postnatal exposure to ethanol. During the first postnatal week the external granule cell layer is thicker in ethanol-treated rats than in controls, and the involution of the external granule cell layer is delayed by ethanol exposure (Kornguth et al., 1979; Borges and Lewis, 1982). Based on the previously described evidence that ethanol either does not affect or inhibits cell proliferation in the external granule cell layer (Bauer-Moffett and Altman, 1977), these data suggest that the initiation of neuronal migration is retarded.

It should be noted that early exposure of *Xenopus laevis* to ethanol produces defects in gastrulation and neurulation (Nakatsugi and Johnson, 1984). Ethanol inhibits the migration of mesodermal cells which in turn causes the formation of multiple, small neural plates. The retardation of the formation of the mesodermal cell layer (and in some cases the total lack of formation of this layer) may underlie defects in neural crest development and the production of craniofacial malformations.

All of the above data are indirect evidence that ethanol causes abnormal neuronal migration. The only direct evidence that ethanol perturbs neuronal migration comes from [^{3}H]thymidine autoradiographic studies of neocortex. In normal rats, neuronal migration is a highly ordered process. Early-generated neurons migrate to deep cortex and succeeding generations of neurons migrate to successively more superficial cortical addresses (Miller, 1988a). Thus, the migration of cortical neurons follows an inside-to-outside sequence. In the rat, the migration of cortical neurons begins on G12 and continues until P6 (Berry and Rogers, 1965; Hicks and D'Amato, 1968). Early-generated neurons take 1–3 days to complete their migration, whereas late-generated neurons must traverse a longer distance and their migration may take as long as 8 days.

Prenatal exposure to ethanol delays the initiation of the migration of neurons destined for a particular layer by 1–2 days (Miller, 1986, 1987, 1988b). Moreover, although the migration of neurons born between G12 and G19 proceeds by the normal inside-to-outside sequence, this sequence degenerates during the latter part of cortical neuronogenesis. Late-generated neurons (those born on G20–G23) are abnormally distributed in all layers of cortex (Fig. 2). For example, a small number of neurons born on G20 are appropriately distributed in layer II, however, a large number of neurons are distributed in layers IV, V, and VI. Some ectopic neurons are even evident in layer I. Despite these changes, cortical lamination in the ethanol-treated rats appears similar to that in the control rats.

The effects of ethanol upon the kinetics of neuronal migration has been explored by tracing the movement of migrating neurons (Miller, 1990). The number of cells that become post-mitotic, i.e., leave the population of proliferating cells, is unaffected by prenatal exposure to ethanol. On the other hand, regardless of when a neuron is generated, the release time (i.e., the time before a post-mitotic neuron begins to migrate from the proliferative zones) is significantly longer in ethanol-treated rats. In addition, ethanol slowed the rate of migration about 25%. The net result of all of these ethanol-induced changes is that neurons take a longer time to complete

Control-G 15   Ethanol-G 15   Control-G 20   Ethanol-G 20

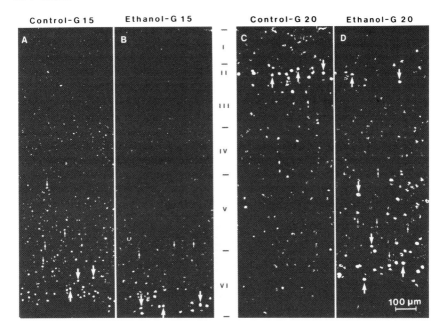

Fig. 2. Distributions of early- and late-generated neurons. These autoradiographs depict the effect of prenatal exposure to ethanol on the ultimate positions of neurons born on G15 and G20. Neurons which are heavily labeled by an injection of [^{3}H]thymidine are noted by large arrows. These are the neurons which divided only once after incorporating the radioisotope. Neurons which are lightly labeled by the same injection are noted by small arrows. Most of these neurons presumably divided two or more times before migrating into cortex and thus, they represent a wave of neurons which were generated at a later time than the heavily-labeled neurons. Early-generated neurons are disposed in deep cortex in both control and ethanol-treated rats. Those in ethanol-treated rats, however, tend to be more deeply distributed than those in control rats. Note that for control and for ethanol-treated rats, alike, lightly-labeled neurons are distributed more superficially than the heavily-labeled neurons. In contrast, late-generated neurons are located in superficial cortex in control rats, Similarly, many late-generated neurons in ethanol-treated rats are also distributed in layer II, but the vast majority are abnormally positioned throughout all layers and particularly the lower half of cortex. Interestingly, the distributions of heavily- and lightly-labeled ectopic neurons are thoroughly intermingled in deep cortex.

their migration. For example, most neurons born on G13 or on G20 in control rats take 4 and 6 days, respectively, whereas the migration of these neurons in ethanol-treated rat take 6 and 8–10 days, respectively.

Neuronal migration is an active process which involves the formation and re-formation of the neuronal cytoskeleton. The effects of ethanol exposure on the cytoskeleton has been examined on neural crest cells and cardiac myocytes (Adickes and Mollner, 1986; Hassler and Moran, 1986). These studies have shown that ethanol leads to the disorganized assembly of contractile elements. In neural crest, actin filaments normally are in a reticular or parallel arrangement around the nucleus and they terminate in the cell membrane in a fine filigree. After being exposed to ethanol, actin filaments are matted and thickened and the filigree is thickened and clumped (Hassler and Moran, 1986). In cardiac muscle, ethanol causes cytoskeletal dysgenesis. The sarcomeres of many cells exposed to ethanol exhibit masses of disorganized myofilaments and scattered clumps of Z-band proteins (Adickes and Mollner, 1986).

The results on the effects of ethanol on contractile elements of the cytoskeleton are particularly interesting in light of the data of Milner and colleagues (Miller et al., 1987; Maciejewski-Lenoir and Milner, 1989). They examined the expression of an mRNA for the Tα1 isotype of α-tubulin, a microtubular component. The patterned, spatiotemporal expression of this mRNA indicates that Tα1 is important in aspects of neuronal migration (Miller et al., 1987). The mRNA for Tα1 is rich neocortex (particularly the proliferative zones and the cortical plate) of normal rats during the first postnatal week, but this mRNA is substantially less abundant in the mature rat. Preliminary studies show that ethanol significantly depresses the expression of this mRNA during the first postnatal week (Maciejewski-Lenoir and Milner, 1989).

In addition to intrinsic features, various extrinsic factors also affect neuronal migration. Neuronal migration involves a complex interaction between migrating neurons and a glial scaffold. The scaffold is formed by radial glia which have elongate fibers that stretch from the proliferative zone(s) to the pial surface (e.g., Rakic, 1972, 1978; Schmechel and Rakic, 1979; Pixley and DeVellis, 1984). Glia with such processes are present throughout the period of neuronal migration after which these cells transform into astrocytes. It was hypothesized that since ethanol causes late-generated neurons to end up in ectopic sites in deep cortex, it might be predicted that ethanol induces radial glia to prematurely lose their contact with the pial surface, i.e., that ethanol accelerates the transformation of the radial glia into astrocytes (Miller, 1986). Preliminary data (Robertson and Miller, 1990) support this hypothesis. Although radial glial fibers are maintained as late as 2 days after the last migrating neurons have arrived at their residence in ethanol-treated and control rats alike, the morphology of these fibers in ethanol-treated rats is abnormal.

Ethanol also may affect the chemical neuronal-glial interactions. Various membrane-bound moieties have been identified as having a role in neuronal migration. Most notable among these are the family of cell adhesion molecules (e.g., Edelman, 1983; Fushiki and Schachner, 1986; Chuong et al.). To date there have been no experiments on the effects of ethanol on the cell adhesion molecules. Various studies, however, have shown that ethanol does affect other membrane-bound proteins, e.g., gangliosides and myelin-basic proteins (Druse, 1986).

CONCLUSIONS

Prenatal and early postnatal exposure to ethanol has dramatic effects on the number and distribution of neurons in the mature central nervous system. These alterations result from disruptions in the early stages of neuronal ontogeny, i.e., cell proliferation and neuronal migration. The effect of the ethanol on a particular structure reflects the level and the timing of the ethanol exposure and the pattern of development within the structure.

Low concentrations of ethanol stimulate cell proliferation and have no effect on cell size (Kennedy and Elliot, 1985; Novicki et al. 1985), whereas high concentrations of ethanol inhibit cell proliferation and increase the size of cycling cells (Borges and Lewis, 1983a; Shireman et al., 1983; Novicki et al., 1985; Kennedy and Mukerji, 1986; Higgins, 1987; Alvarez and Stone, 1988). Such dose-dependent effects may underlie the paradoxical effects of ethanol on cell proliferation in the ventricular zone (depression) versus those in auxiliary cortical germinal zones (stimulation), i.e., the neocortical subventricular zone and the archicortical intrahilar proliferative zone. It is interesting that neural tissue in the ventricular zone is perfused by blood and bathed by cerebrospinal fluid, whereas the auxiliary zones are perfused only by the blood and physically separated from the cerebrospinal fluid. These differences may result in the ventricular zones and the auxiliary zones having different effective exposure to ethanol. If the differential effects of ethanol on the proliferative zones results from the differential bathing of the germinal zones, then it would be predicted that low levels of ethanol (e.g., blood ethanol concentrations below 100 mg/dl) would stimulate cell proliferation in the ventricular zones and have no effect on the auxiliary zones, whereas high levels of ethanol (e.g., blood ethanol concentrations above 300 mg/dl) would inhibit cell proliferation in the ventricular and auxiliary proliferative zones.

An interesting counterpoint to neocortex and the dentate gyrus is the cerebellum. As with neocortex and the dentate gyrus, cerebellar neurons are also derived from two zones. Unlike the neocortex and dentate gyrus, however, cell proliferation in both cerebellar proliferative zones is depressed by exposure to moderate levels of ethanol. The lack of an ethanol-induced stimulation of proliferation in the auxiliary cerebellar proliferative zone, the external granular cell layer, may result from the fact that this zone, like the ventricular zone forms a surface of the brain, and hence, it is perfused by blood and cerebrospinal fluid. Therefore, the effects of ethanol on cell proliferation in the external granule cell layer would be expected to be similar to those on the ventricular zone and not the neo- and archicortical auxiliary proliferative zones.

The alterations in neuronal migration may be secondary to the defects in cell proliferation. For example, although prenatal exposure to ethanol has definable effects on the migration of neocortical neurons, much of this migration of neocortical neurons occurs postnatally (Miller, 1986, 1988b, 1990). Moreover, clusters of ectopic neurons were identified in superficial cortex following an acute exposure to ethanol (Kotkoskie and Norton, 1988). Although these data are only indirect evidence of ethanol-induced disruptions in neuronal migration, they do suggest that the deleterious effects of ethanol on neuronal migration persist after the exposure has ceased.

Despite the overall decrease in the size of brain structures and in changes in cell proliferation and neuronal migration, the numbers of neurons and glia in a wedge of neocortical tissue, i.e., the cell packing density (Miller, 1986; Miller and Potempa, 1990) and the ratio of cerebellar granule cells to Purkinje cells (Bauer-Moffett and Altman, 1977; Borges and Lewis, 1983b; Phillips and Cragg, 1985) are unaffected by ethanol. A parsimonius explanation for these data is that integrity of the developmental unit, the ontogenetic column (Rakic, 1982) is relatively unaffected by ethanol exposure. Although the organization within the column is disrupted by ethanol, the core of stem cells and the radial array of their derivatives apparently are not. Therefore, the microcephaly resulting from an early exposure to moderate levels of ethanol may be caused by a reduction in the stem cell population resulting in a reduction in the total number of ontogenetic columns.

REFERENCES

Abercrombie M (1946): Estimation of nuclear population from microtome sections. Anat Rec 94:239–247.

Adickes ED, Mollner TJ (1986): Ethanol-induced cytoskeletal dysgenesis with dietary protein manipulations. Alcohol Alcohol 21:347–355.

Altman J, Anderson WJ (1972): Experimental reorganization of the cerebellar cortex. I. Morphological effects of elimination of all microneurons with prolonged X-irridation started at birth. J Comp Neurol 146:355–406.

Altman J, Anderson WJ, Wright KA (1969): Early effects of X-irradiation on the cerebellum in infant rates. Decimation and reconstitution of the external granule cell layer. Exp Neurol 24:196–216.

Altman J, Das GD (1966): Autoradiographic and histological studies of postnatal neurogenesis. I. J Comp Neurol 126:337–390.

Alvarez MR, Stone DJ (1988): Hypoploidy and hyperplasia in the developing brain exposed to alcohol in utero. Teratology 37:233–238.

Anderson WJ, Sides GR (1978): Alcohol induced defects in cerebellar development in the rat. In Galanter M (ed): "Currents in Alcoholism. Vol. 5. Biomedical Issues and Clinical Effects of Alcoholism." New York: Grune and Stratton, pp 135–153.

Angevine JB Jr (1965): Time of origin in the hippocampal region: An autoradiographic study in the mouse. Exp Neurol Suppl 2:1–70.

Angevine JB Jr, Sidman RL (1961): Autoradiographic study of cell migration during histogenesis of cerebral cortex in the mouse. Nature 192:766–768.

Atlas M, Bond VP (1965): The cell generation cycle of the eleven-day mouse embryo. J Cell Biol 26:19–24.

Bannigan JG (1987): Autoradiographic analysis of effects of 5-bromodeoxyuridine on neurogenesis in the chick embryo spinal cord. Dev Brain Res 36:161–170.

Bannigan JG, Burke P (1982): Ethanol teratogenicity in mice: A light microscopic study. Teratology 26:247–254.

Barnes De, Walker DW (1981): Prenatal ethanol exposure permanently reduces the number of pyramidal neurons in rat hippocampus. Dev Brain Res 227:333–340.

Bauer-Moffett C, Altman J (1975): Ethanol-reduced reductions in cerebellar growth of infant rats. Exp Neurol 48:378–382.

Bauer-Moffett C, Altman J (1977): The effect of ethanol chronically administered to preweanling rats on cerebellar development: A morphological study. Brain Res 119:249–268.

Bayer SA (1980): Development of the hippocampal region of the rat. I. Neurogenesis examined with ³H-thymidine autoradiography. J Comp Neurol 190:87–114.

Bayer SA, Yackel JW, Puri PS (1982): Neurons in the rat dentate gyrus granular layer substantially increase during early postnatal life. Science 216:890–892.

Benno RH, Williams TH (1978): Evidence for intracellular localization of alpha-fetoprotein in the developing rat brain. Brain Res 142:182–186.

Berry M (1974): Development of the cerebral neocortex of the rat. In Gottlieb G (ed): "Aspects of Neurogenesis." New York: Academic Press, pp 8–67.

Berry M, Rogers AW (1965): The migration of neuroblasts in the developing cerebral cortex. J Anat 99:691–709.

Bonthius DJ, West JR (1990): Alcohol-induced neuronal loss in developing rats: Increased brain damage with binge exposure. Alcohol Clin Exp Res 14:107–118.

Borges S, Lewis PD (1982): A study of alcohol effects on the brain during gestation and lactation. Teratology 25:283–289.

Borges S, Lewis PD (1983a): Effects of ethanol on postnatal cell acquisition in the rat cerebellum. Brain Res 271:388–391.

Borges S, Lewis PD (1983b): The effect of ethanol on the cellular composition of the cerebellum. Neuropathol Appl Neurobiol 9:53–60.

Boulder Committee (1970): Embryonic vertebrate central nervous system: Revised terminology. Anat Rec 166:257–261.

Burns Em, Kruckeberg TW, Stibler H, Cerven E, Borg S (1984): The effects of ethanol exposure during the brain growth spurt in rats. Teratology 29:251–258.

Caviness VS Jr, Crandall JE, Edwards MA (1988): The reeler malformation. Implications for neocortical histogenesis. In Peters A, Jones EG (eds): "Cerebral Cortex. Vol. 7. Development and Maturation of Cerebral Cortex." New York: Plenum, pp 59–89.

Charness ME, Gordon AS, Diamond I (1983): Ethanol modulation of opiate receptors in cultured neural cells. Science 222:1246–1248.

Chuong C-M, Crossin KL, Edelman GM (1987): Sequential expression and differential function of multiple adhesion molecules during the formation of cerebellar cortical layers. J Cell Biol 104:331–342.

Clarke PGH (1985): Neuronal death in the development of the vertebrate nervous system. Trends Neurosci 8:345–349.

Clarren SK, Alvord EC, Sumi SM, Streissguth AP, Smith DW (1978): Brain malformations related to prenatal exposure to ethanol. J Pediatr 92:64–67.

Cragg BG, Phillips SC (1985): Natural loss of Purkinje cells during development and increased loss with alcohol. Brain Res 325:151–160.

Davies DL, Smith DW (1981): A Golgi study of mouse hippocampal CA1 pyramidal neurons following perinatal ethanol exposure. Neurosci Lett 26:49–54.

Diaz J, Samson HH (1980): Impaired brain growth in neonatal rats exposed to ethanol. Science 208:751–753.

Druckney H, Lange A (1972): Carcinogenicity of azomethane dependent on age in BD rats. Fed Proc 31:1482–1485.

Druse MJ (1986): Effects of prenatal alcohol exposure on neurotransmitters, membranes and proteins. In West JR (ed): "Alcohol and Brain Development." New York: Oxford Press, pp 343–372.

Edelman GM (1983): Cell adhesion molecules. Science 219:450–457.

Edwards HG, Dow-Edwards DL (in press): Craniofacial alterations induced by prenatal exposure to ethanol in the rat. Teratology.

Finlay BL, Wikler KC, Sengelaub DR (1987): Regressive events in brain development and scenarios for vertebrate brain evolution. Brain Behav Evol 30:102–117.

Floderus S (1944): Untersuchungen uber den Bau der menschlichen Hypophyse mit besonderer Berucksichtigung der quantitativen mikromorphologischen Verhaltnisse. Acta Pathol Microbiol Scand Suppl 153:587–596.

Fushiki S, Schachner M (1986): Immunocytological localization of cell adhesion molecules L1 and N-CAM and the shared carbohydrate epitope L2 during development of the mouse neocortex. Dev Brain Res 24:153–162.

Gardette R, Courtois M, Bisconte J-C (1982): Prenatal development of mouse central nervous structures: Time of origin and gradients of neuronal production. A Radioautographic study. J Hirnforsch 23:415–431.

Hamburger V, Oppenheim RW (1982): Naturally occurring neuronal death in vertebrates. Neurosci Comm. 1:39–55.

Hassler JA, Moran DJ (1986): The effects of ethanol on embryonic action: A possible role in teratogenesis. Experientia 42:575–577.

Hebel R, Stromberg MW, (1986): "Anatomy of the Laboratory Rat." Baltimore: Williams and Wilkins.

Hicks SP, D'Amato CJ (1968): Cell migration to the isocortex in the rat. Anat Rec 160:619–634.

Hicks SP, D'Amato CJ, Lowe MJ (1959): The development of the mammalian nervous system. I. Malformations of the brain, especially the cerebral cortex, induced in rats by radiation. II. Some mechanisms of the malformations of the cortex. J Comp Neurol 113:435–469.

Higgins PJ (1987): Cell cycle phase-specific perturbation of hepatic tumor cell growth kinetics during short-term in vitro exposure to ethanol. Alcohol Clin Exp Res 11:550–555.

Hinds JW, Ruffett TL (1971): Cell proliferation in the neural tube. An electron microscopic and Golgi analysis in the mouse cerebral vesicle. Z Zellforsch 115:226–264.

His W (1904): Die Entwicklung des menschlichen Gehirns wahrend der ersten Monate. Herzel, Leipzig.

Jacobson M (1978): "Developmental Neurobiology." New York: Plenum.

Jacobson S, Rich J, Tovsky NJ, (1979): Delayed myelination and lamination in cerebral cortex of the albino rat as a result of the fetal alcohol syndrome. In Galanter M (ed): "Currents in Alcoholism/Biomedical Issues and Clinical Effects of Alcoholism. Vol. 5." New York Grune and Stratton, pp. 123–133.

Jones KL, Smith DW, Ulleland CN, Streissguth AP (1973): Pattern of malformation in offspring of chronic alcoholic mothers. Lancet 1:1267–1271.

Kaplan MS, Hinds JW (1977): Neurogenesis in the adult rat: Electron microscopic analysis of light micrographs. Science 197:1092–1094.

Kennedy LA, Elliott MJ (1985): Cell proliferation in the embryonic mouse neocortex following acute maternal alcohol intoxication. Int. J Dev Neurosci 3:311–315.

Kennedy LA, Elliott MJ Laverty WH (1984): Reductions in the plating efficiency of the fetal mouse neural precursor cells following maternal alcohol consumption. Int J Dev Neurosci 2:437–446.

Kennedy LA, Mukerji S (1986): Ethanol neurotoxicity. 1. Direct effects on replicating astrocytes. Neurobehav Toxicol Teratol 8:11–15.

Kent JL, Pert CB, Herkenham M. (1982): Ontogeny of opiate receptors in rat forebrain: Visualization by in vitro autoradiography. Brain Res 254:487–504.

Kershman J (1938): The medulloblast and the medulloblastoma; a study of human embryos. Arch Neurol Psychiatr 40:937–967.

Khatami S, Hoffman PL, Shibuya T, Salafsky B (1987): Selective effects of ethanol on opiate receptor subtypes in brain. Neuropharmacology 26:1503–1507.

Kornguth SE, Rutledge JJ, Sunderland E, Siegel F, Carlson I, Smollens J, Jhl U, Young B (1979): Impeded cerebellar development and reduced serum thyroxine levels associated with fetal alcohol intoxication. Brain Res 177:347–360.

Kotkoskie L, Miller MW (1989): Distribution of callosal projection neurons in somatosensory cortex of rats prenatally exposed to ethanol. Abs. Soc Neurosci 15:1024.

Kotkoskie L, Norton S (1988): Prenatal brain malformations following acute ethanol exposure in the rat. Alcohol Clin Exp Res 12:831–836.

Lancaster FE, Mayur BK, Patsalos PN, Samorajski T, Wiggins RC (1982): The synthesis of myelin and brain subcellular membrane proteins in the offspring of rats fed ethanol during pregnancy. Brain Res 235:105–113.

Leblond CP, Messier B, Kopriwa B (1959): Thymidine-H³ as a tool for the investigation of the renewal of cell populations. Lab Invest 8:276–306.

Levitt P, Cooper ML, Rakic P (1981): Coexistence of neuronal and glial precursor cells in the cerebral ventricular zone of the fetal monkey: An ultrastructural, immunoperoxidase analysis. J Neurosci 1:27–39.

Levitt P, Cooper ML, Rakic P (1983): Early divergence and changing proportions of neuronal and glial precursor cells in the primate cerebral ventricular zone of the monkey: An ultrastructural, immunoperoxidase analysis. Dev Biol 96:472–484.

Lewis PD (1968): Mitotic activity in the primate subependymal layer and the genesis of gliomas. Nature 217:974–975.

Lucchi L, Ruis RA, Govoni S, Trabucchi M (1985): Chronic ethanol induces changes in opiate receptor function and in met-enkephalin release. Alcohol 2:193–195.

Maciejewski-Lenoir D, Milner RJ (1989): Effect of prenatal exposure to ethanol on gene expression during rat brain development. Abs Soc Neurosci 15:1023.

Matsumoto H, Spatz M, Laquer GL, (1972): Quantitative changes with age in the DNA content of methylazoxymethanol-induced microencephalic rat brain. J Neurochem 19:297–306.

Miale IL, Sidman RL (1961): An autoradiographic analysis of histogenesis in the mouse cerebellum. Exp Neurol 4:277–296.

Miller FD, Naus CCG, Durand M, Bloom FE, Milner RJ (1987): Isotypes of α-tubulin are differentially regulated during neuronal maturation. J Cell Biol 105:3065–3073.

Miller MW (1985): Cogeneration of retrogradely labeled corticocortical projection and GABA-immunoreactive local circuit neurons in cerebral cortex. Dev Brain Res 23:187–192.

Miller MW (1986): Effects of alcohol on the generation and migration of cerebral cortical neurons. Science 233:1308–1311.

Miller MW (1987): Effect of prenatal exposure to alcohol on the distribution and time of origin of corticospinal neurons in the rat. J Comp Neurol 257:372–382.

Miller MW (1988a): Development of projection and local circuit neurons in cerebral cortex. In Peters A, Jones EG (eds): "Cerebral Cortex, Vol. 7, Development and Maturation of Cerebral Cortex." New York: Plenum, pp 133–175.

Miller MW (1988b): Effect of prenatal exposure to ethanol on the development of cerebral cortex. I. Neuronal generation. Alcohol Clin Exp Res 12:440–449.

Miller MW (1989): Effect of prenatal exposure to ethanol on the development of cerebral cortex: II. Cell proliferation in the ventricular and subventricular zones of the rat. J Comp Neurol 287:326–338.

Miller MW (1990): Effect of prenatal exposure to ethanol on the rate and schedule of neuronal migration to rat somatosensory cortex. Alcohol Clin Exp Res 14:319.

Miller MW, Dow-Edwards DL (1988): Structural and metabolic alterations in rat cerebral cortex induced by prenatal exposure to ethanol. Brain Res 474:316–326.

Miller MW, Nowakowski RS (1991): Effect of prenatal exposure to ethanol on cell kinetics and growth fraction in the proliferative zones of the fetal rat cerebral cortex. Alcohol Clin Exp Res 15:229–232.

Miller MW, Muller SJ (1989): Structure and histogenesis of the principal sensory nucleus of the trigeminal nerve: Effects of prenatal exposure to ethanol. J Comp Neurol 282:570–580.

Miller MW, Potempa G (1990): Numbers of neurons and glia in mature rat somatosensory cortex: Effects of prenatal exposure to ethanol. J Comp Neurol 293:92–102.

Morgane P, Miller M, Kemper T, Stern W, Forbes W, Hall R, Branzino J, Kissane J, Hawrylew E, Resnick O (1978): Effects of protein malnutrition on developing central nervous systemin rat. Neurosci B 2:137–230.

Nakatsuji N, Johnson KE (1984): Effects of ethanol on the primitive streak stage mouse embryo. Teratology 29:369–375.

Nathaniel EJH, Nathaniel DR Mohamed SA, Nahnybida L, Nathaniel L (1986a) Growth patterns of rat body, brain, and cerebellum in fetal alcohol syndrome. Exp Neurol 93:610–620.

Nathaniel EJH, Nathaniel Dr, Mohamed SA, Nathaniel L, Kowalzik C, Nahnybida L (1986b): Prenatal ethanol exposure and cerebellar development in rats. Exp Neurol 93:601–609.

Nornes HO, Morita M (1979): Time of origin of the neurons in the caudal brain stem of rat. Dev Neurosci 2:101–114.

Norton S, Terranova P, Na JY, Sancho-Tollo M (1988): Daily motor development and cerebral cortical morphology in rats exposed perinatally to alcohol. Alcohol Clin Exp Res 12:130–137.

Novicki DL, Rosenberg MR, Michalpoulos G (1985): Inhibition of DNA synthesis by chemical carcinogens in cultures of initiated and normal proliferating rat hepatocytes. Cancer Res 45:337–344.

Nowakowski RS (1988): Development of the hippocampal formation in mutant mice. Drug Dev Res 15:315–336.

Nowakowski RS, Rakic P (1979): The mode of migration to the hippocampus. A Golgi and electron microscopic analysis in foetal rhesus monkeys. J Neurocytol 8:697–718.

Nowakowski RS, Rakic P (1981): The site of origin and route and rate of migration of neurons to the hippocampal region of the rhesus monkey. J Comp Neurol 196:129–154.

Pearlman AL (1988): The visual cortex of the normal mouse and the reeler mutant. In Peters A, Jones EG (eds): "Cerebral Cortex. Vol. 3. Visual Cortex." New York: Plenum, pp 1–18.

Phillips SC (1985): Age-dependent susceptibility of rat cerebellar Purkinje cells to ethanol exposure. Drug Depend 16:273–277.

Phillips SC, Cragg BG (1982): A change in susceptibility of rat cerebellar Purkinje cells to damage by alcohol during fetal, neonatal and adult life. Neuropathol Appl Neurobiol 8:441–454.

Pinto-Lord MC, Evrard P, Caviness VS Jr (1982): Obstructed neuronal migration along radial glial fibers in the neocortex of the reeler mouse: A Golgi-EM analysis. Dev Brain Res 4:379–393.

Pixley SKR, DeVellis J (1984): Transition between immature radial glial and mature astrocytes studied with a monoclonal antibody to vimentin. Dev Brain Res 15:201–209.

Rakic P (1972): Mode of cell migration to the superficial layers of fetal monkey neocortex. J Comp Neurol 145:61–83.

Rakic P (1978): Neuronal migration and contact guidance in the primate telencephalon. Postgrad Med J 54:25–40.

Rakic P (1982): Early developmental events: Cell lineages, acquisition of neuronal positions, and areal and laminar development. Neurosci Res Prog Bull 20:439–451.

Rakic P, Stensaas LJ, Sayre EP, Sidman RL (1974): Computer-aided three-dimensional reconstruction and quantitative analysis of cells from serial electron microscopic montages of foetal monkey brain. Nature 250:31–34.

Robertson S, Miller MW (1990): Effect of prenatal exposure to ethanol on radial glia and astrocytes in rat somatosensory cortex. Alcohol Clin Exp Res 14:332.

Sauer FC (1935): Mitosis in the neural tube. J Comp Neurol 62:377–405.

Sauer FC (1936): The interkinetic migration of embryonic epithelial nuclei. J Morphol 60:1–11.

Sauer ME (1959): Radioautographic study of the location of newly synthesized deoxyribonucleic acid in the neural tube of the chick embryo: Evidence for intermitotic migration of nuclei. Anat Rec 133:456.

Schaper A (1897): Die Fruhesten differenzierungsvorganger in central nerven system. Arch Entw Mech Org 5:81–132.

Schaper A, Cohen C (1905): Beitraege zur Analyze des tierischen Wachstums. II. Teil: Ueber zellproliferatorische Wachstumszentren and und deren Bezeihung zur Regeneration and Geschwulstbildung. Arch Entw Mech 19:348–445.

Schlessinger AR, Cowan WM, Gottlieb DI (1975): An autoradiographic study of the time of origin and the pattern of granule cell migration in the dentate gyrus of the rat. J Comp Neurol 159:149–176.

Schmechel D, Rakic P (1979): Golgi study of radial glial cells in developing monkey telencephalon- morphogenesis and transformation into astrocytes. Anat Embryol 156:115–152.

Seymour RM, Berry M (1975): Scanning and transmission electron microscope studies of interkinetic nuclear migration in the cerebral vesicles of the rat. J Comp Neurol 160:105–126.

Shimada M, Langman J (1970): Cell proliferation, migration and differentiation in the cerebral cortex of the golden hamster. J Comp Neurol 139:227–244.

Shireman RB, Alexander K, Remsen JF (1983): Effects of ethanol on cultured human fibroblasts. Alcohol Clin Exp Res 7:279–282.

Sidman RL, Miale IL, Feder N (1959): Cell proliferation and migration in the primitive ependymal zone: An autoradiographic study of histogenesis in the nervous system. Exp Neurol 1:322–333.

Smart I (1961): The subependymal layer of the mouse brain and its cell production as shown by radioautography after thymidine-H3 injection. J Comp Neurol 116:325–347.

Smart I (1983): Three dimensional growth of the mouse isocortex. J Anat 137:683–694.

Smolen AJ, Wright LL, Cunningham TJ (1983): Neuron numbers in the superior cervical sympathetic ganglion of the rat: A critical comparison of methods for cell counting. J Neurocytol 12:739–750.

Stanfield BB, Cowan WM (1988): The development of the hippocampal region. In Peters A, Jones EG (eds): "Cerebral Cortex, Vol. 7, Development and Maturation of Cerebral Cortex." New York: Plenum, pp 107–131.

Sulik KK, Johnston MC (1983): Sequence of developmental alterations following acute ethanol exposure in mice: Craniofacial features of the fetal alcohol syndrome. Am J Anat 166:257–269.

Sulik KK, Johnston MC, Webb MA (1981): Fetal alcohol syndrome: Embryogenesis in a mouse model. Science 214:936–938.

Toran-Allerand CD (1980): Coexistence of alpha-fetoprotein, albumin and transferrin immunoreactivity in neurones of the developing mouse brain. Nature 286:733–735.

Trojan J, Uriel J (1979): Localisation intracellulaire de l'alphafoetoproteine et de la serumalbumine dans le systeme nerveux central du Rat au cours du development foetal et postnatal. CR Acad Sci D 289:1157–1160.

Volk B, Maletz J, Tiedemann M, Mall G, Klein C, Berlet HH (1981): Impaired maturation of Purkinje cells in the fetal alcohol syndrome of the rat. Light and electron microscopic investigations. Acta Neuropathol 54:19–29.

Waechter RV, Jaensch B (1972): Generation times of the matrix cells during embryonic brain development: An autoradiographic study in rats. Brain Res 46:235–250.

West JR, Hamre KM, Cassell MD, (1986): Effects of ethanol exposure during the third trimester equivalent on neuron number in rat hippocampus and dentate gyrus. Alcohol Clin Exp Res 10:190–197.

West JR, Hodges CA, Black AC (1981): Prenatal exposure to ethanol alters the organization of hippocampal mossy fiber in rats. Science 211:957–959.

Woodson PM, Ritchley SJ, (1979): Effect of maternal alcohol consumption of fetal brain cell number and cell size. Nutr Res Int 20:225–228.

Yanai J, Waknin S (1985): Comparison of the effects of barbiturate and ethanol given to neonates on the cerebellar morphology. Acta Anat 123:145–147.

**Development of the Central Nervous System:
Effects of Alcohol and Opiates, pages 71–107**
© **1992 Wiley-Liss, Inc.**

5

Effects of Ethanol on Neuronal Morphogenesis

ROBERTA J. PENTNEY AND MICHAEL W. MILLER

*Department of Anatomical Sciences, School of Medicine and Biomedical
Sciences, State University of New York at Buffalo, Buffalo, New York
(R.J.P.); Veterans Administration Medical Center and Department of
Psychiatry, University of Iowa College of Medicine, Iowa City, Iowa
(M.W.M.)*

INTRODUCTION

Common sequelae of exposure to ethanol during early mammalian development are mental retardation, cranial malformation, and microcephaly. These three features are interrelated and result from defects in morphogenesis. Morphometric studies in rodents treated with ethanol during development have showed that the size of the brain may be 12–30% smaller in ethanol-treated rats than in controls; the variability depends upon the method of delivery of the ethanol and the timing of the exposure (Randall et al., 1977; Samson and Diaz, 1981; Lancaster et al., 1982; Spohr and Stoltenburg-Didinger, 1983; Pierce and West, 1987; West et al., 1987; Miller and Potempa, 1990). Different areas within the brain are not altered uniformly. The size of some structures in the central nervous system is virtually unaffected by prenatal exposure to ethanol (Miller and Muller, 1989), whereas other structures, notably cerebral cortex (12%, Miller, 1987b), are significantly smaller. Postnatal exposure to dietary ethanol causes significant reductions in the size of the hippocampus and cerebellum (26.1% and 14.5%, respectively, Pierce and West, 1987).

This chapter will review the literature on the effects of ethanol on the gross and microscopic structure of the neocortex, hippocampus, and cerebellum and the functional consequences of these changes. Many experimental paradigms have been used to examine the effects of ethanol on cortical structures, but the focus in this chapter will be on rodent models in which moderate blood alcohol levels were achieved (100–200 mg/dl). Each structure will be considered separately because information concerning the effects of pre- and postnatal ethanol exposure on their constituent neurons remains incomplete.

NEOCORTEX

General Description

Structure

The mature cortex is a mantle of tissue that covers the outer surface of the brain. All areas of neocortex are laminated, but the cerebral cortex does not have a homogeneous structure. Discrete cortical regions can be discerned based on cytoarchitectonic, hodological, and physiological criteria (Krieg, 1946; Caviness, 1975; Zilles et al., 1980; Miller and Vogt, 1984). Six cortical layers can be differentiated by the size, shape, and packing density of their constituent neurons. For example, layers II and VI contain neurons with small, round cell bodies that are densely packed, whereas layer V contains large cell bodies which are pyriform and distributed in a loosely packed matrix. Motor and somatosensory cortices are neighboring regions, but they can be readily discriminated by the appearance of layer IV. In motor cortex layer IV is obscure, but in somatosensory cortex layer IV is densely packed with small, round neuronal cell bodies.

The various neocortical areas are distinguished in ethanol-treated rats by the same criteria used to identify cytoarchitectonic areas in normal rats (Miller, 1987b). Some neocortical regions apparently are more affected by prenatal exposure to ethanol than others. The volume of somatosensory cortex in ethanol-treated rats was 33% smaller than that in the offspring of pair-fed controls (Miller and Potempa, 1990). On the other hand, the volume of auditory cortex in the same ethanol-treated rats was only 10% smaller than in the control rats (Miller, unpublished results). These data are supported by morphometric analyses that showed that the cortex rostral to the hippocampus (chiefly motor and somatosensory cortex) was particularly susceptible to gestational exposure to ethanol (Zimmerberg and Reuter, 1989).

The lamination of neocortex per se is not affected by gestational exposure to ethanol. Each of the cortical laminae can be readily distinguished by standard criteria in control and ethanol-treated rats, alike (Fig. 1) (Jacobson et al., 1979; Miller, 1986a; Miller and Dow-Edwards, 1988; Norton et al., 1988; Miller and Potempa, 1990). Nevertheless, evidence in ethanol-treated rats showed that the neuronal composition of each layer was abnormally heterogeneous due to the ethanol-induced perturbations in the spatiotemporal patterns of neuronal generation (see Chapter 3). Laminar connectivity was also altered by exposure to ethanol. For example, in layer Vb (the middle ⅗ths of layer V) of the somatosensory cortex of a control rat, 56% of the neurons projected to the spinal cord and 15% projected callosally to the contralateral cortex (Miller, 1987b; Kotkoskie and Miller, 1989). In ethanol-treated rats, 71% and 30% of the layer Vb neurons projected to the spinal cord and to the contralateral cortex, respectively. It is interesting to note, that, since about 90% of all layer Vb neurons are projection neurons, the data for the ethanol-treated rats indicated that some of the layer Vb neurons projected dually to the spinal cord and to the contralateral cortex. Such dual projection neurons are rare in normal rats (Killackey et al., 1989). Therefore, it appears that the normal process of axon elimination is affected by prenatal exposure to ethanol (see below).

Metabolism

The metabolism of mature neocortex, as measured by 2-deoxyglucose autoradiography, is altered by prenatal exposure to ethanol. The glucose utilization of neocortex was as much as 29% lower than control levels in rats that were exposed to ethanol prenatally (Vingan et al., 1986). There was a pattern to this ethanol-induced alteration such that dorsomedial cortex was most severely affected and lateral and ventral cortical regions were not significantly affected. This pattern may reflect the effects of ethanol exposure on the activity and/or structure of cortocopetal projection systems which broadly, but differentially, innervate regions of medial and lateral neocortex. One such example is the cholinergic system (e.g., Mesulam et al., 1983; Saper, 1984).

In a study of the metabolism in cytoarchitectonically distinct cortical areas, Miller and Dow-Edwards (1988) focused on the effects of gestational exposure to ethanol on glucose utilization in motor and somatosensory cortices in mature rats. Overall, glucose utilization was significantly reduced by 21% or more in all segments of motor and somatosensory cortices with the exception of caudal secondary motor cortex, area 6/8 (Fig. 2). The ethanol-induced changes in the laminar pattern of glucose utilization in caudal area 6/8 were distinctly different from those in other motor and somatosensory areas. In most segments of motor and somatosensory cortices, the greatest effect of the ethanol exposure on glucose utilization was in layer IV, and to a lesser extent in layers II/III and V. In contrast, in caudal area 6/8, glucose utilization was most significantly reduced in layer I. These changes may result from ethanol-induced alterations in laminar connectivity. For example, in control rats caudal area 6/8 is virtually devoid of neurons with spinal projections, however, layer V of caudal area 6/8 in ethanol-treated rats is replete with corticospinal neurons (Miller, 1987a). Moreover, it is interesting to note that caudal area 6/8 is unique among the motor areas in that it has connections with visual cortex and has been described as the frontal eye field (Hall and Lindholm, 1974; Neafsay and Siefert, 1982; Miller and Vogt, 1984).

Neuronal Types

The rat neocortex has two types of neurons, projection and local circuit neurons. There are many differences between the two neuronal types (Feldman, 1984; Fairen et al., 1984; Miller, 1988). Three of the notable criteria used widely for differentiating between projection and local circuit neurons are the axonal branching patterns, the density of dendritic spines, and the synaptology of the cell bodies. Projection neurons have axons that travel long distances and pass through the white matter, spinous dendrites, and cell bodies that form only symmetric (Gray type II) synapses (Gray, 1959). On the other hand, local circuit neurons have axons that

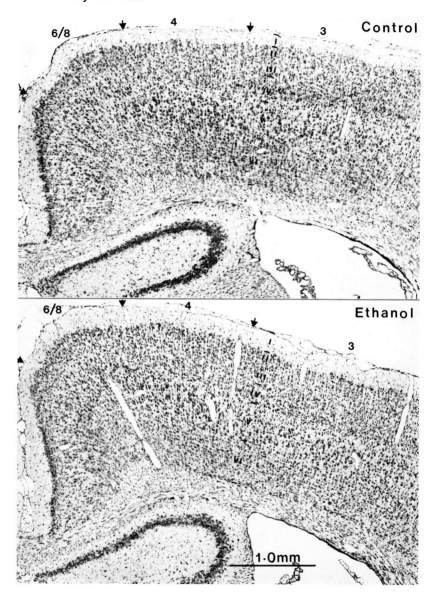

Fig. 1. The laminar organization of three neocortical cytoarchitectonic regions. These coronal sections depict area 4 (primary motor cortex), caudal area 6/8 (secondary motor cortex), and area 3 (primary somatosensory cortex) at the level of the rostral limit of the dorsal hippocampus in the offspring of a pair-fed control rat (top) and of an ethanol-treated rat (bottom). Areal borders are noted by arrows. Cresyl violet stain. (Reproduced from Miller and Dow-Edwards, 1988, with permission.)

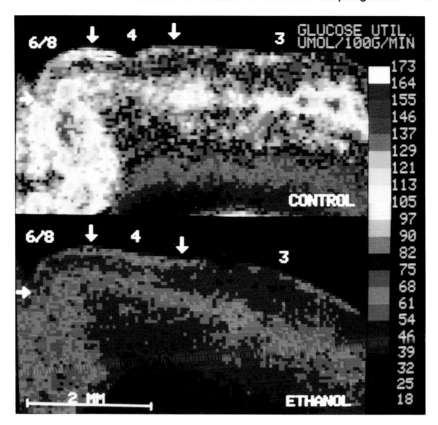

Fig. 2. Glucose utilization in motor-somatosensory cortex. These computer-digit-ized images of the 2-deoxyglucose autoradiographs show the significant differences in metabolic activities of cortex in the offspring of pair-fed control rats (top) and rats which were fed ethanol during gestation (bottom). Three cortical regions are shown, areas 4, 6/8, and 3. Overall, glucose utilization in ethanol-treated rats was 25% lower than that in controls and layer IV in area 3 was the most affected (−29%).

arborize within the vicinity of the dendritic field, sparsely spinous or aspi-nous dendrites, and cell bodies that form symmetric and asymmetric (Gray type I) synapses.

Projection neurons

Projection neurons are distributed in layers II–VI, and they are the most common type of neuron in these laminae. In the visual cortex of normal rats, projection neurons account for 91% of the neurons in layers II–VIa (Peters et al., 1985). Most cortical projection neurons are pyramidal neurons. In fact, the only other type of cortical projection neuron is the spinous stellate neuron; these neurons are rare in the rodent, and their distribution is restricted to layer IV.

The typical pyramidal neuron has a morphology that is characterized by four features. 1) Its cell body is ellipsoidal or pyramid-shaped. 2) Each pyramidal neuron has a single, long spinous dendrite that emanates from the apex of the cell body and ascends toward (and often reaches) layer I. 3) An array of spinous dendrites arises from the base of each cell body. 4) Each neuron has a single axon that originates from the base of the cell body and descends to the white matter.

Cell bodies. The effect of prenatal exposure to ethanol on the size of the cell bodies of pyramidal neurons in each layer of mature cortex has not been determined directly; however, the mean size of all neuronal somata in each layer has been determined (Miller and Potempa, 1990). Since most cortical neurons are pyramidal neurons, these generic data ostensibly provide information on the size of pyramidal neurons. Overall, the mean size of neuronal cell bodies in layers II–VIa was significantly reduced in ethanol-treated rats. The only exceptions were the neurons in layer V. The size of the cell bodies of layer V neurons was unaffected by in utero exposure to ethanol. These data are in accord with previous data that showed that corticospinal neurons, pyramidal neurons in layer V, were of similar size in ethanol-treated and control rats (Miller, 1987b).

A study of the ultrastructure of the somata of layer V neurons in somatosensory cortex of 30-day-old rats provided evidence that exposure to ethanol severely altered the structure of cytoplasmic organelles (Al-Rabiai and Miller, 1989). Qualitatively, the rough endoplasmic reticulum was disrupted and the nuclear envelope was irregular (Fig. 3). Similar results (see below) have been described for hippocampal pyramidal neurons (Smith and Davies, 1990) and cerebellar Purkinje neurons (Volk et al., 1981; Spohr and Stoltenburg-Didinger, 1983). The rough endoplasmic reticulum and the nuclear envelope are contiguous structures that are involved in protein synthesis. Other somatic components essential for protein synthesis were also affected by ethanol exposure; the spaces occupied by lysosomes and by the Golgi complex were significantly reduced in ethanol-treated rats (Al-Rabiai and Miller, 1989). These data suggest that prenatal exposure to ethanol has long-term effects on protein synthesis in rats. In fact, the depressive effect of ethanol upon protein synthesis has been described extensively (Noble and Tewari, 1975; Rawat, 1975, 1985; NIAAA, 1980).

Dendrites. The effects of ethanol on the composition of each cortical layer are indicated by the ratio of the space occupied by the cell body to that occupied by the neuropil. The cell body/neuropil ratio in layers II/III, IV, and VI of somatosensory cortex was significantly lower in 3-month-old ethanol-treated rats than in controls (Miller and Potempa, 1990). The principal cause for this decrease was a significant, ethanol-induced increase in the total volume of the neuropil in these layers. Nearly half of the neuropil is composed of dendrites (Al-Rabiai and Miller, 1989).

Prenatal exposure to ethanol affects the lengths of dendrites, but interestingly, the effect varied with the maturity of the pyramidal neurons. In an ultrastructural study of layer V in somatosensory cortex of 30-day-old rats, it was determined that the coverage by dendrites in ethanol-treated rats was 15% less than in controls (Al-Rabiai and Miller, 1989). This analysis, however, did not discriminate between dendrites from projection and local circuit neurons. There are no light microscopic studies of layer V neurons in somatosensory cortex of 30-day-old rats. Hammer and Scheibel (1981) examined Golgi-impregnated layer V pyramidal neurons in neonates, however. They described an ethanol-induced reduction in the length and complexity of dendrites on these immature pyramidal neurons. These observations were supported by results from an in vitro study which showed that ethanol inhibited neurite elaboration (Dow and Riopelle, 1985). This early stunting of dendritic growth was overcome by the time the rats were 3 months old (Miller et al., 1990). Furthermore, the complexity and extent of the dendritic tree at maturity was significantly greater in ethanol-treated rats than in age-matched controls (Fig. 4).

Parallel results have been reported for layer II/III neurons. Dendrites of these neurons were significantly shorter in immature rats prenatally exposed to ethanol (Shapiro et al., 1984), but in mature rats 8–10 months old, only minor nonsignificant differences were evident (Pentney et al., 1984). Nonetheless, the ratio of the number of branches in the skirt of basal dendrites to the number of primary basal dendrites (those dendrites that emanate directly from the cell body) was consistently greater in ethanol-treated rats. These data suggest that, as with the layer V pyramidal neurons, the early stunting of dendritic growth on layer II/III neurons was overcompensated by a delayed growth of dendrites.

One of the characteristic features of pyramidal neurons is the high density of dendritic spines. Spines are classified into three morphological groups: stubby, thin, and mushroom spines (Peters and Kaiserman-Abramof, 1970). Stubby spines appear as cylinders projecting from dendritic shafts, whereas thin spines have thin necks with small round heads and mushroom spines have thin necks and large, bulbous heads. It has been suggested that spines assume a morphology that is specific to their stage of development (Westrum et al., 1980; Miller, 1981; Miller and Peters, 1981) or state of activity (Crick, 1982). Accordingly, stubby spines are immature spines which are initiating growth from the dendritic shaft, thin spines are mature spines, and mushroom spines are regressing or older spines.

The morphology and density of dendritic spines are affected by prenatal exposure to ethanol. In the neonate and through the first 4 postnatal weeks, the morphology of spines on the pyramidal neurons of ethanol-treated rats appeared similar to that of control rats (Hammer and Scheibel, 1981; Reyes et al., 1983; Stoltenburg-Didinger and Spohr, 1983). The density of dendritic spines during this period was lower in ethanol-treated rats (Hammer and Scheibel, 1981; Reyes et al., 1983; Shapiro et al., 1984). By postnatal day (P) 40, however, dysmorphic spines with tortuous necks and

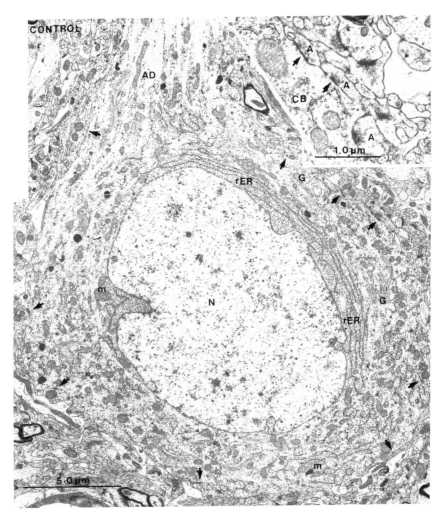

Fig. 3. The ultrastructure of layer V pyramidal neurons from 30-day-old rats. The cell body of a neocortical pyramidal neuron in a control rat (above) has a large, ovoid nucleus (N) with a smooth nuclear envelope and a perikaryon replete in organelles such as mitochondria (m) and Golgi apparatus (G). Note the highly ordered rough endoplasmic reticulum (rER) which is characterized by parallel arrays of cisternae. A large dendrite (AD) arises from the apex of the cell body. The inset depicts a magnified segment of the perikaryon. The cell body forms symmetric synapses

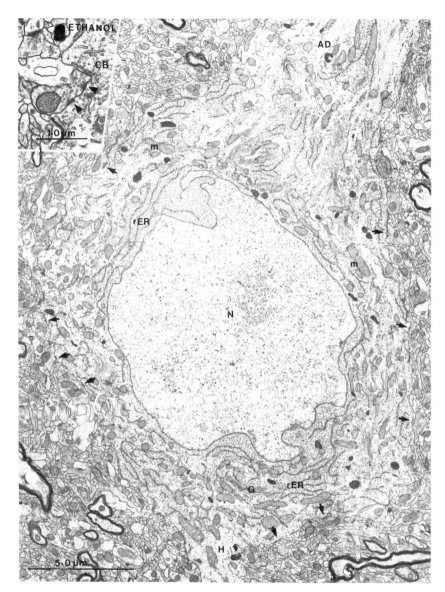

(arrows) with multiple axon terminals (A). Each terminal makes a simple synaptic contact with the cell body. In pyramidal neurons of rats prenatally exposed to ethanol (above), the nuclear envelope is irregular and cisternae of the rough endo-plasmic reticulum appear disorganized. In ethanol-exposed rats, axosomatic syn-apses are frequently associated with complex profiles consisting of two synaptic sites (arrowheads). H, axon hillock. (Reproduced from Al-Rabiai and Miller, 1989, with permission.)

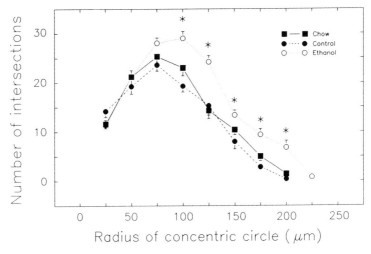

Fig. 4. Effect of ethanol on the complexity of the basal dendrites of intracellularly labeled corticospinal neurons. This graph describes the number of intersections of branches of basal dendrites with a series of concentric circles spaced 25 μm apart (Sholl analysis). The center of the circles was coincident with the center of the cell body. Each value represents the mean of 10 neurons and T-bars signify the standard errors of the means. Asterisks (*) denote statistically significant differences ($P < 0.05$) between the control and ethanol-exposed rats. (Reproduced from Miller et al., 1990, with permission.)

enlarged heads were common in the ethanol-treated rats (Fig. 5) (Stoltenburg-Didinger and Spohr, 1983; Miller et al., 1990). These abnormal spines were similar to the mushroom-shaped spines on pyramidal neurons in normal mature rat cortex and the dysmorphic spines identified in the brains of mentally retarded humans (Marin-Padilla, 1972, 1974; Purpura, 1974). Moreover, the density of spines on the apical shafts of pyramidal neurons of ethanol-treated rats was greater than in controls (Stoltenburg-Didinger and Spohr, 1983; Miller et al., 1990). These data were supported by electron microscopic studies of layers I and V of rat somatosensory cortex which showed an ethanol-induced increase in the frequency of axospinous synapses (Jones and Colangelo, 1985b; Al-Rabiai and Miller, 1989) despite no changes in the volume of the neuropil either in layer I or in Layer V (Miller and Potempa, 1990).

Presumably, the abnormalities in spine morphology and density affect their function. For example, if spines normally move actively within the cortical neuropil, this movement would be seriously hampered by the enlarged head and longer neck seen in the ethanol-treated rats. If spines normally recycle over time, ethanol-induced increases in spine density and in frequency of dysmorphic spines would reflect an altered recycling process. That is, the rate of spine turnover should decrease as many spines

CHOW   CONTROL   ETHANOL

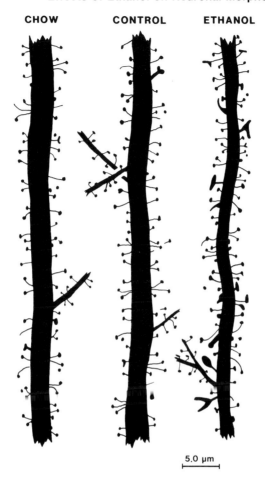

5.0 µm

Fig. 5. The morphology of dendritic spines on apical dendrites of layer Vb corticospinal neurons from chow-fed, pair-fed control, and ethanol-exposed rats. Dysmorphic spines are prominent in the ethanol-exposed rat. (Reproduced from Miller et al., 1990, with permission.)

develop abnormally into dysmorphic spines that cannot be reincorporated into the dendritic shaft for reuse in the formation of new spines. Viewed in another way, if spine production is unaffected by ethanol exposure and continues at a constant basal rate, but recycling is reduced, then the density of spines should rise. The net result of a decrease in turnover would likely be a reduction in neuronal plasticity.

Axons. The axons of pyramidal neurons have long projections to structures such as the spinal cord via the pyramidal tract and the contralateral cortex via the corpus callosum. Corticospinal axons are one of the major extracortical projection systems. In mature normal rats, these axons arise from cell bodies in layer Vb of discrete cortical areas (Hicks and D'Amato, 1977; Wise et al., 1979; Leong, 1983; Miller, 1987a). The vast majority of these cell bodies were distributed in the primary and secondary motor cortex and in primary and secondary somatosensory cortex, cortical areas that are related to the movement and sensation of all parts of the body other than the face (Hall and Lindholm, 1974; Donoghue and Wise, 1982; Gioanni and Lamarche, 1985). A small number of corticospinal neurons were in areas of visual, auditory, and limbic cortices.

Prenatal exposure to ethanol produced marked alterations in the distribution and number of corticospinal neurons (Miller, 1987b; Miller et al., 1990). As in control rats, cortiocospinal neurons in mature ethanol-treated rats were distributed in layer Vb of motor, somatosensory, visual, auditory, and limbic cortices. The biggest ethanol-induced changes were the addition of an abnormal field of corticospinal neurons in caudal secondary motor cortex (a region that is largely devoid of corticospinal neurons in normal rats) and the abnormally distributed corticospinal neurons in layers II/III, IV, Va, Vc, and VI. It is likely that both of these alterations lead to incorrect connectivity of spinal projection neurons and to abnormal cortical output which underlie ethanol-induced motor dysfunction.

In the regions of motor and somatosensory cortices which normally contain spinal projection neurons, the density of corticospinal neurons was significantly greater in ethanol-treated rats than in controls (Miller, 1987b). For example, the density of corticospinal neurons in layer Vb of primary somatosensory cortex of ethanol-treated rats was 27% greater than in controls. On the other hand, the size of somatosensory cortex was reduced significantly by 31% (Miller and Potempa, 1990). Thus, it is estimated that there was no net change in the number of corticospinal neurons. These data were supported by a quantitative analysis of the composition of the pyramidal tract. The absolute number of axons in the pyramidal tract were similar in ethanol-treated and control rats (Al-Rabiai and Miller, 1989). It should be kept in mind that although the absolute number of corticospinal neurons is not affected by ethanol exposure, because of the ethanol-induced microcephaly, the ethanol-treated animal effectively has more corticospinal neurons than control animals.

The exuberance of the corticospinal projection in mature, ethanol-treated rats may result from the arrest of the corticospinal system in a developmentally immature state. Early in their development, layer V neurons throughout neocortex project axons into the spinal cord (Stanfield et al., 1982; O'Leary and Stanfield, 1985, 1986). Over time, most layer V neurons in areas other than motor and somatosensory cortices lose their spinal axons. It has been suggested that ethanol interferes with this pruning process so that more cortical neurons retain their projections to the spinal cord.

Recent intracellular recording/labeling studies show that corticospinal neurons in mature normal rats have distinct morpho-physiological characteristics (Miller et al., 1990). These cells are pyramidal neurons with 1) dendrites that ramify within layers I, IV, and V, and 2) axons that do not ascend beyond layer IV but have extremely long horizontal collaterals (up to 2.6 mm) that arborize within layers V and VI. Electrophysiologically, corticospinal neurons apparently have an uncommon firing pattern. On stimulation, these neurons responded with a burst of action potentials rather than with a single action potential like most other cortical projection neurons (Connors et al., 1982, 1983; Landry et al., 1984; McCormick et al., 1985; Miller et al., 1990; Chagnac-Amitai et al., 1990).

The distinctive nature of corticospinal neurons is lost in ethanol-treated rats (Miller et al., 1990). Many of the layer Vb pyramidal neurons in ethanol-treated rats exhibited morpho-physiological characteristics similar to corticospinal neurons in control rats. On the other hand, some layer Vb corticospinal neurons did not. Not only did these corticospinal neurons have long axons that branched within the infragranular laminae, they also had axons that ascended to layers I and II/III, and on stimulation, these neurons had regular spiking behaviors.

Many neurons in motor and somatosensory cortex project axons to the contralateral cortex. In fact, the corpus callosum is the largest tract in the mammalian central nervous system. Callosal neurons serve as a means to coordinate movements and sensations that cross the midline so that the body can function as a unit and not as two separate halves.

There is debate about how susceptible the corpus callosum is to early exposure to ethanol. On one end of the spectrum, it was reported that prenatal exposure to ethanol caused agenesis of the corpus callosum in mice (Chernoff, 1977). More recent data have questioned this finding for although agenesis of the corpus callosum occurred in ethanol-treated BALB/c mice, the occurrence of this deformity was as common in ethanol-treated mice as it was in pair-fed and chow control rats (Wainwright et al., 1985). The cross-sectional sagittal area of the corpus callosum in neonatal C57BL/6 mice and in neonatal rats prenatally exposed to ethanol was not significantly different from that in pair-fed controls (Wainwright and Gagnon, 1985; Wainwright et al., 1985; Zimmerberg and Scalzi, 1989). Other data show that the size of the corpus callosum in 20-day-old BALB/c mouse fetuses was significantly smaller in ethanol-treated mice than in controls; however, this difference was gone by the third postnatal week (Fritz, 1984).

Two studies have examined the effect of gestational exposure to ethanol on the distribution of the cell bodies of callosal projection neurons. Jacobson et al. (1979) reported that there was no change in the distribution of callosal neurons; in both control and ethanol-treated rats, callosal neurons were distributed in layers II/III and V. Using a more sensitive tract tracing technique, Kotkoskie and Miller (1989) showed further that the density of callosal neurons in layers V and VI of ethanol-trated rats was as much as 2.5 fold greater than that observed in controls, whereas the density of labeled neurons in layer II/III was 2–3 fold less in ethanol-treated rats than in controls.

In addition to long projections, pyramidal neurons also form a vast network of local connections. The axons of projection neurons form asymmetric synapses (LeVay, 1973; Parnavelas et al., 1978; Miller and Peters, 1981; Winfield et al., 1981). These synapses are considered to mediate excitation (Peters et al., 1976). The presynaptic elements in most asymmetric synapses in rat neocortex arise from the collaterals of pyramidal neurons (White, 1989). Analyses of the cortical neuropil showed that prenatal exposure to ethanol led to an increased number of asymmetric synapses and an increase in the volume occupied by axonal varicosities (Al-Rabiai and Miller, 1989). Axonal varicosities contain synaptic sites. Moreover, the numbers of varicosities along the axons of intracellularly labeled corticospinal neurons was greater in ethanol-treated rats than in controls (Miller and Rhoades, unpublished results).

In early stages of synaptogenesis, the presynaptic grid is a simple, circular plate (Miller and Peters, 1981; Jones and Colangelo, 1985a). During normal maturation, synaptic grids, notably those associated with axospinous synapses, often mature into a more complex geometry, e.g., an annular or horseshoe-shaped grid (Peters and Kaiserman-Abramof, 1969; Cohen and Siekevitz, 1978; Calverly and Jones, 1987). In the case of axospinal synapses, the complexity of the synapse varies with spine size. Small spine heads are associated with simple synaptic junctions, whereas large spines are associated with presynaptic elements exhibiting geometrically complex grids (Peters and Kaiserman-Abramof, 1969). The frequency of complex synapses in rats that were at least 30 days old and exposed to ethanol pre- or postnatally, was greater than in control rats (Jones and Colangelo, 1985a; Al-Rabiai and Miller, 1989). It is appealing to speculate that the increase in the frequency of complex synapses correlates with the increase in the frequency of dysmorphic spines with abnormally enlarged heads and that this overdevelopment of the synaptic grid results form the abnormal stabilization of the spine or maintenance of a spine beyond the time when it would normally have been recycled (see above).

Local circuit neurons

Fewer data are available regarding the effect of prenatal ethanol exposure on the structure and function of local circuit neurons than for pyramidal neurons. Local circuit neurons can be classified into at least three morphological classes: stellate neurons, bitufted neurons, and bipolar neurons (Feldman and Peters, 1978). These discriminations are based upon somato-dendritic morphology. Stellate neurons have round cell bodies with dendrites radiating from all aspects. Bitufted neurons have relatively large, fusiform cell bodies with a spray of dendrites arising from the opposite poles of the cell body. In contrast, bipolar neurons have small ellipsoidal cell bodies with a single dendrite originating from the apical and basal somatic poles. Local circuit neurons are considered to be essential for the integration of information within mammalian neocortex.

Cell bodies. Apparently, most local circuit neurons use γ-aminobutyric acid (GABA) as a neurotransmitter (Houser et al., 1984; Sillito, 1984). Therefore, many studies of local circuit neurons in rat cortex have exploited immunohistochemical techniques to identify GABAergic neurons. With such an approach, the distribution, number, and size of the cell bodies of local circuit neurons were determined in control and ethanol-treated rats (Miller, unpublished results). GABA-immunoreactive neurons were distributed in all layers of the somatosensory cortex of mature normal rats; however, the greatest concentration was in layer II/III. This distribution of GABA-positive neurons was altered by prenatal exposure to ethanol. The change largely resulted from a decrease in the numbers of immunoreactive neurons in layer II/III and an increase in the density of GABA-positive neurons in layer VI. It should be noted that prenatal exposure to ethanol caused an increase in the cortical content of GABA (Sytinsky et al., 1975; Rawat, 1977) particularly in the frontal region (Ledig et al., 1988). In light of the immunohistochemical data, it appears that this ethanol-induced increase in GABA content resulted from an increase in the mean GABA content per neuron. All three types of local circuit neurons were identified in the cortices of ethanol-treated rats. As a result of the ethanol exposure, however, the mean size of the cell bodies of GABA-positive neurons in each layer was reduced 15%.

The fine structure of the cell bodies of local circuit neurons was changed by prenatal exposure to ethanol in a manner similar to that of pyramidal neurons (Al-Rabiai and Miller, 1989). That is, the orderly parallel arrays of cisternae of the rough endoplasmic reticulum that were readily identified in cortical local circuit neurons of control rats, were severely disrupted. In addition, the volume of the somata that was occupied by the Golgi apparatus and by lysosomes was significantly less in ethanol-treated rats. Thus, it appeared that protein synthesis in local circuit neurons was affected by prenatal exposure to ethanol.

Regardless of their stage of development, the axons of most local circuit neurons form symmetric synapses with the somata of other local circuit neurons and pyramidal neurons (e.g., Peters and Kaiserman-Abramof, 1970; Ribak, 1978; Peters and Fairen, 1978; Miller and Peters, 1981; Miller, 1986b). In fact, these axons provide the only synaptic input to the cell bodies of pyramidal neurons, shown to form exclusively symmetric synapses. Prenatal exposure to ethanol produced a significant increase in the number and density of symmetric synapses on somata of local circuit (130%) and pyramidal neurons (30%) in layer V of somatosensory cortex of 30-day-old rats (Al-Rabiai and Miller, 1989). In contrast, the density of symmetric axodendritic synapses was decreased 47% by prenatal exposure to ethanol. This apparent ethanol-induced redistribution of symmetric synapses opposed the changes in the density of asymmetric synapses (see above).

The net effect of the ethanol-induced reorganization of cortical synaptology apparently has functional consequences. Symmetric synapses have been described as serving an inhibitory function whereby the membrane excitability of the postsynaptic neuron is reduced (Sillito, 1984). The increased inhibitory input to the cell bodies at least partially closes the gate of the electrical activity. This inhibition occurs regardless of the potential increase in excitatory activity in the periphery. This may explain the reduction in laminar glucose utilization (Miller and Dow-Edwards, 1988) described above.

Corticopetal Systems

The most thorough examinations of the effect of ethanol on the development of corticopetal systems have focused on the monoaminergic and cholinergic afferents. Although a fuller treatment of the effects of ethanol on these systems is offered in Chapter 6, as these afferents influence cortical development they are also discussed here briefly.

Each of these afferent systems arises almost exclusively from subcortical structures. Catecholaminergic axons originate in the locus ceruleus in the brainstem (Levitt and Moore, 1978; Lindvall and Bjorklund, 1984), serotonergic afferents emanate from the raphe nuclei in the midbrain (Moore et al., 1978; Lindvall and Bjorklund, 1984), and cholinergic afferents arise from the basal forebrain (Mesulam et al., 1983; Saper, 1984). Lesion of these afferents leads to physiological and anatomical changes in cerebral cortex (e.g., Blue and Parnavelas, 1982; Felten et al., 1982; Shaw et al., 1984; Bear and Singer, 1986). Although controversial, it has been suggested that these systems are important in promoting neuronal morphogenesis and in maintaining neuronal plasticity (e.g., Lauder and Krebs, 1978; Kasamatsu et al., 1979, 1981; Bear and Daniels, 1983; Haydon et al., 1984; Shaw et al., 1984; Bear and Singer, 1986; Chubakov et al., 1986; Trombley et al., 1986; D'Amato et al., 1987).

Prenatal exposure alters the monoaminergic and cholinergic systems. The cortical content of catecholamines, serotonin and acetylcholine and/or receptors for these neurotransmitters are affected by gestational exposure to ethanol (e.g., Elis et al., 1976, 1978; Krsiak et al., 1977; Rawat, 1977; Boggan et al., 1979; Borg et al., 1983; Rathbun and Druse, 1985; Riley et al., 1986). Since the cortical content of these neurotransmitters arises chiefly, if not solely, from ascending afferents, it appears that ethanol exposure affects the arborization of the subcortical afferents.

Ethanol exposure also causes the depletion of the serotonergic input to cortex, albeit transient. Significant differences between the cortical levels of serotonin in ethanol-treated rats and controls disappear by P90 (Chapter 6). Apparently, serotonin serves as a trophic factor which induces or promotes neuritic outgrowth (Haydon et al., 1984, 1987; McCobb et al., 1988). Conceivably, these changes in the serotonergic content underlie the temporal, ethanol-induced changes in the length of dendrites on pyramidal neurons. The reduced length of the dendrites during the first 3 postnatal weeks may result from the normally low levels of serotonin in cortex. Likewise, after the levels of serotonin in ethanol-treated rats recover to the levels observed in normal, age-matched rats, there is an increase in the lengths of the dendrites to normal or even supranormal levels.

HIPPOCAMPAL FORMATION

General Description

The dentate gyrus and hippocampus have a simpler cortical organization than neocortex. In both structures, a single layer of neuronal cell bodies is bordered above and below by neuropil-rich zones containing few neuronal somata. In the hippocampus, the cellular zone is composed primarily of pyramidal neurons, and in the dentate gyrus, the cellular zone is occupied by granule neurons.

The hippocampal formation has a characteristic appearance in sectioned material. The layer of granule neurons in the dentate gyrus has a curvature that resembles a horseshoe or arrowhead, depending upon the location of the section within the hippocampal formation (Fig. 6). The apical dendrites of granule neurons extend from the convexity of the horseshoe toward the cortical surface bordering the hippocampal fissure. The mossy fibers, the axons of the granule cells, project into the concavity of the hilus and from there into the hippocampus (field CA3) where they terminate. A number of polymorphic neurons and local circuit neurons, integral to the dentate gyrus, are also situated within the hilus just below the granule neurons.

The layer of pyramidal neurons in the hippocampus also has a characteristic curvature that somewhat resembles an enlarged mirror-image of the curved dentate gyrus. The neuronal layer of the hippocampus can be subdivided into four linearly adjacent regions or fields, identified as CA1 through CA4 (Lorente de No, 1934). These subdivisions are based on cytoarchitectural differences that can be recognized in cresyl violet-stained sec-

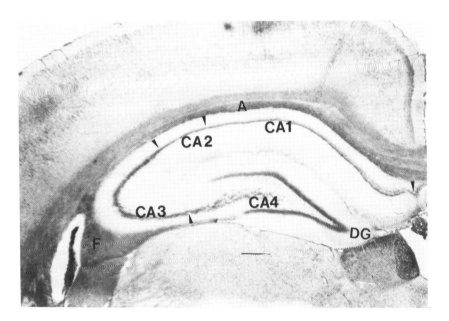

Fig. 6. Dorsal hippocampus in normal rat brain. The four fields of the hippocampus can be appreciated in this coronal section. Arrowheads indicate approximate boundaries of fields CA1-CA4. DG, dentate gyrus; A, alveus; F, fimbria. Toluidine blue stain. Bar = 20 μm.

tions. The CA4 field, within the hilus of the dentate gyrus (i.e., the intrahilar zone of the dentate gyrus), merges with the groups of polymorphic neurons that belong to the dentate gyrus. Distal to the dentate gyrus, field CA3 is contiguous with field CA3, a region easily recognized by its large pyramidal neurons. The large CA3 neurons are gradually replaced distally by the smaller pyramidal neurons of field CA1. Between CA3 and CA1, there is a small transitional zone designated as CA2.

The pyramidal neurons extend apical dendrites toward the hippocampal fissure. The neuropil-rich layer surrounding the apical dendrites is composed of two to three sublaminae of afferent fibers that are arranged parallel to the layer of pyramidal neurons. Afferents from the entorhinal cortex project through the superficial stratum (stratum moleculare/lacunosum) and terminate on distal portions of the apical dendrites. Afferents that originate from neurons in the septum and in the contralateral hippocampus (stratum radiatum) terminate at all other levels along the apical dendrites in fields CA1/CA2. In field CA3, however, a deeper stratum containing the mossy fibers from the ipsilateral dentate gyrus (stratum lucidum) can be identified between the stratum radiatum and the layer containing the cell bodies of the pyramidal neurons (stratum pyramidale). Mossy fibers terminate on uniquely branched spines present on the trunks of apical dendrites of the pyramidal neurons. Dendrites also radiate from the base of each pyramidal neuron, and afferents that project from neurons in the septum and contralateral hippocampus to these basal dendrites form a separate infrapyramidal layer (stratum oriens). Axons of pyramidal neurons also arise from the base of the cell body or from a dendritic trunk. They pass through the stratum oriens and enter the alveus, a thin sheet of fibers over the ventricular surface of the hippocampus. Fibers from the alveus merge at the fimbria for efferent distribution. Collaterals (Schaffer collaterals) that branch from these axons in CA3 also innervate pyramidal neurons in fields CA1/CA2 ipsilaterally.

The overall structure features of the hippocampal formation appeared unaltered by early exposure to ethanol. The laminar organization in the dentate gyrus and hippocampus appeared normal. Quantitative measurements in the dentate gyrus show that prenatal exposure to ethanol causes no significant differences in the number of granule cells (Barnes and Walker, 1981); however, postnatal exposure to ethanol produces a significant increase in the number of granule cells (West et al., 1986). In the hippocampus, the areas of all sublaminae were reduced by ethanol exposure, but the stratum oriens and the stratum moleculare/lacunosum were most severely affected. Prenatal ethanol exposure (G10–G21) caused a significant reduction (20%, Barnes and Walker, 1981) in cell number in field CA1 of the dorsal hippocampus, and postnatal ethanol exposure (P4-P10) caused a significant reduction in area of the midtemporal hippocampus (26.1%, Pierce and West, 1987). These data are detailed in Chapter 5. Their importance in the present context is that they suggest that underlying changes in neuronal morphology had occurred.

Neuronal Types

Pyramidal neurons

Cell bodies. Early exposure to ethanol produced conspicuous cytoplasmic alterations in the somata of the CA1 neurons. The cytoplasm in the ethanol-treated mice had fewer free polyribosomes, causing these neurons to appear paler than those in control mice, and the Golgi apparatus was less well developed than in neurons of control animals (Fig. 7) (Smith and Davies, 1990). These changes showed that cytoplasmic organelles essential for protein synthesis were altered in the neurons of the ethanol-treated mice. It is likely, therefore, that protein synthesis was also disrupted in these neurons, a conclusion that is consistent with the effects of ethanol on neocortical neurons (Al-Rabiai and Miller, 1989).

Dendrites. The growth of the dendritic trees of hippocampal pyramidal neurons of rodents has been studied in detail following exposure to ethanol

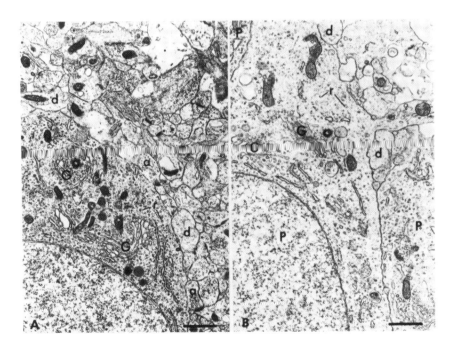

Fig. 7. Ultrastructure of hippocampal pyramidal neurons. In a pyramidal neuron from a control mouse (**A**), the Golgi apparatus (G) is robust and free polyribosomes (r) are numerous. The perikaryal surface is studded with dendritic (d) and axonal (a) profiles. In contrast, pyramidal neurons from an ethanol-exposed mouse (**B**) exhibit a less well developed Golgi apparatus and there are fewer free polyribosomes. Perikaryal surfaces (P) of pyramidal neurons in the ethanol-exposed mouse are more closely apposed to each other than to dendritic or axonal profiles. Bars = 0.5 μm. (Reproduced from Smith and Davies, 1990, with permission.)

from G12 to P7. During the first postnatal week, there were no structural differences between these neurons in pups from chow-fed, pair-fed, or ethanol-fed mothers (Davies, 1982). On P14, however, basal dendritic arbors of Golgi-Cox impregnated CA1 pyramidal neurons of ethanol-treated mice were markedly shorter and had fewer branches than those in control mice. The total length of the basal dendritic arbors in these neurons was significantly reduced (20%) by ethanol exposure (Davies and Smith, 1981). By P21, the dendrites of pyramidal neurons of ethanol-treated and control mice were again indistinguishable (Davies, 1982). Davies and Smith (1981) interpreted their results as indicative of either a delay in development or a deviant mode of development of pyramidal neurons in field CA1 followed by a period of compensatory growth. Interestingly, these types of dendritic alterations were not detected in neurons elsewhere in the hippocampal formation.

The ultrastructure of the stratum pyramidale and the stratum oriens of CA1 in mice treated with ethanol between G12 and P7 was examined on P14 (Smith and Davies, 1990). The neuronal somata in the chow-fed control mice (the only control in this study) were separated by a plexus of dendritic profiles but those in the ethanol-exposed mice were tightly packed together with only a few dendritic processes present between them. There were also fewer dendritic profiles in the stratum oriens of the ethanol-exposed mice, and these profiles were irregularly shaped. Presynaptic terminals in contact with dendrites in the ethanol-treated mice were also smaller and vesicles within them were frequently clumped.

Spines on Golgi-impregnated neurons were not quantified by Davies and Smith (1981), but Davies (1982) reported that the basal dendrites of hippocampal neurons were densely studded with spines in both control and ethanol-exposed mice on P21. The spines appeared to be of normal length and were not deformed, and qualitative observations suggested that spine densities were greater in the ethanol-exposed mice than in the control mice. The latter observation is consistent with the quantitative analyses by Stoltenburg-Didinger and Spohr (1983) and Miller et al. (1990) that spine densities on the apical shafts of neocortical pyramidal neurons of ethanol-treated rats were increased above control values. In the neocortex, however, the increases in spine density occurred later (P40) in development and were associated with the appearance of dysmorphic spines.

Dysmorphic spines were not reported by Davies and Smith (1981) or by Davies (1982). Abel et al. (1983), however, found that after 14 weeks of postnatal development there was a decrease in the number of Type 1 (thin) spines and a corresponding increase in the number of Type 2 (mushroom) spines on dendrites in rats exposed to ethanol during gestation. The numbers of Type 3 (stubby) spines were low in all rats. They also reported that at that time there were fewer spines on CA1 pyramidal neurons in the ethanol-exposed rats. These data suggest that ethanol exposure during gestation can alter both spine production and spine turnover in the hippocampus.

Granule neurons

Dendrites. Dendritic arbors of granule neurons in the dentate gyrus of mice were unaltered by ethanol (Davies and Smith, 1981), and Hoff (1985, 1988) reported that synaptogenesis was not affected by ethanol exposure since there were no significant differences in overall synaptic density on either P10 or P20. Other phases of synaptic development, however, were affected by ethanol, a conclusion based on studies of photomontages of tangential sections through the molecular layer (Hoff, 1988). Synaptic profiles were classified as simple or complex in shape and each profile formed a symmetric or asymmetric synapse. Presynaptic terminals with multiple synaptic junctions were also tabulated. Multiple synapses were described as triads composed of two presynaptic profiles forming synapses with a single dendritic spine.

Ethanol exposure was associated with significant reductions in the density of multiple synaptic junctions on P10 (a 10 fold decrease) and in the density of complex synapses on P20 (approximately 50% fewer) (Hoff, 1985). The development of complex synaptic geometry has been directly associated with synaptic maturation (Peters and Kaiserman-Abramof, 1969; Cohen and Siekevitz, 1978; Calverly and Jones, 1987), and a reduction in the number of complex synapses in the ethanol exposed rats indicated that synaptic maturation was delayed in the dentate granule neurons. Since there were no significant differences in overall synaptogenesis, however, it is probable that the onset of synaptic turnover was also delayed (Hoff, 1988). These results were the opposite of those described in neocortex where the number of complex synapses increased with age (Jones and Colangelo, 1985a; Al-Rabiai and Miller, 1989), implying that synaptic turnover was impeded by prenatal ethanol exposure.

Development of dendritic structure in CA3 neurons was normal in ethanol-treated mice (Davies and Smith, 1981). Unfortunately, neither synaptogenesis nor the effects of perinatal ethanol on this critical stage of neuronal maturation have been studied in CA3.

Axons. Early exposure to ethanol results in mossy fiber hypertrophy (West et al., 1981; West and Hamre, 1985). In Timm-stained sections of the hippocampus of control rats, mossy fiber projections from granule neurons were distributed in the hilus of the dentate gyrus, the stratum lucidum of CA3, and a small infrapyramidal bundle near the hilus. In rats treated with ethanol either prenatally throughout gestation (West et al., 1981) or postnatally on P1–P10 (West and Hamre, 1985), mossy fibers were present both intra- and infrapyramidally throughout field CA3 as well as the hilus. A detailed discussion of this aberrant mossy fiber projection is found in Chapter 5.

Reasons for the altered mossy fiber distribution to CA3 pyramidal neurons are not immediately apparent. An ethanol-induced loss of normal target cells or a decrease in synaptic sites on normal target cells might cause afferents to seek out new available synaptic sites within CA3. But data indicating that CA3 neurons decrease in number following perinatal ethanol exposure or that they undergo maturational delay as a result of ethanol treatment have not been forthcoming. Determinations of cell number from measurements of cell density in a single or a few sections indicated that ethanol treatment had no effect on cell numbers in field CA3 (Barnes and Walker, 1981; West et al., 1986), but the total numbers of pyramidal cells in field CA3 were not determined (West et al., 1986). This is an important consideration since Miller and Potempa (1990) demonstrated that the total number of neurons in primary somatosensory cortex was significantly reduced by prenatal ethanol treatment due to decreases in the overall volume of area 3 and the volume of the individual layers, even though laminar cell packing density was unaltered. Thus, although no differences in cell number may be evident in measurements of cell density in single sections, significant differences in cell number may result from reductions in the volume of a nucleus or cortical region.

Severe ethanol-related reductions in the area of the stratum oriens, the stratum radiatum, and the stratum moleculare/lacunosum (approximately 34%, 20%, and 32%, respectively) may contribute to hypertrophic growth of the mossy fiber projection to field CA3 (Pierce and West, 1987).

CEREBELLAR CORTEX
General Description

The mature cerebellar cortex has a relatively simple organization with three readily demarcated laminae. The granule cell layer (densely populated with the small cell bodies of granule neurons) and the molecular layer (a neuropil-rich layer, sparsely populated by local circuit interneurons) sandwich the Purkinje cell layer (formed by a single layer of Purkinje neurons). The entire cortex overlies the white matter which is composed of myelinated axons (Fig. 8). During its development, the cerebellar cortex becomes separated into lobules by transverse fissures that appear early in ontogeny.

Neuronal Types
Purkinje neurons

Purkinje neurons are among the largest and most elaborate neurons in the central nervous system and they have extensively branched dendritic arbors. These neurons are oriented perpendicular to the longitudinal axes of the cerebellar lobules and to the parallel fibers. In addition to the excitatory input from numerous parallel fibers, each Purkinje neuron receives powerful excitation from a single climbing fiber, an extrinsic afferent that makes multiple synaptic contacts with specialized spines on the main dendritic branches. Purkinje neurons receive inhibitory input from local circuit neurons, the basket and stellate cells, distributed in the molecular layer.

Cell bodies. Reports from several studies have shown that ethanol-related deficits in Purkinje cell number occurred in the cerebellum of rodents following ethanol exposure during gestation (Phillips and Cragg, 1982) and during the early postnatal period (Bauer-Moffett and Altman, 1977; Phillips and Cragg, 1982; Volk, 1984; Yanai and Waknin, 1985).

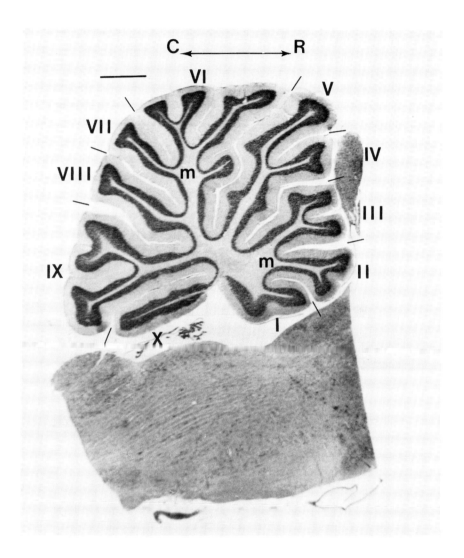

Fig. 8. Midsagittal section of a normal cerebellar vermis. At this magnification the layer of granule neurons (continuous, convoluted dark band) and the molecular layer (pale, convoluted surface layer) are readily distinguished. Lobules are denoted by Roman numerals. m, medullary layer; R, rostral; C, caudal. Cresyl violet stain. Bar = 200 μm.

Ultrastructural features of Purkinje neurons of rats exposed to ethanol were studied by Volk (1984), Spohr and Stoltenburg-Didinger (1985), and Mohamed et al. (1987a). In spite of differences in the timing of ethanol administration during development and in the lobules of the cerebellar vermis that were selected for study, similar results were obtained in these studies.

The somata of Purkinje neurons of ethanol-treated rats generally appeared to be less mature than those of control rats. On P4, there were fewer ribosomes, mitochondria, and vesicles in neurons of the ethanol-treated rats. On P7 (Volk, 1984), P8 (Spohr and Stoltenburg-Didinger, 1985), and P10 (Mohamed et al., 1987a), the nuclei in neurons of the ethanol-treated rats were smaller and more irregular in shape than in the controls. There were also unusual accumulations of free ribosomes basally within the cytoplasm of the ethanol exposed neurons, and the primary dendrites had fewer and less well developed organelles. By P12 (Volk, 1984; Spohr and Stoltenburg-Didinger, 1985) and P14 (Mohamed at al., 1987a), Purkinje neurons of the ethanol-treated rats differed chiefly in having less well developed rough endoplasmic reticulum and more numerous free ribosomes than in the controls. The immature appearance of cytoplasmic organelles in these neurons was consistent with ethanol-related changes described above in neocortical neurons (Al-Rabiai and Miller, 1989), that suggest that prenatal exposure to ethanol depresses protein synthesis through a disruptive action on organelles essential for protein synthesis.

Volk (1984) reported that by P17 differences in the ultrastructural appearance of the cytoplasm of Purkinje neurons of the experimental and control rats were no longer detectable. An ethanol-induced inhibition of protein synthesis may, however, persist through lengthy and critical periods of postnatal development of the cerebellar cortex. Spohr and Stoltenburg-Didinger (1985) found that on P21 a severe delay in maturation of Purkinje neurons was still apparent in their preparations, and some Purkinje neurons still retained an extremely immature appearance characteristic of control neurons on P8. Furthermore, Mohamed et al., (1987a) found that even on P42 the Purkinje neurons in offspring of ethanol-treated mothers exhibited a marked reduction in the development of rough endoplasmic reticulum compared with neurons from control rats. It is likely that discrepancies in the timing of maturational changes in Purkinje neurons and in the duration of ethanol-related effects, noted above, stem from differences in the timing and duration of ethanol treatment as well as from differences in the lobules that were selected for study. Nonetheless, all of these studies show clearly that ethanol exposure during gestation caused a severe retardation of maturation in rat Purkinje neurons associated with disruption of organelles responsible for protein synthesis, an effect that could persist at least throughout early development.

Ethanol-related effects on ultrastructural features of the somata of Purkinje neurons were less severe in mice. The smooth endoplasmic reticulum in Purkinje neurons of ethanol-treated mice appeared to be less prominent and, surprisingly, free polyribosomes were less numerous than in chow-fed controls (Smith and Davies, 1990). Reasons for the discrepancy between the effects of ethanol in mice and in rats have not been provided as yet.

Dendrites. Spohr and Stoltenburg-Didinger (1985) showed that on P12 lateral perisomatic processes were almost entirely absent from Golgi-impregnated neurons in control rats but were still demonstrable in neurons of ethanol-exposed rats, a sign of retarded development. Furthermore, Smith and Davies (1990) found that, on P14, dendrites of Golgi-impregnated Purkinje neurons in ethanol-exposed mice were truncated and in some regions denuded of spines. The developing dendritic arbors of the Purkinje neurons were also oriented abnormally so that the typical fan shape was lacking.

Ultrastructural features of Purkinje cell dendrites in ethanol-exposed mice were consistent with the appearance of these neurons in Golgi-impregnated material (Smith and Davies, 1990). Microtubules and smooth endoplasmic reticulum in the large dendrites were less prominent in the ethanol-treated mice, and orientation of the mitochondria within the cytoplasmic matrix of the dendrites appeared to be more random than in the controls. There were more profiles of parallel fiber bundles between the dendrites of Purkinje neurons in the molecular layer in the chow controls than in the ethanol-exposed mice. Glial sheaths around the larger dendrites of Purkinje neurons in the control mice allowed contact between presynaptic structures and the dendrites, but in the ethanol-exposed mice the glial processes were distended, appearing to isolate the dendrites completely from the surrounding neuropil. There was a trend toward fewer dendritic thorns in synaptic contact with parallel fibers in the ethanol-exposed mice, but this reduction was not statistically significant (Smith and Davies, 1990).

There were prominent effects of ethanol exposure on synaptic maturation in rats that had been exposed to ethanol throughout gestation and the neonatal period (Volk, 1984). On P12, there were fewer active synaptic zones in the middle of the molecular layer of the cerebellar cortex in the ethanol-treated rats than in the controls; there were irregularities in the presynaptic dense projections; and there were smaller postsynaptic bands in the active zones of synapses (Fig. 9). These results are consistent with the report by Noronha and Druse (1982) that perinatal ethanol exposure of rats, between G1 and P3, was associated with glycoprotein abnormalities in synaptic plasma membranes isolated from brain homogenates on P10, P17, and P24.

An impairment of climbing fiber maturation was also apparent in offspring of ethanol-treated rat mothers (Mohamed et al., 1987b). In control pups, climbing fiber maturation was nearly complete by P14. Almost all climbing fiber synapses occurred on the smooth dendrites of Purkinje neurons by that time, with very few remaining on somatic spines. In contrast, numerous climbing fiber synapses with somatic spines could still be seen in the ethanol-exposed pups on P14. There were also fewer basket cell axons that synapsed with the Purkinje cell somata and the initial segment of the Purkinje cell axon in ethanol-exposed pups on P14, suggesting that basket cell maturation was also retarded either directly by ethanol expo-

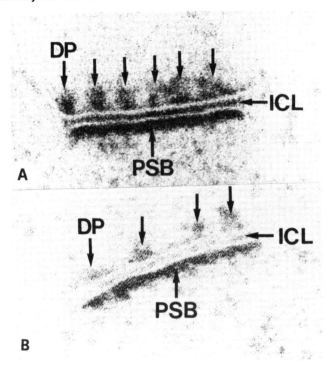

Fig. 9. Synapses in the molecular layer of the cerebellum. **A:** An axodendritic synaptic terminal (vermis, lobule VIII) of a 12-day-old control rat is characterized by a series of electron dense projections of the vesicular grid of the active zone (DP), a distinct intercleft line (ICL), and a robust postsynaptic band (PSB). **B:** In the axodendritic synaptic terminal of an age-matched ethanol-exposed rat, the DP are weakly stained and irregularly located, the ICL is nearly missing, and the PSB is wanting. Stained with ethanolic phosphotungstic acid. X 70,000. (Reproduced from Volk, 1984, with permission.)

sure or indirectly through the slower disappearance of climbing fiber synapses with Purkinje cell somata.

Axons. There are no data available currently relative to the effects of prenatal or early postnatal ethanol exposure on the axonal processes of Purkinje neurons.

Granule neurons

The cell bodies of the granule neurons are 5–8 μm in diameter and each extends two to seven short dendrites. Thin nonmyelinated axons of granule neurons project into the molecular layer of the cortex where each forms a T-shaped bifurcation. The resulting parallel fibers extend some distance in the longitudinal axis of each lobule and make synaptic contact with dendritic arbors of a number of Purkinje neurons. One of the major inputs to the granule cells is by way of the myelinated axons known as mossy fibers. These fibers arise from a variety of extra-cerebellar sources and from the intrinsic cerebellar nuclei and they terminate in rosettes which form synapses with the dendrites of granule neurons (Palay and Chan-Palay, 1974).

Cell bodies. The mean maximal cross-sectional area and the mean maximal diameter of the cell body were significantly smaller in mice which had been exposed to ethanol between G12 and P7 (Smith et al., 1986).

Dendrites. Smith et al. (1986) found differences in dendritic maturation in granule neurons of ethanol-exposed C57BL/6J mice. The distal portions of the dendrites of granule neurons normally mature from a simple "club-like" stage to a "claw-like" stage during their first week of development. By P14, the "claw-like" dendritic structures attain a digitiform appearance. The maturation of these dendrites corresponds to the development of mossy fiber rosettes. Granule neurons in chow-fed mice had developed the normal complex digitiform dendritic terminals by P14, but granule neurons in both the pair-fed controls and the ethanol-exposed mice had less mature dendritic structures. Dendrites of granule neurons in pair-fed controls were moderately retarded in development with appendages that were still claw-shaped, indicating that the dietary vehicle used to administer the ethanol delayed dendritic maturation. The maximum diameter and area of the granule cell bodies in the pair-fed mice, however, did not differ from those in the chow-fed mice. The granule neurons in the ethanol-exposed mice, on the other hand, were severely affected. These neurons still had "club-shaped" dendritic appendages or dendrites that were just beginning to develop the claw-like form (Fig. 10). Morphometric measurements of these neurons showed also that both the mean dendritic length and dendritic field area were significantly reduced in these neurons (Smith et al., 1986).

Axons. From a study of the ultrastructural features of the molecular layer of the cerebellar cortex of C57BL/6J mice, it was concluded that the development of parallel fibers was also altered by ethanol exposure (Smith and Davies, 1990). In control mice, parallel fibers were prominently aggregated into compact bundles. In ethanol-tested mice, parallel fiber bundles were fewer and more widely spaced (Fig. 11). The intervening glial cell cytoplasm separating the parallel fiber bundles was also more prominent in the ethanol-exposed mice. Mohamed et al. (1987b) noted that parallel fiber varicosities contacted two to three times more Purkinje cell spines in ethanol-exposed rats than in controls. This observation was interpreted by these investigators as evidence that parallel fibers were reduced in number in the ethanol-treated animals. On the other hand, these findings would also be consistent with a quantitative increase in dendritic spines on Purkinje neurons of ethanol-exposed pups without any change in the number of parallel fibers. In view of the ethanol-induced increases in spine density that are known to occur in neocortical neurons (Stoltenburg-Didinger and

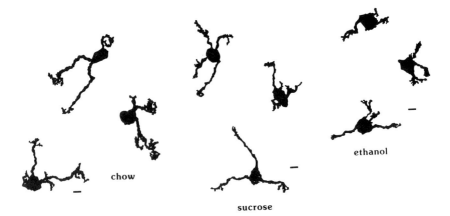

Fig. 10. Granule neurons of 14-day-old mouse pups. The dendrites are longer in neurons of control mice (from both chow- and sucrose-fed mothers) than in neurons of ethanol-exposed mice. Moreover, the appearance of these dendrites is affected by early exposure to ethanol. In neurons of mice from chow-fed mothers, the terminal arborizations of these dendrites are complex, fine finger-like (digitiform) processes. In neurons of mice from sucrose-fed mothers, the development of such processes is somewhat retarded for they appear to be "claw-like". The neurons of mice from ethanol-fed mothers are most adversely affected by the prenatal diet. The dendrites of granule neurons are severely retarded in development and appear "club-like". Bars = 10 μm. (Reproduced from Smith et al, 1986, with permission.)

Spohr, 1983; Miller et al., 1990), this alternative explanation must be entertained.

CONCLUSIONS

Ethanol-induced changes in the development of neuronal structure and function underlie the motor and learning deficits associated with early exposure to alcohol. Be it in the neocortex, hippocampal formation, or cerebellar cortex, neuronal maturation, connectivity, and electrophysiology are altered by ethanol.

The effect of ethanol appears to be greatest on the so-called "regressive" developmental events such as the pruning of exuberant axonal projections. Such abnormalities may result from methanol-induced removal or disruption of tightly governed control mechanisms which maintain the delicate balance required for normal neuronal morphogenesis. At least in the case of neocortex, it must be kept in mind that the structural and functional abnormalities in the mature structure are epiphenomena for the rats were only exposed to ethanol prenatally and neocortical morphogenesis occurs largely after birth. Thus, these findings highlight an important fact that the manipulation of the environment during the early stages of ontogeny can have long lasting effects upon the structure and function of the central nervous system.

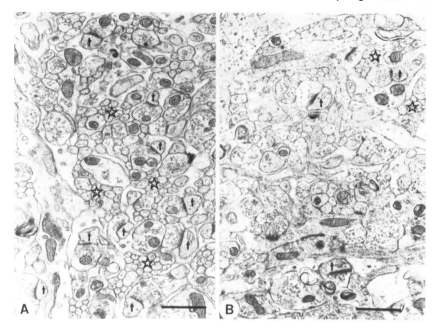

Fig. 11. Neuropil of the molecular layer of the cerebellum. Fewer synaptic profiles are present on dendritic thorns (t) of Purkinje neurons in the ethanol-exposed mouse (**B**) than in the control mouse (**A**). There are also fewer and less well organized bundles of parallel fibers (star denotes bundle) in the neuropil of the ethanol-exposed mouse. Bars = 1 μm. (Reproduced from Smith and Davies, 1990, with permission.)

It has been reported frequently that neurons of ethanol-treated animals appear to be less mature than those of age-matched controls. One way in which ethanol may retard maturation of neurons is through a depression of circulating thyroxin levels. Thyroxin normally causes an increase in mitochondrial protein synthesis and a decrease in protein degradation, and reductions in serum thyroxin are known to occur in rats treated with ethanol during pregnancy (Kornguth et al., 1979; Nathaniel et al., 1986). Ethanol-induced deficits in circulating levels of thyroxin during critical periods in development might, therefore, be expected to depress protein synthesis severely in affected cells. Ultrastructural studies, however, show that the delayed cytoplasmic maturation is also characterized by disruption of organelles involved in protein synthesis. Ethanol-induced structural modification of organelles involved in protein synthesis are likely to cause alterations in the transcription of the RNA in developing cortical neurons with production of inappropriate or abnormal proteins that may have long-lasting effects on structure and function in the central nervous system. It remains to be shown that modified levels of circulating thyroxin are directly responsible for any of the structural changes in organelles that are associated with ethanol treatment.

Despite the great advances in our understanding of the effects of ethanol on neuronal morphogenesis, a number of important questions still need to be addressed. Ethanol affects the cytoplasmic maturation of neurons in various cortical structures, but morphologically distinct subpopulations, e.g. CA1 and CA3 hippocampal pyramidal neurons or Purkinje neurons in the various lobules differ in their sensitivity to ethanol. The bases for such differences need to be studied more extensively. It is likely that embryological, biochemical, pharmacological, and ultrastructural characteristics specific to each subpopulation are responsible for these differences.

REFERENCES

Abel EL, Jacobson S, Sherwin BT (1983): In utero alcohol exposure: Functional and structural brain damage. Neurobehav Toxicol Teratol 5:363–366.

Al-Rabiai S, Miller MW (1989): Effect of prenatal exposure to ethanol on the ultrastructure of layer V of mature rat somatosensory cortex. J Neurocytol 18:711–729.

Barnes DE, Walker DW (1981): Prenatal ethanol exposure permanently reduces the number of pyramidal neurons in rat hippocampus. Dev Brain Res 1:333–340.

Bauer-Moffett C, Altman J (1977): The effect of ethanol chronically administered to preweanling rats on cerebellar development: A morphological study. Brain Res 119:249–268.

Bear MF, Daniels JD (1983): The plastic response to monocular deprivation persists in kitten visual cortex after chronic depletion of norepinephrine. J Neurosci 3:407–416.

Bear MF, Singer W (1986): Modulation of visual cortical plasticity by acetylcholine and noradrenaline. Nature 320:172–176.

Blue ME, Parnavelas JG (1982): The effect of neonatal 6-hydroxydopamine treatment on synaptogenesis in the visual cortex of the rat. J Comp Neurol 205:199–205.

Boggan WO, Randall CL, Wilson-Burrows C, Parker LS (1979): Effect of prenatal ethanol on brain serotonergic systems. Trans Am Soc Neurochem 10:186.

Borg S, Kvande H, Mossberg D, Valverius P, Sedvall G (1983): Central nervous system noradrenaline metabolism and alcohol consumption in man. Pharmacol Biochem Behav 18:375–378.

Calverley RKS, Jones DG (1987): A serial-section study of perforated synapses in rat neocortex. Cell Tissue Res 247:565–572.

Caviness VS (1975): Architectonic map of neocortex of the normal mouse. J Comp Neurol 164:247–264.

Chagnac-Amitai Y, Luhmann HJ, Prince DA (1990): Burst generating and regular spiking layer five pyramidal neurons of rat neocortex have different morphological features. J Comp Neurol 296:598–613.

Chernoff GF (1977): The fetal alcohol syndrome in mice: An animal model. Teratology 15:223–230.

Chubakov AR, Gromova EA, Konovalov GV, Sarkisova EF, Chumasov EI (1986): The effects of serotonin on the morphofunctional development of rat cerebral neocortex in tissue culture. Brain Res 369:285–297.

Cohen RS, Siekevitz P (1978): Form of the postsynaptic density: A serial section study. J Cell Biol 78:36–46.

Connors BW, Gutnick MJ, Prince DA (1982): Electrophysiological properties of neocortical neurons in vitro. J Neurophysiol 48:1302–1320.

Connors BW, Bernardo LS, Prince DA (1983): Coupling between neurons of the developing rat neocortex. J Neurosci 3:773–782.

Crick F (1982): Do dendrites twitch? Trends Neurosci 5:44–46.

D'Amato RJ, Blue ME, Largent BL, Lynch DR, Ledbetter DJ, Molliver M, Snyder SH (1987): Ontogeny of the serotonergic projection to rat neocortex: Transient expression of a dense innervation to primary sensory areas. Proc Natl Acad Sci USA 84:4322–4326.

Davies DL (1982): Morphologic changes in hippocampal CA1 pyramidal cells following perinatal ethanol administration. Doctoral Dissertation, Dept. Anatomy, Louisiana State University.

Davies DL, Smith DE (1981): A Golgi study of mouse hippocampal CA1 pyramidal neurons following perinatal ethanol exposure. Neurosci Lett 26:49–54.

Donoghue JP, Wise SP (1982): The motor cortex of the rat: Cytoarchitecture and microstimulation mapping. J Comp Neurol 212:76–88.

Dow KE, Riopelle RJ (1985): Ethanol toxicity: Effects on neurite formation and neurotrophic factor production in vitro. Science 228:591–593.

Elis J, Krsiak M, Poschlova N, Masek K (1976): The effect of alcohol administration during pregnancy on the concentration of noradrenaline, dopamine and 5-hydroxytryptamine in the brain of offspring of mice. Activitas Nerv Supp 18:220–221.

Elis J, Krsiak M, Poschlova N (1978): Effect of alcohol given at different periods of gestation on brain serotonin in offspring. Activitas Nerv Supp 20:287–288.

Fairen A, DeFelipe J, Regidor J (1984): Nonpyramidal neurons. General account. In Peters A, Jones EG (eds): "Cerebral Cortex. Vol. 1. Cellular Components of Cerebral Cortex." New York: Plenum Press, pp 201–253.

Feldman ML (1984): Morphology of the neocortical pyramidal neuron. In Peters A, Jones EG (eds): "Cerebral Cortex. Vol. 1. Cellular Components of Cerebral Cortex." New York: Plenum Press. pp. 128–189.

Feldman ML, Peters A (1978): The forms of non-pyramidal neurons in the visual cortex of the rat. J Comp Neurol 179:761–794.

Felten DL, Hallman H, Jonsson G (1982): Evidence for a neurotrophic role of noradrenaline neurons in the postnatal development of rat cerebral cortex. J Neurocytol 11:119–135.

Fritz G (1984): Effect of alcohol consumption during pregnancy and lactation on the development of the brain and behaviour in BALB/c CRBL mice. Master's thesis. University of Waterloo, Waterloo, Ontario.

Gioanni Y, Lamarche M (1985): A reappraisal of rat motor cortex organization by intracortical microstimulation. Brain Res 344:49–61.

Gray EG (1959): Axo-somatic and axodendritic synapses of the cerebral cortex: An electron microscopic study. J Anat 93:420–433.

Hall RD, Lindholm EP (1974): Organization of motor and somatosensory neocortex in the albino rat. Brain Res 66:23–38.

Hammer RP, Scheibel AB (1981): Morphologic evidence for a delay of neuronal maturation in fetal alcohol exposure. Exp Neurol 56:298–311.

Haydon PG, McCobb DP, Kater SB (1984): Serotonin selectively inhibits growth cone motility and synaptogenesis of specific identified neurons. Science 226:561–564.

Haydon PG, McCobb DP, Kater SB (1987): The regulation of neurite outgrowth, growth cone motility, and electrical synaptogenesis by serotonin. J Neurobiol 18:197–215.

Hicks SP, D'Amato CH (1977): Locating corticospinal neurons by retrograde axonal transport of horseradish peroxidase. Exp Neurol 56:410–420.

Hoff SF (1985): Synaptogenesis in the dentate gyrus in rats is not permanently altered by prenatal ethanol exposure. Alcohol Clin Exp Res 9:192.

Hoff SF (1988): Synaptogenesis in the hippocampal dentate gyrus: Effects of in utero ethanol exposure. Brain Res Bull 21:47–54.

Houser CR, Vaughn JE, Hendry SHC, Jones EG, Peters A (1984): GABA neurons in the cerebral cortex. In Jones EG, Peters A (eds): "Cerebral Cortex. Vol. 2. Functional Properties of Cortical Cells." New York: Plenum Press. pp 63–87.

Jacobson S, Rich J, Tovsky NJ (1979): Delayed myelination and lamination in the cerebral cortex of the albino rat as a result of the fetal alcohol syndrome. In Galanter M (ed): "Currents in Alcoholism. Vol. 5. Biomedical Issues and Clinical Effects of Alcoholism." New York: Grune and Stratton, pp 123–133.

Jones DG, Colangelo W (1985a): Ultrastructural investigation into the influence of ethanol on synaptic maturation in rat neocortex. I. Qualitative assessment. Dev Neurosci 7:94–106.

Jones DG, Colangelo W (1985b): Ultrastructural investigation into the influence of ethanol on synaptic maturation in rat neocortex. II. Quantitative assessment. Dev Neurosci 7:107–119.

Kasamatsu T, Pettigrew JD, Ary M (1979): Restoration of visual cortical plasticity by local microperfusion of norepinephrine. J Comp Neurol 185:163–182.

Kasamatsu T, Pettigrew JD, Ary M (1981): Cortical recovery from effects of monocular deprivation: Acceleration with norepinephrine and suppression with 6-hydroxydopamine. J Neurophysiol 45:254–266.

Killackey HP, Koralek K-A, Chiaia NL, Rhoades RW (1989): Laminar and areal differences in the origin of the subcortical projection neurons of the rat somatosensory cortex. J Comp Neurol 282:428–445.

Kornguth SE, Rutledge JJ, Sunderland E, Siegel F, Carlson I, Smollens J, Juhl Y, Young B (1979): Impeded cerebellar development and reduced serum thyroxine levels associated with fetal alcohol intoxication. Brain Res 177:347–360.

Kotkoskie LA, Miller MW (1989): Distribution of callosal projection neurons in somatosensory cortex of rats prenatally exposed to ethanol. Abs Soc Neurosci 15:1024.

Krieg WJS (1946): Connections of the cerebral cortex. I. The albino rat. A. Topography of the cortical areas. J Comp Neurol 84:221–275.

Krsiak M, Elis J, Poschlova N, Masek K (1977): Increased aggressiveness and lower brain serotonin levels in offspring of mice given alcohol during gestation. J Stud Alcohol 38:1696–1704.

Lancaster FE, Mayur BK, Patsalos PN, Samorajski T, Wiggins RC (1982): The synthesis of myelin and brain subcellular membrane proteins in the offspring of rats fed ethanol during pregnancy. Brain Res 309:209–216.

Landry P, Wilson CJ, Kitai ST (1984): Morphological and electrophysiological characteristics of pyramidal tract neurons in the rat. Exp Brain Res 57:177–190.

Lauder JM, Krebs H (1978): Serotonin as a differentiation signal in early neurogenesis. Dev Neurosci 1:15–30.

Ledig M, Ciesiels L, Simler S, Lorentz JG, Mandel P (1988); Effect of prenatal and postnatal alcohol consumption on GABA levels of various brain regions in the rat offspring. Alcohol Alcohol 23:63–67.

Leong SK (1983): Localizing the corticospinal neurons in neonatal, developing and mature albino rat. Brain Res 265:1–9.

LeVay S (1973): Synaptic patterns in the visual cortex of the cat and monkey: Electron microscopy of Golgi preparations. J Comp Neurol 150:53–86.

Levitt P, Moore RY (1978): Noradrenaline neuron innervation of the neocortex in the rat. Brain Res 139:219–231.

Lindvall O, Bjorklund A (1984): Cerebral cortex: Architecture, intracortical connections, motor projections. In Descarries L, Reader TR, Jasper HH (eds): "Physiology of the Nervous System." London: Oxford University Press, pp 288–330.

Lorente de No R (1934): Studies on the structure of cerebral cortex. II. Continuation of the study of the ammonic system. J Psychologie Neurologie 46:113–117.

Marin-Padilla M (1972): Structural abnormalities of the cerebral cortex in human chromosomal aberrations: A Golgi Study. Brain Res 44:625–629.

Marin-Padilla M (1974): Structural organization of the cerebral cortex (motor area) in human chromosomal aberrations. A Golgi Study. I. D1 (13-15) trisomy, Patau Syndrome. Brain Res 66:375–391.

McCobb DP, Haydon PG, Kater SB (1988): Dopamine and serotonin inhibition of neurite elongation of different identified neurons. J Neurosci Res 19:19–26.

McCormick DA, Connors BW, Lighthall JW, Prince DA (1985): Comparative electrophysiology of pyramidal and sparsely spinous stellate neurons of the neocortex. J Neurophysiol 54:782–806.

Mesulam M-M, Mufson EJ, Levy AI, Wainer BH (1983): Central cholinergic pathways in the rat- an overview based on an alternative nomenclature (Ch1-Ch6). Neuroscience 10:1185–1201.

Miller M (1981): Maturation of rat visual cortex. I. A quantitative study of Golgi-impregnated pyramidal neurons. J Neurocytol 10:859–878.

Miller M, Peters A (1981): Maturation of rat visual cortex. II. A combined Golgi-electron microscope study of pyramidal neurons. J Comp Neurol 203:555–573.

Miller MW (1986a): Effects of alcohol on the generation and migration of cerebral cortical neurons. Science 233:1308–1311.

Miller MW (1986b): The migration and neurochemical differentiation of γ-aminobutyric acid (GABA)-immunoreactive neurons in rat visual cortex as demonstrated by a combined immunocytochemical-autoradiographic technique. Dev Brain Res 28:41–46.

Miller MW (1987a): Effect of prenatal exposure to alcohol on the distribution and the time of origin of corticospinal neurons in the rat. J Comp Neurol 257:372–382.

Miller MW (1987b): The origin of corticospinal projection neurons in rat. Exp Brain Res 67:339–351.

Miller MW (1988): Development of projection and local circuit neurons in neocortex. In Peters A, Jones EG (eds): "Cerebral Cortex. Vol. 7. Development and Maturation of Cerebral Cortex." New York: Plenum Press, pp 133–175.

Miller MW, Chiaia NL, Rhoades RW (1990): An intracellular recording and injection study of corticospinal neurons in rat somatsensory cortex: effect of prenatal exposure to ethanol. J Comp Neurol 297:91–105.

Miller MW, Dow-Edwards DL (1988): Structural and metabolic alterations in rat cerebral cortex induced by prenatal exposure to ethanol. Brain Res 474:316–326.

Miller MW, Muller SJ (1989): Structure and histogenesis of the principal sensory nucleus of the trigeminal nerve: Effects of prenatal exposure to ethanol. J Comp Neurol 282:570–580.

Miller MW, Potempa G (1990): Numbers of neurons and glia in mature rat somatosensory cortex: effects of prenatal exposure to ethanol. J Comp Neurol 293:92–102.

Miller MW, Vogt BA (1984): Direct connections of rat visual cortex with sensory, motor, and association cortices. J Comp Neurol 226:184–202.

Mohamed SA, Nathaniel EJ, Nathaniel DR, Snell L (1987a): Altered Purkinje cell maturation in rats exposed prenatally to ethanol. I. Cytology. Exp Neurol 97:35–52.

Mohamed SA, Nathaniel EJH, Nathaniel DR, Snell L (1987b): Altered Purkinje cell maturation in rats exposed prenatally to ethanol. II. Synaptology. Exp Neurol 97:53–69.

Moore RY, Halaris AE, Jones BE (1978): Serotonin neurons of the midbrain raphe: Ascending projections. J Comp Nerol 180:417–438.

Nathaniel EJH, Nathaniel DR, Mohamed S, Nathaniel L, Kowalzik C, Nahnybida L (1986): Prenatal ethanol exposure and cerebellar development in rats. Exp Neurol 93:601–609.

National Institute of Alcohol Abuse and Alcoholism (1980): Alcohol and protein synthesis: Ethanol, nucleic acid, and protein synthesis in the brain and other organs. Res Monogra No. 10.

Neafsay EJ, Siefert C (1982): A second forelimb area exists in the rat frontal cortex. Brain Res 232:151–156.

Noble EP, Tewari S (1975): Ethanol and brain ribosomes. Fed Proc 34:1942–1947.

Noronha AB, Druse MJ (1982): Maternal ethanol consumption and synaptic membrane glycoproteins in offspring. J Neurosci Res 8:83–97.

Norton S, Terranova P, Na JY, Sancho-Tello M (1988): Early motor development and cerebral cortical morphology in rats exposed perinatally to alcohol. Alcohol Clin Exp Res 12:130–136.

O'Leary DDM, Stanfield BB (1985): Occipital cortical neurons with transient pyramidal tract axons extend and maintain collaterals to subcortical but not to intracortical targets. Brain Res 336:326–333.

O'Leary DDM, Stanfield BB (1986): A transient pyramidal tract projection from the visual cortex in the hamster and its removal by selective collateral elimination. Dev Brain Res 27:87–89.

Palay SL, Chan-Palay V (1974): "Cerebellar Cortex." New York: Springer-Verlag.

Parnavelas JG, Bradford R, Mounty EJ, Lieberman AR (1978): The development of non-pyramidal neurons in the visual cortex of the rat. Anat Embryol 155:1–14.

Pentney RJ, Cotter JR, Abel E (1984): Quantitative measures of mature neuronal morphology after in utero ethanol exposure. Neurobehav Toxicol Teratol 6:59–65.

Peters A, Fairen A (1978): Smooth and sparsely spined stellate neurons in the visual cortex of the rat: A study using a combined Golgi-electron microscope technique. J Comp Neurol 181:129–172.

Peters A, Kaiserman-Abramof IR (1969): The small pyramidal neuron of the rat cerebral cortex: The synapses upon dendritic spines. Z Zellforsch Mikrosk Anat 100:487–506.

Peters A, Kaiserman-Abramof IR (1970): The small pyramidal neuron of the rat cerebral cortex: The perikaryon, dendrites, and spines. Am J Anat 127:321–356.

Peters A, Kara DA, Harriman KM (1985): The neuronal composition of area 17 of rat visual cortex. III. Numerical considerations. J Comp Neurol 238:263–274.

Peters A, Sanford SL, Webster H deF (1976): "The Fine Structure of the Nervous System. The Neurons and Supporting Cells." Philadelphia; Saunders.

Phillips SC, Cragg BG (1982): Change in susceptibility of rat cerebellar Purkinje cells to damage by alcohol during fetal, neonatal, and adult life. Neuropathol Appl Neurobiol 8:441–454.

Pierce DR, West JR (1987): Differential deficits in regional brain growth induced by postnatal alcohol. Neurotoxicol Teratol 9:129–141.

Purpura DP (1974): Dendritic spine "dysgenesis" and mental retardation. Science 18:1126–1128.

Randall CL, Taylor WJ, Walker DW (1977): Ethanol-induced malformations in mice. Alcohol Clin Exp Res 1:219–224.

Rathbun W, Druse MJ (1985): Dopamine, serotonin, and acid metabolites in brain regions from the developing offspring of ethanol-treated rats. J Neurochem 44:-57–62.

Rawat AK (1975): Ribosomal protein synthesis in the fetal and neonatal rat brain as influenced by maternal ethanol consumption. Res Common Chem Pathol Pharmacol 12:723–732.

Rawat AK (1977): Developmental changes in the brain levels of neurotransmitters as influenced by maternal ethanol consumption in the rat. J Neurochem 28:-1175–1182.

Rawat AK (1985): Nucleic acid and protein synthesis inhibition in developing brain by ethanol in the absence of hypothermia. Neurobehav Toxicol Teratol 7:161–166.

Reyes E, Rivera JM, Saland LC, Murray HM (1983): Effects of maternal administration of alcohol on fetal brain development. Neurobehav Toxicol Teratol 5:263–267.

Ribak CE (1978): Aspinous and sparsely-spinous stellate neurons in the visual cortex of rats contain glutamic acid decarboxylase. J Neurocytol 7:461–478.

Riley EP, Barron S, Hannigan JH (1986): Response inhibition deficits following prenatal alcohol exposure. A comparison to the effects of hippocampal lesions in rats. In West JR (ed): "Alcohol and Brain Development." New York: Oxford University Press, pp 71–102.

Samson HH, Diaz J (1981): Altered development of brain by neonatal ethanol exposure: Zinc levels during and after exposure. Alcohol Clin Exp Res 5:563–569.

Saper CB (1984): Organization of cerebral cortical afferent systems in the rat: I. Magnocellular basal nucleus. J Comp Neurol 222:313–342.

Shapiro MB, Rosman NP, Kemper TL (1984): Effects of chronic exposure to alcohol on the developing brain. Neurobehav Toxicol Teratol 6:351–356.

Shaw C, Needler MC, Cynader M (1984): Ontogenesis of muscarinic acetylcholine binding sites in cat visual cortex: Reversal of specific laminar distribution during the critical period. Dev Brain Res 14:295–299.

Sillito AM (1984): Functional considerations of the operations of GABAergic inhibitory processes in the visual cortex. In Jones EG, Peters A (eds): "Cerebral Cortex. Vol. 2. Functional Properties of Cortical Cells." New York: Plenum Press. pp 91–117.

Smith DE, Davies DL (1990): Effect of perinatal administration of ethanol on the C1 pyramidal cell of the hippocampus and the Purkinje cell of the cerebellum: An ultrastructural survey. J Neurocytol 19:708–717.

Smith DE, Foundas A, Canale J (1986): Effect of perinatally administered ethanol on the development of the cerebellar granule cell. Exp Neurol 92:491–501.

Spohr HL, Stoltenburg-Didinger G (1983): Zum problem der abortiven alkoholembryopathie. Monatsschr Kinderheilkd 131:96–99.

Spohr HL, Stoltenburg-Didinger G (1985): Morphological aspects of experimental alcohol fetopathy: Purkinje cell development and synaptic maturation in Wistar rats exposed to alcohol pre- and postnatally. In Rydberg U, Alling C, Engel J (eds): "Alcohol and the Developing Brain." New York: Raven Press, pp 109–124.

Stanfield BB, O'Leary DDM, Fricke C (1982): Selective collateral elimination in early postnatal development restricts cortical distribution of rat pyramidal tract neurons. Nature 298:371–373.

Stoltenburg-Didinger G, Spohr HL (1983): Fetal alcohol syndrome and mental retardation: Spine distribution of pyramidal cells in prenatal alcohol-exposed rat cerebral cortex. A Golgi study. Dev Brain Res 1:119–123.

Sytinsky IA, Guzikov BM, Gomarko MV, Eremin VP, Komovalo NN (1975): Gamma-aminobutyric acid (GABA) system in brain during acute and chronic ethanol intoxication. J Neurochem 25:43–48.

Trombley P, Allen EE, Soyke J, Blaha CD, Lane RF, Gordon B (1986): Doses of 6-hydroxydopamine sufficient to deplete norepinephrine are not sufficient to decrease plasticity in the visual cortex. J Neurosci 6:266–273.

Vingan RD, Dow-Edwards DL, Riley EP (1986): Cerebral metabolic alterations in rats following prenatal alcohol exposure: A deoxyglucose study. Alcohol Clin Exp Res 10:22–26.

Volk B (1984): Cerebellar histogenesis and synaptic maturation following pre- and postnatal alcohol administration. Acta Neuropathol (Berl) 63:57–65.

Volk B, Maletz J, Tiedemann M, Mall G, Klein C, Berlet HH (1981): Impaired maturation of Purkinje cells in the fetal alcohol syndrome of the rat. Acta Neuropathol (Berl) 54:19–29.

Wainwright P, Gagnon M (1985): Moderate prenatal ethanol exposure interacts with strain in affecting brain development in BALB/c and C57BL/6 mice. Exp Neurol 88:84–94.

Wainwright P, Ward GR, Blom K (1985): Combined effects of moderate ethanol consumption and a low protein diet during gestation on brain development in BALB/c mice. Exp Neurol 90:422–433.

West JR, Hamre KM (1985) Effects of alcohol exposure during different periods of development: Changes in hippocampal mossy fibers. Dev Brain Res 17:280–284.

West JR, Hamre KM, Cassell MD (1986): Effects of ethanol exposure during the third trimester equivalent on neuron number in rat hippocampus and dentate gyrus. Alcohol Clin Exp Res 10:190–197.

West JR, Hodges CA, Black AC (1981): Prenatal exposure to ethanol alters the organization of hippocampal mossy fibers in rat. Science 211:957–959.

West JR, Kelly SJ, Pierce DR (1987): Severity of alcohol-induced deficits in rats during the third trimester equivalent is determined by the pattern of exposure. Alcohol Alcohol, Suppl 1:461–465.

Westrum LE, Jones DH, Gray EG, Barron J (1980): Microtubules, dendritic spines, and spine apparatuses. Cell Tissue Res 208:171–181.

White EL (1989): "Cortical Circuits: Synaptic Organization and Cerebral Cortex. Structure, Function and Theory." Cambridge MA: Birkhauser Boston.

Winfield DA, Brooke RNL, Sloper JJ, Powell TPS (1981): A combined Golgi-electron microscope study of synapses made by the proximal axon and the recurrent collaterals made of a pyramidal cell in the somatic sensory cortex of the monkey. Neuroscience 6:1217–1230.

Wise SP, Murray EA, Coulter JD (1979): Somatotopic organization of corticospinal and corticotrigeminal neurons in the rat. Neuroscience 4:65–78.

Yanai J, Waknin S (1985): Comparison of the effects of barbiturate and ethanol given to neonates on the cerebellar morphology. Acta Anat 123:145–147.

Zilles K, Zilles B, Schliecher A (1980): A quantitative approach to cytoarchitectonics. VI. The areal pattern of the cortex of the albino rat. Anat Embryol 159:335–360.

Zimmerberg B, Reuter JM (1989): Sexually dimorphic behavioral and brain asymmetries in neonatal rats- effects of prenatal alcohol exposure. Dev Brain Res 46:281–290.

Zimmerberg B, Scalzi LV (1989): Commissural size in neonatal rats: Effects of sex and prenatal alcohol exposure. Int J Dev Neurosci 7:81–86.

Development of the Central Nervous System:
Effects of Alcohol and Opiates, pages 109–138
© 1992 Wiley-Liss, Inc.

6

Effects of Ethanol During Development on Neuronal Survival and Plasticity

GLENN R. WARD AND JAMES R. WEST

Alcohol and Brain Research Laboratory, Department of Anatomy, University of Iowa College of Medicine, Iowa City, Iowa

INTRODUCTION

Although exposure to ethanol in utero can produce anatomical and physiological abnormalities in a variety of organ systems, its devastating functional consequences in the central nervous system (CNS) have led researchers to focus their attention primarily on the CNS effects (see Chapter 2). In humans, varying degrees of behavioral and intellectual impairment are fixtures of fetal alcohol syndrome (FAS) (Clarren and Smith, 1970; Streissguth et al., 1978; Shaywitz et al., 1980; Steinhausen et al., 1984; Streissguth, 1986), often occurring in the absence of other obvious abnormalities (Streissguth, 1986), and prenatal ethanol exposure may now be the leading known cause of mental retardation in North America (Abel and Sokol, 1987). Given the grave personal and social tragedy associated with prenatal ethanol-induced retardation (e.g., Dorris, 1989), coupled with the economic burden to society of a problem of this magnitude (Abel and Sokol, 1987), interest in the CNS effects is not only understandable but necessary if this problem is to be alleviated.

Of course, direct observation and study of the developing human brain is somewhat problematic. Effects of prenatal ethanol exposure on the CNS have usually been inferred from performance on general behavioral and intelligence tests, whereas the limited direct evidence of neuroanatomical deficits has been obtained from a few autopsies of FAS infants and children. For the most part, these represent the most severely affected cases, so this work tells us little of the underlying structural changes which are associated with the more commonly reported functional impairments. Therefore, it is not surprising that researchers have come to rely upon animal models of FAS, particularly those involving rodents, to elucidate the mechanisms by which prenatal ethanol exposure can affect the structure of the developing brain.

The relevance of animal models depends partly upon an understanding of the differences in the temporal pattern of CNS development across species. Although humans and other mammals exhibit a period of rapid brain growth—the so-called brain growth spurt—during which the brain is especially vulnerable to adverse developmental influences (Dobbing, 1981; West, 1987), this period differs in relation to the timing of birth among species (Dobbing and Sands, 1979; Dobbing, 1981). In humans, the brain growth spurt encompasses the third trimester of pregnancy as well as early postnatal life, while in rats and mice the same period occurs exclusively during the early postnatal period. Thus, if the laboratory rat is to be a useful tool for understanding the effects of ethanol during this period of rapid brain growth in humans, the alcohol treatment must be implemented during neonatal and early postnatal development. Therefore, although the following discussion will include studies of either prenatal or postnatal exposure, the underlying assumption will be that *all* are models of prenatal exposure in humans.

By far the most consistent finding in animal studies of early ethanol exposure is a reduction in brain weight. However, while brain weight reductions following gestational exposure have been reported in end-of-term fetuses (Weinberg, 1985; Cassells et al., 1987) and at weaning (Wainwright et al., 1985), these deficits have usually been accompanied by reductions in body weight. On the other hand, early postnatal exposure (i.e., during the brain growth spurt) causes profound reductions in brain weight which can occur in the absence of any effect on body weight (Bauer-Moffett and Altman, 1975, 1977; Samson, 1986; Kelly et al., 1987), and which can persist into adulthood, even after only one day of exposure in rats (Burns et al., 1986). While normal variability in brain weight among individuals or groups does not appear to be correlated with functional variability (Wahlsten, 1977), the fact that the behavioral and intellectual deficits resulting from early ethanol exposure in humans are associated with reductions in the size of the brain implies that at least part of these deficits result from impaired brain development. Nevertheless, effects on brain weight tell us little about the changes, at the microscopic level, by which early ethanol exposure may lead to functional deficits in offspring. An understanding of the mechanisms by which these functional deficits are produced requires, among other things, insight into the effects of ethanol on the development of various cell populations within the CNS.

In the CNS, the most harmful effect of ethanol is its potentially lethal effect on individual cells which, due to the characteristic plasticity of the developing nervous system, can have consequences during early development which may differ from its consequences in adulthood. In the earliest stages of development, of course, depletions in neuronal populations may be offset by the addition of newly generated cells, or responsive changes in associated afferent and efferent systems may result. Furthermore, the potential for plasticity itself may be adversely affected by ethanol exposure, resulting in responsive changes which may not mimic those following cell depletion in other situations. Therefore, the following discussion reviews research directed toward understanding the morphological effects of early ethanol exposure in the CNS at the cellular level with particular attention to effects on cell survival in various regions of the brain and to effects on neuronal plasticity.

ETHANOL EFFECTS ON CELL SURVIVAL

In FAS research, effects on cell survival have been inferred from reductions in the numbers of cells in a particular population following early ethanol exposure. Generally, these reductions in cell number can be produced in two ways: through changes in the rate of cell generation or through changes in the rate of cell death (Jacobson, 1978; Oppenheim, 1981). Furthermore, when considering specific neuron types in particular regions of the brain, cell number can be a function of a number of other factors as well. For example, a normal complement of specific neuron types may indeed by generated but may fail to differentiate fully or to migrate to the "proper" location in the brain, and the timing of the proliferative stage may be affected by ethanol such that the number of a particular type of neuron may be reduced early in development but, because of a delay in the cessation of neuronal proliferation, may no longer differ from the normal complement when the proliferative period has ended (see Chapter 4). Therefore, alterations in cell number in a specific brain region could conceivably result from one or more of at least four causes: 1) changes in the rate of cell generation; 2) changes in the duration of cell generation; 3) changes in the pattern of cell migration; and 4) changes in the rate of cell death. Although the term "cell survival" implies primarily the last of these changes, in many cases there will be no compelling reason to exclude a possible influence, or even a major role, of the other potential causes of ethanol-induced cell depletion

The Neocortex

The effects of early ethanol exposure on the neocortex are reviewed in detail elsewhere in this volume (see Chapters 4 and 5) and will be discussed very briefly here. Ethanol exposure during gestation in rats has been reported to result in both a decreased number (Miller and Potempa, 1990) and redistribution (Miller et al., 1991) of neocortical neurons, and these perturbations appear to be the result of complex interactions between temporal and spatial factors in cortical development. Specifically, prenatal ethanol exposure was reported to delay the onset of neocortical neurogenesis and extend the period of proliferation by 2 days (Miller, 1986, 1989). Furthermore, from gestation days 13–19, the period of most active proliferation, fewer neurons were generated in the fetuses exposed to ethanol, but this decrease was partially offset by a dramatic but transient increase in the number of neurons generated after day 19. This late proliferative surge may be due to differential effects of ethanol on the two major neocortical proliferative zones. Following injections of [^{3}H] thymidine, the ventricular zone, the major site of neurogenesis during the early proliferative period, was reported to be thinner and to exhibit fewer labeled cells in ethanol-exposed brains than in controls, while the subventricular zone, the prominent proliferative zone during the later stages of neurogenesis, was reported to be thicker in the ethanol-exposed group, and to exhibit more labeled cells as well as more cells exhibiting mitotic figures (Miller, 1989).

These changes in the respective rates of neurogenesis in these two proliferative zones may account for both the altered numbers of neurons and the altered distribution of the neurons in the neocortex of rats prenatally exposed to ethanol. Although all layers of neocortex exhibited significant ethanol-induced reductions in neuronal number (Miller and Potempa, 1990), there was a laminar redistribution of neurons derived from each proliferative zone, and this redistribution of neurons appeared to be caused by impaired migration of late-generated neurons. Instead of migrating outward from the subventricular zone to the outer cortical layers (layers II and III), many of these late-generated neurons remained in the deeper layers (Miller, 1986, 1988; Miller et al., 1991). Such an effect on migration could be due to at least two factors: 1) withdrawal, before migration is complete, of the pially extended radial glial processes along which the immature neurons migrate; or 2) deficits in the ability of the late-generated neurons to respond appropriately to glial factors (Miller, 1988). These findings suggest that alterations in cell number may be due to ethanol-induced changes in a number of processes including both cell proliferation and migration, and they underscore the importance of considering a multifactorial interpretation of ethanol's effects on specific brain regions.

Brainstem and Olfactory Bulb

One study has reported effects of prenatal ethanol exposure in rats on a pontine nucleus in the brainstem (Miller and Muller, 1989). Ethanol exposure throughout most of gestation reduced the number of neurons in the principal sensory nucleus (PSN) of the trigeminal nerve, and the effect was restricted mainly to the smaller rather than larger neurons. As in the neocortex, ethanol delayed the onset and prolonged the period of neurogenesis of PSN neuronal precursors by approximately 1 day. In this case, however, unlike in the neocortex, there was no late proliferative surge, which may be due to the fact that PSN neurons are derived exclusively from the ventricular zone while the late proliferative surge appears to occur mainly in the subventricular zone (Miller, 1989).

Another report has suggested that granule cells in the olfactory bulb may be vulnerable to the toxic effects of ethanol. In this study (Nyquist-Battie and Gochee, 1985), ethanol administered from gestational day 13 to postnatal day 21 led to reductions in the volume of the granule cell layer, but not of the mitral cell layer. The timing of the exposure was during the period of olfactory bulb development in which mitral cells have completed neurogenesis but granule cells are still being generated (Hinds, 1968). Although the authors suggested that the reduced size of the granule cell layer was due to an ethanol-induced reduction in the number of granule cells present rather than a change in the density of the cells, it must be noted that their study did not measure granule cell number directly. Interestingly, the density of both granule-to-mitral and mitral-to-granule synapses in the external plexiform layer was increased by the ethanol treatment, which suggests either a compensatory increase in synaptogenesis in this layer to offset a reduced number of granule cells, or a greater packing density of granule cells, without a concurrent decrease in cell number, in the ethanol group. Because neither of these explanations can be eliminated by the data provided in this report, the cause of the decreased volume of the granule cell layer remains unclear.

Hippocampus

There are three reasons why the hippocampus has been a major investigative focus in FAS research. 1) The hippocampus exhibits a relatively simple cytological organization with a layer of large, prenatally generated neurons (the pyramidal cells) and smaller, postnatally generated granule cells. 2) This structure is reported to be vulnerable to the effects of long-term ethanol abuse in adulthood (McLardy, 1975; Riley and Walker, 1978; Walker et al., 1980, 1981; Phillips, 1989). 3) The fact that the hippocampus is believed to play a major role in the regulation of behavior and the fact that hippocampal damage is associated with deficits in response inhibition (Altman et al., 1973) and learning and memory (Douglas, 1967; Solomon, 1979; Olton, 1983), suggests that similar behavioral deficits noted in FAS cases may be mediated, in part, by effects of ethanol on the development of this structure (Riley et al., 1986; Wigal and Amsel, 1990).

There have been few investigations into early ethanol-induced cell loss in the hippocampal formation. In studies of ethanol exposure during gestation, when hippocampal pyramidal cells are being generated, the number of pyramidal cells in certain hippocampal regions was reported to be reduced in ethanol-exposed offspring at 21 (Wigal and Amsel, 1990) and 60 (Barnes and Walker, 1981) days of age. In a series of studies in which we administered ethanol during the brain growth spurt (i.e., postnatal days 4–9), our laboratory investigated the effects of ethanol on the survival of cells which have already ceased their proliferation and migration. We used an artificial-rearing technique in which a feeding tube was implanted intragastrically into neonatal rats (Diaz and Samson, 1980; Samson and Diaz, 1982; West et al., 1986, 1989) so that the amount and the constituents of the diet could be controlled precisely. Furthermore, since peak blood alcohol concentration (BAC) is a function of both the *amount* of ethanol administered to the subject, and the rate at which it enters, and is eliminated from, the bloodstream (Sellers et al., 1980), this technique allowed for the control of peak BACs in the pups by adjusting either the *amount* of ethanol administered each day (Pierce and West, 1986a; Bonthius and West, 1988) or the *pattern* of administration (i.e., the number of consecutive daily feedings over which the ethanol was administered) (Pierce and West, 1986b; Bonthius et al., 1988; Bonthius and West, 1990) (Fig. 1). For example, a specific dosage of ethanol can be administered gradually over a number of days, producing low but relatively constant BACs, or it can be administered over a very brief period, as in the case of injection or intubation, producing high BACs for relatively short periods of time (Bonthius et al., 1988; West et al., 1989). Through the use of this artificial-rearing technique, we found that a feeding regimen in which the daily dosage of ethanol was administered over all 12 feedings (West et al., 1986), or was condensed into four consecutive feedings (Pierce et al., 1989), did not reduce hippocampal pyramidal cell number, while a regimen in which the daily dosage was further condensed into only two feedings did lead to significant reductions (Bonthius and West, 1990). It should be noted that a recent study from another laboratory which administered ethanol in every feeding via an artificial-rearing technique, and subsequently produced relatively low BACs, did not find significant reductions in pyramidal cell number (Wigal and Amsel, 1990).

There appear to be distinct regional differences in vulnerability to early ethanol effects in the hippocampus. In one of the prenatal studies mentioned above (Barnes and Walker, 1981), and the postnatal study which reported significant pyramidal cell loss following condensed exposure (Bonthius and West, 1990), the reductions occurred almost exclusively in pyramidal field CA1, while the number of cells in fields CA2 and CA3 remained unaltered. Furthermore, in one study in which no significant cell reduction occurred (Pierce et al., 1989), there was still a trend toward fewer CA1 cells in the ethanol-exposed group.

With regard to the effects of ethanol on the dentate gyrus granule cells, which are primarily generated postnatally, the results are less clear. In one prenatal study in which ethanol was administered throughout gestation (Wigal and Amsel, 1990), the number of mature but not immature granule cells was reduced, while another study which did not distinguish between mature and immature granule cells (Barnes and Walker, 1981), reported no difference following exposure to ethanol during only the second half of gestation (i.e., days 10–21). On the other hand, we observed a significant increase in the number of granule cells in 10-day-old rats following postnatal exposure in an early study using the method of continuous ethanol administration (West et al., 1986), but not in later experiments in which the ethanol was administered in a condensed fashion (Pierce et al., 1989; Bonthius and West, 1990).

Cerebellum

The cerebellum may be particularly vulnerable to ethanol-induced growth deficiency (Bauer-Moffett and Altman, 1975, 1977; Phillips and Cragg, 1982; Borges and Lewis, 1983; Cragg and Phillips, 1985; Pierce et al., 1989; Bonthius and West, 1990). Furthermore, as in the case of the hippocampus, cerebellar cells are reported to be adversely affected by chronic ethanol consumption in adults (Pentney, 1982; Tavares and Paula-Barbosa, 1982; Pentney and Quigley, 1987). Therefore, it is not surprising that a major focus of studies of ethanol-induced cell loss has been on deficits in cerebellar Purkinje cell number. Purkinje cells, the major output neurons of the cerebellar cortex, appear to be particularly vulnerable to ethanol exposure during development. The number of Purkinje cells is

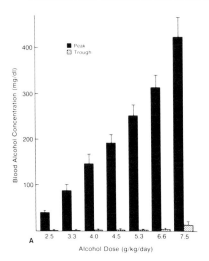

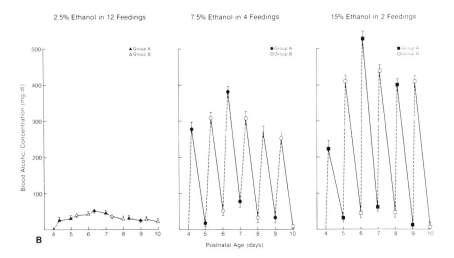

Fig. 1. Effect of manipulation of ethanol dosage and pattern of administration on BACs in artificially-reared Sprague-Dawley rat pups. **A:** The effect of various dosages of ethanol administered in four consecutive feedings each day (followed by eight feedings of normal milk formula), beginning on postnatal day 4. Peak BACs (mean and SEM) were obtained 1 hour after the end of the last alcohol feeding on day 6, and trough values were obtained 30 minutes prior to the start of the first alcohol feeding on day 7. (Reproduced from Bonthius and West, 1988, with permission.) **B:** The effect of 6.6 g/kg/day ethanol administered in the form of either a 2.5% (v/v) fraction in every feeding (left panel), a 7.5% fraction in four consecutive feedings (middle panel), or a 15% fraction in two feedings (right panel). Groups A and B refer to the fact that each animal had blood removed on alternate days. (Reproduced from Bonthius et al., 1988, with permission.)

known to be reduced following prenatal (Phillips and Cragg, 1982) or post-natal (Bauer-Moffett and Altman, 1975, 1977) exposure, with greater re-ductions reported following postnatal (Phillips and Cragg, 1982) or combined pre- and postnatal exposure (Cragg and Phillips, 1985). Further-more, peak BAC appears to be an important variable. Prenatal studies which have reported maternal BACs of less than 160 mg/dl (Volk et al., 1981; Borges and Lewis, 1983) have not found reduced numbers of Purkinje cells, while one study which did find significant reductions reported peak maternal BACs of up to 390 mg/dl (Phillips and Cragg, 1982). The effects of postnatal exposure also appear to be dependent on peak BAC. Studies which have reported Purkinje cell loss following postnatal ethanol expo-sure are also those which have reported peak BACs of at least 190 mg/dl (Bauer-Moffett and Altman, 1975, 1977; Phillips and Cragg, 1982; Volk, 1984a; Cragg and Phillips, 1985; Bonthius and West, 1990), and one study which failed to find any reductions administered the postnatal ethanol treatment via the maternal drinking water (Borges and Lewis, 1983). Al-though they did not report BACs in this study, a previous report from the same laboratory noted that this method produced BACs of only 44 mg/dl in the pups (Borges and Lewis, 1982).

If peak maternal and neonatal BAC is, indeed, an important variable in ethanol-induced Purkinje cell loss, then the duration of exposure may also be important. In this regard, it is interesting to note that at least one study (Yanai and Waknin, 1985) reported significant reductions in Purkinje cell number following administration, in neonatal rats, of only 2.0 g/kg/day ethanol, which is considerably less than the amount given in many studies which find no adverse effects (i.e., see Bond, 1981). However, the dosage in this study was given in a single injection, which is known to produce higher peak BACs than other forms of administration (Wallgren and Barry, 1970), suggesting that the peak BAC may have been more critical than the dura-tion of ethanol exposure. Unfortunately, since the authors did not report the BACs of their subjects, such an explanation for this discrepancy in findings must remain speculative.

A related issue is the minimum period of time in which the ethanol treatment must be carried out before significant Purkinje cell loss occurs. While prenatal exposure to sufficiently high maternal BACs can lead to cell depletion, additional postnatal exposure may augment this loss (Cragg and Phillips, 1985), suggesting that the extent of cell loss may be dependent upon the duration of exposure. With regard to postnatal exposure, how-ever, the first postnatal week may be a critical period of vulnerability. In neonatal rats, ethanol exposure on postnatal days 3 and 4 leads to a reduc-tion in Purkinje cell number on day 5 (Bauer-Moffett and Altman, 1975, 1977), and further exposure (up to and including day 21) does not appear to lead to further reductions beyond those produced on these 2 days, nor does 2 weeks of prenatal exposure (Cragg and Phillips, 1985). Another study reported cerebellar cell loss in adult rats following ethanol exposure on a single day (day 6), but did not identify loss according to the types of cells (Burns et al., 1986). In any event, it appears that even very brief exposure to high concentrations of ethanol can lead to permanent reductions in cell number in certain areas of the cerebellum.

Within the cerebellum, there appear to be clear regional differences in the degree of Purkinje cell reduction due to ethanol exposure, and these differences are reported to be associated with the maturational state of the region. Although, morphologically, the cerebellum is a relatively homogeneous structure, certain cerebellar lobules in the rat can be distinguished during development by differences in their respective rates of maturation (Altman, 1982). A number of reports (Bauer-Moffett and Altman, 1975, 1977; Phillips and Cragg, 1982) have noted that the early-maturing lobules (i.e., lobules I, IX, and X) generally exhibit greater reductions than do the relatively late-maturing lobules (i.e., lobules V, VI, and VII), suggesting that there is a stage of development during which Purkinje cells are particularly vulnerable to the toxic effects of ethanol. In this regard, it is unfortunate that some reports published since that time have not calculated Purkinje cell loss according to lobule (Cragg and Phillips, 1985; Phillips, 1985; Yanai and Waknin, 1985) or have chosen to analyze only a limited number of specific lobules (Volk, 1984a,b; Pierce et al., 1989).

Although the finding that prenatal exposure can also reduce Purkinje cell number (Phillips and Cragg, 1982; Cragg and Phillips, 1985) indicates that ethanol-induced effects on Purkinje cell neurogenesis may occur, it should be pointed out that, since Purkinje cells are generated exclusively prenatally, the effects of early postnatal ethanol exposure cannot be attributed to effects on cell generation. Rather, in this particular case, ethanol appears to kill cells which have already formed. On the other hand, certain cerebellar cell types are generated postnatally and one of these, the granule cells, also has been the subject of a number of studies of early ethanol exposure. Once again, ethanol-induced cell depletion was found to be a function of the lobule in which the cells reside, with the early-maturing lobules exhibiting greater reductions than did the late-maturing lobules (Bauer-Moffett and Altman, 1975, 1977). Although, in these studies, the pattern of loss of granule cells paralleled that of the Purkinje cells, in at least two reports the loss of the two types of cells appeared to be independent of each other. In one study of exposure to low levels of ethanol during gestation and lactation (Borges and Lewis, 1983), significant granule cell loss was seen in the absence of any Purkinje cell loss while, in another study of postnatal exposure in mice to either of two doses of ethanol, the higher dose (3.0 g/kg daily in a single injection) caused deficits in both types of cells while the lower dose (2.0 g/kg) affected Purkinje cells but not granule cells (Yanai and Waknin, 1985).

Overall, the results of these studies suggest that the effect of ethanol on neuronal loss in the cerebellum is a function of a number of factors including peak BAC, the timing of the exposure, and the region of the cerebellum being investigated. One drawback to the studies outlined above is the fact that no laboratory has attempted to address these various factors using a single paradigm. Although the results of the studies just described appear to exhibit certain patterns, conclusions must be limited by the fact that few of the studies shared a common methodology. Therefore, we decided to assess the effects of various patterns of administration of ethanol to rat pups of various postnatal ages on the Purkinje cells of each cerebellar lobule. Furthermore, given that early undernutrition itself can have neuroteratogenic effects, we incorporated a nutritional control group into our design, something which was not done in the previous studies described in this section.

Generally, our results have confirmed the implications of the earlier work (Pierce et al., 1989; Bonthius and West, 1990). For example, Purkinje cell loss has been found to result from ethanol exposure when it is administered in either a quantity or a pattern which leads to high BACs. Specifically, a dose of 6.6 g/kg/day administered throughout a 24-hour period on days 4 through 9, and resulting in low but steady BACs (less than 50 mg/dl), does not lead to Purkinje cell loss (Bonthius and West, 1990), while the same amount, provided in only four of the 12 daily feedings, results in high peak BACs (480 mg/dl) and significant Purkinje cell loss (Pierce et al., 1989). Furthermore, a lower dose of ethanol (4.5 g/kg/day) compressed into only four or two feedings produced a significant degree of Purkinje cell loss (Bonthius and West, 1990), supporting the theory that lower doses of alcohol consumed over a relatively brief period of time can be more teratogenic than higher doses consumed more slowly.

As the earlier work (Burns et al., 1986; Cragg and Phillips, 1985) has suggested, ethanol exposure of even very short duration can result in significant cerebellar cell loss if the pattern of consumption is such that it results in high BACs. We found reductions in Purkinje cell number in 10-day-old rats following intubation of 6.6 g/kg ethanol in two consecutive feedings on postnatal day 4 only (Goodlett et al., 1990b). Again, this effect was dose dependent: 3.3 g/kg ethanol administered in the same fashion did not reduce overall cell number.

When the pattern of Purkinje cell loss seen in these studies was examined more closely, the variability between individual cerebellar lobules was quite dramatic. As first reported by Bauer-Moffett and Altman (1975, 1977), the greatest degree of cell loss occurred in the early-maturing lobules (Pierce et al., 1989; Bonthius and West, 1990), and this effect was found following both condensed and continuous exposure. For example, when the ethanol administration was condensed in a way that produced very high BACs, significant cell loss was seen in all lobules although the greatest loss was found in the most mature ones. However, if the same daily dosage was administered over a greater number of feedings, thereby resulting in lower BACs, cell loss no longer occurred in the late-maturing lobules VII and VIII (Bonthius and West, 1990).

We then set out to clarify further the association between maturational status and regional vulnerability to ethanol's effects. Although regional differences in the maturity of cerebellar tissue have been recognized for the past two decades, they have generally been described in terms of the development of the granule cell layer (Altman, 1969, 1982). Except for a brief mention in one study (Altman, 1972), little has been published on differences in Purkinje cell morphology between different cerebellar regions. Since the data presented above suggest that Purkinje cell vulnerability may be related to differences in maturational status, further elucidation of those differences would be of great benefit to researchers in the field. We have found that Purkinje cells residing in late-maturing regions of the cerebellum differ from those residing in the early-maturing region on post-natal day 10 in a number of respects. The latter exhibit features character-istic of more mature cells: their somata are larger and more regular in their shape, they possess distinct, round nuclei, and they lack the apical cones and perisomatic processes which are characteristic of less mature cells (Bonthius and West, 1990). Furthermore, they differ greatly in the extent of dendritic development. Purkinje cells in lobules I, II, IX, and X exhibit relatively extensive patterns of dendritic growth compared with those in lobules VI and VII (Goodlett et al., 1990a). Also consistent with previous reports (Altman, 1972) was the observation that differences also exist between various regions *within* many of the lobules. For instance, the cells within the proximal portion of lobules VII and VIII are clearly more mature than those in the more distal portions, while the cells lining the proximal portion of the primary fissure in lobules V and VI are more mature than those in the more distal aspects of those lobules (Fig. 2). These findings suggest that, when discussing differential rates of maturation in the cerebellum, lobular distinctions are still imprecise. Rather, it is more appropriate to envision late- and early-maturing *regions* which, them-selves, may encompass no more than a portion of specific lobules.

Our studies have also confirmed earlier findings regarding ethanol's effects on cerebellar granule cells. In the granular layer, which is formed rapidly during the early postnatal period the number of granule cells is

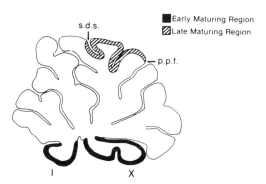

Fig. 2. Schematic diagram of midsagittal section of the cerebellum of a 10-day-old rat. Hatched bar indicates late-maturing regions, and solid bar indicates early-maturing region. s.d.s., second declival sulcus; p.p.f., prepyramidal fissure; I and X, lobules I and X, respectively. (Reproduced from Bonthius and West, 1990, with permission.)

reduced by early postnatal ethanol exposure, and the correlation between granule and Purkinje cell loss in each lobule is highly significant (Pierce et al., 1989; Bonthius and West, 1990). It is interesting to note that the number of granule cells in the external granular layer (EGL), which consists of proliferating granule cells which then migrate inward to the granular layer, is reduced to a much lesser extent by this treatment than is the number in the granular layer.

Conclusions

The findings discussed in the preceding sections suggest that the effects of early ethanol exposure on neuronal survival are complex, affecting not only the process of neurogenesis, but also the processes of migration and cell death. Unfortunately, it is difficult to draw general conclusions from these data since much of the research has been carried out on only a handful of cell populations. Most of our information regarding effects on neurogenesis and migration comes from studies of the neocortex, while information about cell depletion in tissues in which neurogenesis is, for the most part, complete, has come from studies of the hippocampus and cerebellum. Therefore, in many cases, it is impossible to determine whether the effects described here are general effects, or whether they are specific to the region under observation.

Effects on neurogenesis and neuronal migration have been most thoroughly studied directly in the neocortex. Although other studies have reported cerebellar Purkinje cell loss (Phillips and Cragg, 1982; Cragg and Phillips, 1985) and hippocampal pyramidal cell loss (Barnes and Walker, 1981; Wigal and Amsel, 1990) following ethanol exposure during the period of neurogenesis of these populations, it is impossible to tell whether this depletion was due to impaired neurogenesis or whether the cells had indeed been generated but had failed to migrate to their final positions in the molecular layers of the cerebellum and hippocampus, respectively, or died after migration had occurred. Only when the ethanol was administered postnatally (Pierce et al., 1989; Bonthius and West, 1990), after neurogenesis and migration had ceased, could ethanol's effects on these two processes be eliminated as the cause of cell depletion. In this latter case, we may conclude that the ethanol effect was due to one or more of at least two possible mechanisms: 1) a direct toxic effect on postmitotic Purkinje cells and hippocampal pyramidal cells; or 2) a secondary effect due to reductions in the numbers of granule cells. Although the studies just described cannot distinguish between these two possibilities, it should be noted that at least two studies (Borges and Lewis, 1983; Yanai and Waknin, 1985) reported independent effects on granule and Purkinje cells, which would not support the hypothesis that effects on Purkinje cells are secondary to effects on granule cells. Clearly, more work must be done before the exact mechanism of ethanol-induced Purkinje and granule cell loss can be elucidated.

The situation is even more complex in the case of the granule cells of the cerebellum and hippocampus since each population is being generated throughout the early postnatal period. The cerebellar granule cells are formed predominantly in the EGL, from which they migrate inward, through the molecular layer, to the granular cell layer where their maturation and survival depend upon the formation of efferent connections with Purkinje cell dendrites. Since both granular layers exhibit some granule cell depletion, wiht the greatest loss occurring in the granular layer in the lobules exhibiting the greatest Purkinje cell loss (Pierce et al., 1989; Bonthius and West, 1990), ethanol may exert its effects on a number of levels, ranging from deficits in mitotic activity and errors in migration to the increased loss of efferent targets. Interestingly, in the dentate gyrus of the hippocampal formation, there was an increase in the number of granule cells following early postnatal ethanol exposure (West et al., 1986), and this increase was associated with a significant reduction in cells in the hilar region, which is a secondary site of proliferation of the granule cells before they migrate to the dentate gyrus. However, the hilar region contains many cell types and, since the types were not identified in this study, it is not known whether or not the reduction was associated with increased migration of granule cells from the hilar region to the dentate gyrus. On the other hand, there was a positive correlation between the number of cell fragments in the hilus and that in the dentate gyrus whereas, if increased hilus-to-dentate migration were occurring, one would expect to see a negative correlation. Miller (1989) has suggested that this increase in granule cell number following postnatal exposure is consistent with the theory that ethanol affects primary and secondary proliferative zones in different ways, actually increasing neurogenesis in the hilar region. If so, this would be in accordance with the findings regarding both the late proliferative surge in the neocortex (Miller, 1986, 1989), and the lack of such a surge in the PSN, which is derived from a single proliferative zone (Miller, 1989).

The hypothesis that ethanol may differentially influence the two proliferative zones in the CNS is an interesting one and deserves to be examined in greater detail. It is important to note that, although the increased proliferation in the subventricular zone was only seen in the ethanol-exposed brains, this alone is not evidence for a direct effect of ethanol on this tissue. It is often the case in teratology research that, when developmental alterations occur in sequence over time, the secondary alterations occur not as a direct effect of the presence of the teratogen, but in response to the primary changes which were, themselves, caused by exposure to the teratogen. Since ethanol was administered throughout the whole proliferative period in each of these studies, the enhanced mitotic activity seen in the subventricular zone could have been in response to the ethanol-induced reduction and delay in mitotic activity in the ventricular zone. The possibility that this proliferative surge is a compensatory event cannot be discounted based on the evidence as it now stands. Furthermore, it is important to note that this hypothesis was derived from a series of studies utilizing the same dosage of ethanol, one which produced moderate BACs, and it is unclear whether this effect would be observed at higher BACs. For example, in the study reporting differential effects of ethanol on the hilar region and dentate gyrus of the hippocampus (West et al., 1986), only the ethanol regimen which produced relatively low BACs led to increases in dentate gyrus granule cell number. Once again, it is clear that BAC must be included as a variable in FAS research before hypotheses can be adequately tested.

The importance of considering both the dosage *and* the pattern of ethanol administration in FAS research cannot be overemphasized. It should be remembered that changes in the pattern of administration of ethanol do more than alter peak and trough BACs: they also alter the degree and duration of physiological withdrawal from ethanol. In recent years, attention has focused increasingly on the potentially harmful effects on the CNS of ethanol withdrawal in adults, and Purkinje cell loss is one of the effects which has been reported (Phillips and Cragg, 1984). One study in which rats had been subjected to a period of ethanol withdrawal during the brain growth spurt reported no additional brain weight deficits when compared with a group exposed to ethanol but not to withdrawal (Samson et al., 1982). However, since these authors did not examine cerebellar structure, the possible contribution of withdrawal-induced changes to early ethanol-induced Purkinje cell loss remains unanswered. Given the fact that infants of alcoholic mothers are often seen to undergo signs of ethanol withdrawal shortly after birth (Hanson et al., 1976; Pierog et al., 1977), the potentially harmful effects of withdrawal during the brain growth spurt warrant greater attention.

Finally, the issue of regional vulnerability should be considered further since it implies that the toxic effects of ethanol are dependent not only on such factors as the amount and intensity of ethanol administered, but also on certain properties of the neurons themselves. Within the hippocampus, pyramidal cells in different regions can differ from each other on a number of variables. For instance, while CA3 cells receive afferent inputs from the dentate gyrus granule cells, CA1 cells receive much of their input from Schaffer collaterals and from the commissural projection of the CA3 pyramidal cells (Andersen, 1975), and the formation of these afferent connections is known to occur at different times (Zimmer and Haug, 1978). Furthermore, CA3 neurons are much larger than those in CA1 (Chronister and White, 1975). On the other hand, little has been reported on differences in rates of maturation between these two regions. Studies using ^{3}H-thymidine have found that the period of generation of CA1 pyramidal cells continues later than it does in the rest of the pyramidal cell layer (Angevine, 1965; Schlessinger et al., 1978; Bayer, 1980), although time of origin does not necessarily correlate with the timing of morphological and functional maturation. Given the fact that differential vulnerability of pyramidal cells may be mediated by morphological or maturational differences, clarification of these issues should warrant greater attention in future studies. In the cerebellum, the available evidence suggests that there are spatial differences in vulnerability correlated with the maturational state of the neurons. This issue is compounded by the fact that, within the cerebellum, there is a narrow temporal window—in rats, the middle of the first postnatal week—during which Purkinje cells are particularly vulnerable to the effects of ethanol. Since the research described here found the most severe effects on Purkinje cell number in the early-maturing lobules, and since these effects could be produced by exposure on a single day, a reasonable explanation would be that it was the state of maturation of those particular Purkinje cells which determined their vulnerability. Determining which aspects of cellular maturation contribute to this vulnerability should be a priority in future studies.

ETHANOL EFFECTS ON PLASTICITY

Morphological aspects of neuronal plasticity are included in this review since they are relevant to any discussion of ethanol's effects on cell production and survival. If ethanol can have lethal effects on some members of a population of cells, then it is reasonable to ask whether there is a responsive change in surviving cells which represents an *adaptation* to the altered developmental environment. Unfortunately, plasticity is a term for which an unambiguous definition remains elusive (i.e., Jacobson, 1978; Lund, 1978). Whereas neuronal survival is operationally defined according to the relatively clear criterion of relative cell number, a definition of plasticity often relies upon a subjective interpretation of the functional significance of a particular morphological alteration. For instance, abnormal patterns of dendritic branching could be due to ethanol-induced aberrations in growth, or they could be due to an adaptive response by the maturing neuron to ethanol-induced changes in afferent systems. Therefore, it is not always clear whether the developmental alterations described in the following sections are true examples of developmental plasticity or are simply examples of direct toxic effects of ethanol on developing tissue.

On the other hand, we *can* examine the effects of ethanol on plasticity per se by observing postlesion reorganization and sprouting in the CNS of animals which were exposed to ethanol early in development. Though sparse, such a literature does exist, and it will be reviewed here because it provides insight into the way ethanol can affect the ability of mature nervous tissue to respond morphologically to changes in the surrounding milieu.

Neocortex

We have already seen that there is a late proliferative surge in the neocortex which offsets the ethanol-induced reductions in neurogenesis in the ventricular zone. As stated earlier, it is unclear whether this is truly a compensatory response of the subventricular zone to the altered state of the cortex due to the ethanol treatment or whether it is, instead, simply a direct stimulatory effect of ethanol. In any event, although increased cell proliferation in response to prior cell depletion might be termed a type of plastic response, most researchers have limited their discussion of developmental plasticity in the CNS to changes in axonal migration, synaptogenesis, or the pruning of axons (e.g., Miller, 1987). Interestingly, little is known about such changes in the neocortex. Due perhaps to the relative ease with which it can be studied, most researchers have relied instead upon measures of dendritic arborization when examining ethanol-induced changes, and the results have been inconclusive. For example, while some studies have reported decreases in the extent and density of dendritic branching (Hammer and Scheibel, 1981; Schapiro et al., 1984) following prenatal ethanol exposure, others have found no difference either on measures of dendritic extent (Pentney et al., 1984a,b) or on measures of synaptic density (Druse et al., 1986; Lancaster et al., 1989). On the other hand, the findings of two recent studies suggest that there may be increases in the density of axodendritic synapses in layer V corticospinal neurons in somatosensory cortex following prenatal ethanol exposure. In one study (Al-Rabiai and Miller, 1989), prenatal ethanol was reported to increase the density of afferents to projection cortical neurons in layer V of adult rats. Although axon density *per se* was not measured in this study, the overproduction of afferents was inferred from the fact that asymmetric synapses were more dense in the ethanol-exposed group. In a second study (Miller et al., 1991), prenatal ethanol exposure produced an increase in both the density of dendritic branching and the number of dendritic spines in this neuronal population.

Olfactory Tubercle

Following ablation of the olfactory bulb in rats, dopaminergic synapses in the olfactory tubercle undergo reorganization and sprouting and one study (Gottesfeld et al., 1989) has reported effects of prenatal ethanol exposure on this response. While deafferented rats generally exhibit lesion-induced plasticity in the olfactory tubercle in the form of axonal sprouting, increased density of postsynaptic dopamine receptors, and potentiation of postsynaptic adenylate cyclase activity (Gilad and Reis, 1979; Lingham and Gottesfeld, 1986), all of these changes are suppressed in rats which were prenatally exposed to ethanol (Gottesfeld et al., 1989). Since prenatal ethanol exposure leads to aberrant olfactory bulb development (Nyquist-Battie and Gochee, 1985), it is reasonable to ask whether prelesion synaptic morphology was already altered in these animals to such an extent that little postlesion reorganization was possible. In fact, sham-lesioned, ethanol-exposed controls did not differ from their pair-fed counterparts on any of the indices measured with the exception of dopaminergic D_1 and D_2 receptor binding, which was actually *reduced* in the ethanol-exposed rats both before and after the lesion. Therefore, prenatal ethanol appeared to exert long-term effects on dopaminergic synapses which included, but was not exclusive to, effects on plasticity.

Hippocampus

A number of studies have dealt with the effects of ethanol on development of the mossy fibers: the axons of the dentate gyrus granule cells which constitute a major excitatory efferent to CA3 hippocampal pyramidal cells (Andersen, 1975). These axons extend, in a narrow band, along the pyramidal cell layer in a direction transverse to the longitudinal (septo-hippocampal) axis. Axons reaching as far as the distal point of pyramidal subfield

CA3a then turn and extend in a temporal direction (Blackstad et al., 1970; Gaarskjaer, 1978, 1981; Swanson et al., 1978; West et al., 1982; West, 1983). In normal rats, Timm-stained terminal fields of these fibers constitute a suprapyramidal band, while a shorter infrapyramidal band is seen proximal to the hilus (Blackstad et al., 1970; Gaarskjaer, 1978, 1981; Swanson et al., 1978), although sparse staining in the distal infrapyramidal region has been reported in a few studies (West et al., 1982; West, 1983). Following prenatal (West et al., 1981; West and Hodges-Savola, 1983) or early postnatal (West and Hamre, 1985) exposure, however, a band of intra- and infrapyramidal staining, much more extensive than the pattern seen in normal rats, is found in field CA3a at the midtemporal level (Fig. 3).

Since the Timm-staining procedure used in the preceding studies shows only the presence of axon terminals, it was not clear from these studies whether the aberrant staining truly represented dentate granule cell axon terminals, and, if so, by what pathways these terminals entered the intra- and infrapyramidal layers. A study using anterograde transport of horseradish peroxidase (HRP), which allows for the visualization of mossy fiber axons, showed that these aberrant fields did indeed represent terminal fields of the dentate gyrus granule cell axons, and also indicated that this pattern was a result of altered axonal migration across the pyramidal cell layer in CA3a rather than an extension of the naturally occurring infrapyramidal bundles from CA3c (West and Pierce, 1984). Specifically, there was no evidence of axons extending from their normal infrapyramidal position in field CA3c or from the infrapyramidal bundles normally seen in more dorsorostral positions (West, 1983). Rather, the mossy fiber

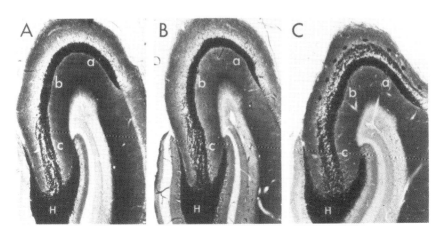

Fig. 3. Horizontal sections of midtemporal region of hippocampus in (A) normal adult rat; (B) artificially-reared adult rat; and (C) artificially-reared, ethanol-exposed adult rat. H, hilar region of dentate gyrus; a, b, and c, pyramidal cell layer CA3a, CA3b and CA3c, respectively. Note intra- and infrapyramidal staining in (C) (arrows). (Reproduced from West and Hamre, 1985, with permission.)

axons appeared to originate as part of the suprapyramidal bundle, from which they diverged in a direction transverse to the longitudinal axis of the hippocampus.

Once again, the occurrence and extent of this mossy fiber hyperdevelopment was found to be dependent upon a number of factors. The duration of ethanol exposure appears to be critical since prenatal exposure is effective only when it is continued throughout the period of gestation (West et al., 1981; West and Hodges-Savola, 1983; West and Pierce, 1984): if carried out during only the first or second 10 days of gestation, aberrant mossy fiber development is not seen (West and Hamre, 1985). On the other hand, early postnatal exposure for only 10 days did lead to mossy fiber hyperdevelopment (West and Hamre, 1985). Furthermore, the infrapyramidal terminal field was more extensive following exposure during the first 10 postnatal days than it was following exposure throughout the 21 days of gestation. This is not to say, however, that mossy fiber terminal field reorganization is more sensitive to the influence of ethanol during the early postnatal period than it is during gestation. For example, it should be noted that early postnatal exposure to ethanol of a shorter duration (days 4–9) did not produce aberrant mossy fibers (Kelly and West, unpublished observations). Also, the fact that methods of ethanol administration differ vastly between prenatal and postnatal models of exposure means that the pups in the postnatal exposure group may have been exposed to much higher BACs than were the fetuses in the prenatal groups. Given that BAC is clearly a critical factor in FAS research, this issue needs to be addressed.

Ethanol-induced mossy fiber hyperdevelopment could be the result of a number of alterations in the hippocampus. Specifically, any delay or permanent alteration in the migration of pyramidal cells could lead to the formation of synaptic connections deep to the pyramidal layer in the stratum oriens, although this would not explain the effects of postnatal ethanol exposure, since migration of these neurons was completed by the time of the exposure. Also, any treatment which reduced the number of pyramidal cells present could produce a compensatory response by afferent terminals which would then form synapses with basilar dendrites of surviving pyramidal cells. However, as we saw in the previous section, pyramidal cells in field CA3, the region in which the aberrant terminal fields are found, appear to be relatively resistant to the toxic effects of ethanol. On the other hand, if ethanol was found to reduce the density of the pyramidal cell dendritic field, then this too could conceivably lead to increased synaptogenesis in the region of the basilar dendrites, and a few studies have investigated ethanol effects on dendritic arborization and synaptogenesis in the hippocampus. One report (Abel et al., 1983) noted reduced numbers of spines on both the apical and basilar dendrites of CA1 pyramidal cells in prenatally ethanol-exposed adult rats, as well as a shift in the type of spines observed. Specifically, ethanol-treated rats exhibited greater numbers of spines with short, thin necks and large end bulbs, and fewer spines with long, thin necks and small end bulbs. Another study of combined pre- and postnatal exposure (Davies and Smith, 1981) found reduced numbers and lengths of basilar dendrites of CA1 pyramidal cells in 14-day-old rat pups, and these deficits were associated with reduced perikaryal diameters. In this latter study, ethanol was administered postnatally via the maternal diet, and the resulting BACs in the pups were low relative to the prenatal maternal BACs (<25 and 110 mg/dl, respectively), suggesting that the neuronal changes were due primarily to the prenatal exposure.

Another possibility is that this hyperdevelopment is due to alterations in the source of the afferents: the dentate gyrus granule cells. As described in an earlier section, early postnatal exposure to ethanol caused an increase in the number of granule cells in the dentate gyrus (West et al., 1986) and this increase conceivably could lead to increased axonal proliferation with the subsequent formation of synapses in regions in which they are not normally found. Alternatively, ethanol could adversely affect the normal pruning of granule cell axons in the hippocampus. It has been shown that, in some regions of the brain, there is an initial overproduction of axons innervating a particular area which is followed by a selective "pruning" of axons (Stanfield et al., 1982). In the case of corticospinal neurons, ethanol has been hypothesized to reduce the extent of this pruning process (Miller, 1987). Future studies should elaborate what role, if any, these processes play in the ethanol-induced mossy fiber hyperdevelopment in the hippocampus.

Given the profound effects on the development of the granule cell efferents, we also examined the effects of early ethanol exposure on the development of the major afferent fibers of the dentate gyrus: the perforant pathway from the entorhinal cortex (Dewey and West, 1985a) and the commissural projection from the contralateral hilar region (Dewey and West, 1985b). Following the same pattern of prenatal exposure which produced the aberrant mossy fiber development in earlier studies, adult rats exhibited perforant pathway terminal fields which were normal in terms of their size and organization, as well as a normal spatial pattern of the commissural pathway terminal field. However, although the ethanol effect on axon terminal development appeared to be specific only to the efferents of the dentate gyrus (the mossy fiber system), there were long-term effects on lesion-induced plasticity in the dentate gyrus afferent pathways. Following unilateral entorhinal lesions in adult rats which had been exposed to ethanol prenatally, terminal sprouting in the commissural/associational (C/A) zone was significantly enhanced relative to that seen in lesioned controls (West et al., 1984; Dewey and West, 1985c). Therefore, although commissural fiber terminal fields were not affected directly by early ethanol exposure, long-term alterations in lesion-induced plasticity of these fibers did result.

The nature of this abnormal pattern of plasticity is unclear. The potential for axon sprouting in the dentate gyrus in rats is known to decrease with age (West, 1984). Therefore, the abnormal sprouting response exhibited by the ethanol-exposed animals could be a sign of immaturity in the relative afferent systems, although the degree of sprouting is also a function of postsynaptic events (Frotscher, 1983). Nevertheless, it is evident that at least some long-term aspects of CNS plasticity can be affected by ethanol exposure early in development.

Cerebellum

One problem with interpreting the significance of the studies of ethanol's effects on neuronal plasticity discussed so far has been the lack of understanding of the mechanisms involved. In most cases, this is due to the fact that little is known about the range of ethanol's associated effects on the relevant systems. On the other hand, we have seen that relatively more is known about ethanol's effects on the cerebellum, both with regard to factors related to the practical aspects of ethanol administration, and to factors relating to the structure of the region. Furthermore, a great deal is known about the formation of neuronal connections within the cerebellum under both normal and abnormal conditions. For instance, Purkinje cell synaptogenesis and dendritic arborization have been studied extensively and, in normal rats, are known to follow a specific sequence of events (Altman, 1972, 1982; Bloom, 1982). The first synapses to form are asymmetrical synapses between perisomatic processes and climbing fiber terminals. These connections disappear after approximately 1 week, replaced by symmetrical synapses between basket cell axons and the Purkinje cell perikarya. Throughout this period, the primary dendrites are forming from the apical cone, and elaborate secondary and tertiary branches have begun to develop, and the parallel fibers from "en passant" synaptic connections with these dendrites.

This well organized sequence of events makes this system especially attractive for researchers interested in the developmental effects of environmental agents because it provides the opportunity to study possible interactive effects between various temporal and spatial events between the different cerebellar cell types. For example, studies of neurological mutations (e.g., Landis and Sidman, 1978; Herrup and Mullen, 1982; Herrup and Wilczynski, 1982; Herrup, 1983) and the effects of X-irradiation (e.g., Altman and Anderson, 1972, 1973; Altman, 1976a, b) have provided researchers with a wealth of knowledge regarding the interdependence of the varied developmental events in the cerebellum. Therefore, the cerebellum may be an excellent structure in which to seek patterns of plastic responding by afferent and efferent systems to ethanol administration during development directly, and to ethanol-induced morphological alterations in associated cell populations. Unfortunately, organized investigation of such plastic changes has yet to be carried out, with the majority of studies done so far restricted to general measures of synaptogenesis and dendritic branching.

With regard to synaptogenesis, studies have generally reported ethanol-induced reductions in the number of synapses at early ages (Volk, 1984b), which may be due to developmental delay (Mohamed et al., 1987). On the other hand, the effects on dendritic branching are less clear, with one study reporting less dense dendritic arborization, as determined from electron micrographs of 12-day-old rats (Volk, 1984b), while a series of Golgi studies found no differences in Purkinje cell arborization (Pentney et al., 1984a, b) or in the number and density of dendritic spines (Pentney et al., 1984b) between ethanol-exposed and control adult rats. At least one study has reported that the dendritic trees of the cerebellar granule cells in 14-day-old mouse pups did not differ in dendritic length between ethanol-exposed and pair-fed controls, but the overall area of the dendritic field was decreased in the ethanol pups (Smith et al., 1986).

It must be noted that none of these studies of synaptogenesis and dendritic branching took into account the regional differences in cerebellar vulnerability to ethanol which were shown earlier to merit important consideration. Although some of the studies did identify the lobules from which the tissue was obtained (Pentney et al., 1984a, b; Volk, 1984a, b; Mohamed et al., 1987), the actual location in that lobule was not defined. Therefore, the relationship between the results reported in these studies and the well-established Purkinje cell loss described previously remains elusive. Clearly, much work remains to be done in order to elaborate further the effects of ethanol on neuronal maturation within the cerebellum.

Conclusion

As in the case of cell survival, few general conclusions can be drawn regarding the effects of ethanol exposure during development on neuronal plasticity. While early ethanol exposure can lead to reorganization of axons, this effect appears to be specific to certain structures, and even to certain fiber pathways within those structures. Furthermore, while ethanol during development may lead to enhanced postlesion axon sprouting in some regions of the brain, it may inhibit such a response in other regions. Such varied effects could reflect a general disorganizing effect of ethanol on cell responding which would be manifested in either reduced or enhanced sprouting, depending upon the characteristics of associated tissues. In this case, it would not be the effect of early ethanol exposure on neuronal plasticity per se which varied, but rather the effect of ethanol on the development of the environment in which the neuron resides. This issue remains unresolved at present, since little concerted effort has been made to relate the few examples of plasticity seen with known effects of ethanol on changes in the associated cell populations. In the case of the hippocampus, where much of the work on plasticity has been carried out, little work has been conducted on the effects of ethanol on the relevant cell populations while, in the case of the cerebellum, relatively more is known regarding cell depletion but little is known of neuronal plasticity.

Finally, since most of our information pertaining to ethanol's early effects on plasticity comes from studies using single doses of ethanol, we know very little about the relationship between BAC and neuronal plasticity. Given the indisputable importance of BAC in the studies of cell depletion described earlier, this omission should be corrected by future research.

GENERAL DISCUSSION

It should be clear that few general conclusions can be drawn regarding ethanol's effects during development on neuronal survival and plasticity. Although ethanol can produce developmental abnormalities via effects on neuronal survival, it should be evident from the preceding review that such a statement requires further qualification. For the sake of clarity, such qualifications could be assigned to either a consideration of the particular properties of ethanol when its potential teratogenic nature is being studied, or to the complex multifactorial nature of neurobiological development.

Ethanol, as a teratogen, has at least two properties which are particularly relevant to the preceding discussion. First, because it is a relatively small molecule, it rapidly diffuses across biological membranes and equilibrates throughout the body water (Kalant et al., 1980). Therefore, since it is present in all tissues in both the mother and fetus, the health of the fetus can be threatened not only by the direct effects of ethanol, but by effects on the integrity of the maternal system as well, particularly with regard to placental transport (Fisher et al., 1982; Gordon et al., 1985), especially of amino acids (Henderson et al., 1981), and oxygen supply to the fetus (Altura et al., 1983). Because studies of ethanol's effects during the brain growth spurt in rats have used an artificial-rearing method which bypasses these maternal variables, extrapolation to effects in humans requires certain caveats. For instance, if impairment of nutrient utilization by the developing cell is a factor in ethanol-induced cell death in the studies described here, then the problem may be compounded in humans, where adequate nutrition to the fetus during the brain growth spurt could not be assured.

Once it enters the developing organism, ethanol may influence cells in many ways, including effects on such integral functions as protein synthesis (Kennedy, 1984; Pennington et al., 1983) and maintenance of membrane structure and function (Segarnick et al., 1982; Sun and Sun, 1985; Taraschi and Rubin, 1985). This pervasive influence of ethanol is an important consideration in any discussion of its effects on development because it implies the likelihood that any experimental findings which shed light on "the mechanism" of ethanol teratogenicity may: 1) not be generalizable beyond the tissue or organ studied in that particular case, and 2) represent only one of many factors which contribute to this teratogenicity. Ethanol can affect the proliferation, migration, long-term survival, and response to injury, of neurons, and there is no compelling reason to believe that it could not affect all of these processes in the same neuronal population.

A second property of ethanol which must be considered is the fact that its administration is complex and highly variable, incorporating a number of medical, social and psychological variables. There is no such thing as a standard "amount" of ethanol to which a fetus is exposed. Rather, the amount consumed interacts with such factors as duration and pattern of consumption, and the fetus is, in turn, exposed to the product of this interaction. Thus, the many apparent discrepancies among research findings in areas such as cerebellar cell loss could be explained only by addressing the complex nature of ethanol administration. The continual reliance upon such unidimensional aspects of ethanol as the *amount* administered, therefore, will certainly obstruct rapid progress in fetal alcohol research.

The other consideration which must be made when interpreting FAS research is the multifactorial nature of neurobiological development. Many FAS researchers have dealt with the complex nature of FAS, and of development itself, by continuing to seek to identify ever increasing numbers of its component parts, and the literature now abounds with reports simply identifying specific organs, systems, and cell populations which can be altered by ethanol exposure. These studies have been valuable in establishing beyond a reasonable doubt that ethanol can, indeed, be teratogenic. However, in the quest to understand the mechanisms underlying ethanol's teratogenicity, this approach has been of rather questionable utility. What may be needed now is an approach which recognizes that a developing system ". . . emerges from successive interactions . . ." (Oyama, 1985, p. 22) and that those interactions may interact with each other. While it is indeed necessary to identify the various tissues and organs which are affected by early ethanol exposure, it is important to remember that what contributes to the complexity of development is not the *number* of its component events, but rather ". . . the diversity of the interactions among its component events" (Stent, 1985, p. 216). According to this view, fruitful strategies in FAS research would seek to identify interactive effects of ethanol with other temporal and spatial factors in development. We have seen that ethanol may affect Purkinje cells at one stage of development but not at other stages, or may differentially affect pyramidal cells residing in different regions of the brain. These findings suggest that there are important relationships between these neurons and other events in the CNS which make them vulnerable to ethanol-induced aberrations. Clearly, the future goal of FAS research should be to identify the nature of these relationships.

ACKNOWLEDGMENTS

This study was supported by research grants AA05523 and AA07313 from the National Institute on Alcohol Abuse and Alcoholism.

REFERENCES

Abel EL, Jacobson S, Sherwin BT (1983): In utero alcohol exposure: Functional and structural brain damage. Neurotoxicol Teratol 5:363–366.

Abel EL, Sokol RM (1987): Incidence of fetal alcohol syndrome and economic impact of FAS-related anomalies. Drug Alcohol Dep 19:51–70.

Al-Rabai S, Miller MW (1989): Effect of prenatal exposure to ethanol on the ultrastructure of layer V of mature rat somatosensory cortex. J Neurocytol 18:711–729.

Altman J (1969): Autoradiographic and histological studies of postnatal neurogenesis. III. Dating the time of production and onset of differentiation of cerebellar microneurons in rats. J Comp Neurol 136:269–294.

Altman J (1972): Postnatal development of the cerebellar cortex in the rat. II. Phases in the maturation of the Purkinje cells and of the molecular layer. J Comp Neurol 145:399–464.

Altman J (1976a): Experimental reorganization of the cerebellar cortex. V. Effects of early X-irradiation schedules that allow or prevent the acquisition of basket cells. J Comp Neurol 165:31–48.

Altman J (1976b): Experimental reorganization of the cerebellar cortex. VI. Effects of X-irradiation schedules that allow or prevent cell acquisition after basket cells are formed. J Comp Neurol 165:49–64.

Altman J (1982): Morphological development of the rat cerebellum and some of its mechanisms. Exp Brain Res, Suppl 6:8–49.

Altman J, Anderson WJ (1972): Experimental reorganization of the cerebellar cortex. I. Morphological effects of elimination of all microneurons with prolonged X-irradiation started at birth. J Comp Neurol 146:355–406.

Altman J, Anderson WJ (1973): Experimental reorganization of the cerebellar cortex. II. Effects of elimination of most microneurons with prolonged X-irradiation started at four days. J Comp Neurol 149:123–152.

Altman J, Brunner RL, Bayer SA (1973): The hippocampus and behavioral maturation. Behav Biol 8:557–596.

Altura BM, Altura BT, Carella A, Chatterjee M, Halevy S, Tejani N (1983): Alcohol produces spasms of human umbilical blood vessels: Relationship to fetal alcohol syndrome (FAS). Eur J Pharmacol 86:311–312.

Andersen P (1975): Organization of hippocampal neurons and their interconnections. In Isaacson RL, Pribram KH (eds): "The Hippocampus, Vol. 1." New York: Plenum Press, pp 155–175.

Angevine JB Jr (1965): Time of neuron origin in the hippocampal region: An autoradiographic study in the mouse. Exp Neurol, Suppl 2:1–70.

Barnes DE, Walker DW (1981): Prenatal ethanol exposure permanently reduces the number of pyramidal neurons in rat hippocampus. Dev Brain Res 1:333–340.

Bauer-Moffett C, Altman J (1975): Ethanol-induced reductions in cerebellar growth of infant rats. Exp Neurol 48:378–382.

Bauer-Moffett C, Altman J (1977): The effect of ethanol chronically administered to preweanling rats on cerebellar development: A morphological study. Brain Res 119:249–268.

Bayer SA (1980): Development of the hippocampal region in the rat: I. Neurogenesis examined with ^{3}H-thymidine autoradiography. J Comp Neurol 190:87–114.

Blackstad TW, Brink K, Hem J, Jeune B (1970): Distribution of hippocampal mossy fibers in the rat. An experimental study with silver impregnation methods. J Comp Neurol 138:433–450.

Bloom FE (1982): Prospects from retrospect. In Schmitt FO, Bird SJ, Bloom FE (eds): "Molecular Genetic Neuroscience." New York: Raven Press, pp 467–475.

Bond NW (1981): Prenatal alcohol exposure in rodents: A review of its effects on offspring activity and learning ability. Aust J Psych 33:331–344.

Bonthius DJ, Goodlett CR, West JR (1988): Blood alcohol concentration and severity of microencephaly in neonatal rats depend on the pattern of alcohol administration. Alcohol 5:209–214.

Bonthius DJ, West JR (1988): Blood alcohol concentration and microencephaly: A dose-response study in the neonatal rat. Teratology 37:223–231.

Bonthius DJ, West JR (1990): Alcohol-induced neuronal loss in developing rats: Increased brain damage with binge exposure. Alcohol Clin Exp Res 14:107–118.

Borges S, Lewis PD (1982): A study of alcohol effects on the brain during gestation and lactation. Teratology 25:283–289.

Borges S, Lewis PD (1983): The effect of ethanol on the cellular composition of the cerebellum. Neuropathol Appl Neurobiol 9:53–60.

Burns EM, Kruckeberg TW, Kanak MF, Stibler H (1986): Ethanol exposure during brain ontogeny: Some long-term effects. Neurotoxicol Teratol 8:383–389.

Cassells B, Wainwright P, Blom K (1987): Heredity and alcohol-induced brain anomalies: Effects of alcohol on anomalous prenatal development of the corpus callosum and anterior commissure in BALB/c and C57BL/6 mice. Exp Neurol 95:587–604.

Chronister RB, White LE (1975): Fiberarchitecture of the hippocampal formation: Anatomy, projections, and structural significance. In Isaacson RL, Pribram KH (eds): "The Hippocampus. Vol. I: Structure and Development." New York: Plenum Press pp 9–39.

Clarren SK, Smith DW (1978): The fetal alcohol syndrome. N Engl J Med 298:1063–1067.

Cragg B, Phillips S (1985): Natural loss of Purkinje cells during development and increased loss with alcohol. Brain Res 325:151–160.

Davies DL, Smith DE (1981): A Golgi study of mouse hippocampal CA1 pyramidal neurons following prenatal ethanol exposure. Neurosci Lett 26:49–54.

Dewey SL, West JR (1985a): Perforant pathway lamination in the dentate gyrus is unaffected by prenatal ethanol exposure. Alcohol 2:221–225.

Dewey SL, West JR (1985b): Organization of the commissural projection to the dentate gyrus is unaltered by heavy ethanol exposure during gestation. Alcohol 2:617–622.

Dewey SL, West JR (1985c): Direct evidence for commissural axon sprouting in adult rats exposed to ethanol in utero. Brain Res Bull 14:339–348.

Diaz J, Samson HH (1980): Impaired brain growth in neonatal rats exposed to ethanol. Science 208:751–753.

Dobbing J (1981): The later development of the brain and its vulnerability. In Davis JA, Dobbing J (eds): "Scientific Foundations of Paediatrics." London: Heinemann, pp 331–336.

Dobbing J, Sands J (1979): Comparative aspects of the brain growth spurt. Early Hum Dev 3:79–83.

Dorris M (1989): "The Broken Cord." New York: Harper and Row, Publishers, Inc.

Douglas RJ (1967): The hippocampus and behavior. Psych Bull 67:416–442.

Druse MJ, Rathbun WE, McNulty JA, Nyquist-Battie C (1986): Maternal ethanol consumption: Lack of effect on synaptogenesis in layer I of the motor cortex in 19-day-old rat offspring. Exp Neurol 94:497–508.

Fisher SE, Atkinson M, Burnap JK, Jacobson S, Sehgal PK, Scott W, Van Thiel DH (1982): Ethanol-associated selective fetal malnutrition: A contributing factor in the fetal alcohol syndrome. Alcohol Clin Exp Res 6:197–201.

Frotscher M (1983): Dendritic plasticity in response to partial deafferentation. In Seifert W (ed): "Neurobiology of the Hippocampus." New York: Academic Press.

Gaarskjaer FB (1978): Organization of the mossy fiber system of the rat studied in extended hippocampi. I. Terminal area related to number of granule and pyramidal cells. J Comp Neurol 178:49–72.

Gaarskjaer FB (1981): The hippocampal mossy fiber system of the rat studied with retrograde tracing techniques. Correlation between topographic organization and neurogenetic gradients. J Comp Neurol 203:717–735.

Gilad GM, Reis DJ (1979): Collateral sprouting in central mesolimbic dopaminergic neurons: Biochemical and immunocytochemical evidence of changes in the activity and distribution of tyrosine hydroxylase in terminal fields and cell bodies of A10 neurons. Brain Res 160:17–36.

Goodlett CR, Hamre KM, West JR (1990a): Regional differences in the timing of dendritic outgrowth of Purkinje cells in the vermal cerebellum demonstrated by MAP2 immunocytochemistry. Dev Brain Res 53:131–134.

Goodlett CR, Marcussen BL, West JR (1990b): A single day of alcohol exposure during the brain growth spurt induces brain weight restriction and cerebellar Purkinje cell loss. Alcohol 7:107–114.

Gordon BHJ, Streeter ML, Rosso P, Winick M (1985): Prenatal alcohol exposure: Abnormalities in placental growth and fetal amino acid uptake in the rat. Biol Neonate 47:113–119.

Gottesfeld Z, Garcia CJ, Lingham RB, Chronister RB (1989): Prenatal ethanol exposure impairs lesion-induced plasticity in a dopaminergic synapse after maturity. Neuroscience 29:715–723.

Hammer RP, Scheibel AB (1981): Morphologic evidence for a delay of neuronal maturation in fetal alcohol exposure. Exp Neurol 74:587–596.

Hanson JW, Jones KL, SmithDW (1976): Fetal alcohol syndrome. Experience with 41 patients. JAMA 235:1458–1460.

Henderson GI, Turner D, Patwardhan RV, Lumeng L, Hoyumpa AM, Schenker S (1981): Inhibition of placental valine uptake after acute and chronic maternal ethanol consumption. J Pharmacol Exp Ther 216:465–472.

Herrup K (1983): Role of staggerer gene in determining cell number in cerebellar cortex. I. Granule cell death is an indirect consequence of staggerer gene action. Dev Brain Res 11:267–274.

Herrup K, Mullen RJ (1981): Role of the staggerer gene in determining Purkinje cell number in the cerebellar cortex of mouse chimeras. Dev Brain Res 1:475–485.

Herrup K, Wilczynski SL (1982): Cerebellar cell degeneration in the leaner mutant mouse. Neuroscience 7:2185–2196.

Hinds JW (1968): Autoradiographic study of histogenesis in the mouse olfactory bulb. I. Time of origin of neurons and neuroglia. J Comp Neurol 134:287–304.

Jacobson M (1978): "Developmental Neurobiology." New York: Plenum Press.

Kalant H, Khanna JM, Israel Y (1980): The alcohols. In Seeman P, Sellers EM, Roschlau WHE (eds): "Principles of Medical Pharmacology." Toronto: University of Toronto Press, pp 245–253.

Kelly SJ, Pierce DR, West JR (1987): Microencephaly and hyperactivity in adult rats can be induced by neonatal exposure to high blood alcohol concentrations. Exp Neurol 96:580–593.

Kennedy LA (1984): The pathogenesis of brain abnormalities in the fetal alcohol syndrome: An integrating hypothesis. Teratology 29:363–368.

Lancaster F, Delaney C, Samorajski T (1989): Synaptic density of caudate-putamen and visual cortex following exposure to ethanol in utero. Int J Dev Neurosci 7:581–589.

Landis DMD, Sidman RL (1978): Electron microscopic analysis of postnatal histogenesis in the cerebellar cortex of staggerer mutant mice. J Comp Neurol 179:831–864.

Lingham RB, Gottesfeld Z (1986): Deafferentation elicits increased dopamine-sensitive adenylate cyclase and receptor binding in the olfactory tubercle. J Neurosci 6:2208–2214.

Lund RD (1978): "Development and Plasticity of the Brain." New York: Oxford University Press.

McLardy T (1975): Hippocampal zinc and structural deficit in brains from chronic alcoholics and some schizophrenics. J Orthomol Psychiatry 4:32–40.

Miller MW (1986): Effects of alcohol on the generation and migration of cerebral cortical neurons. Science 233:1308–1311.

Miller MW (1987): Effect of prenatal exposure to alcohol on the distribution and time of origin of corticospinal neurons in the rat. J Comp Neurol 257:372–382.

Miller MW (1988): Effect of prenatal exposure to ethanol on the development of cerebral cortex: I. Neuronal generation. Alcohol Clin Exp Res 12:440–449.

Miller MW (1989): Effects of prenatal exposure to ethanol on neocortical development: II. Cell proliferation in the ventricular zones of the rat. J Comp Neurol 287:326–338.

Miller MW, Chiaia NL, Rhoades RW (1991): An intracellular recording and injection study of corticospinal neurons in rat somatosensory cortex: Effect of prenatal exposure to ethanol. J Comp Neurol (in press.).

Miller MW, Muller SJ (1989): Structure and histogenesis of the principal sensory nucleus of the trigeminal nerve: Effects of prenatal exposure to ethanol. J Comp Neurol 282:570–580.

Miller MW, Potempa G (1990): Numbers of neurons and glia in mature rat somatosensory cortex: Effects of prenatal exposure to ethanol. J Comp Neurol 293:92–102.

Mohamed SA, Nathaniel EJ, Nathaniel DR, Snell L (1987): Altered Purkinje cell maturation in rats exposed prenatally to ethanol: II. Synaptology. Exp Neurol 97:53–69.

Nyquist-Battie C, Gochee A (1985): Alterations in the development of the main olfactory bulb of the mouse after ethanol exposure. Int J Dev Neurosci 3:211–222.

Olton DS (1983): Memory functions and the hippocampus. In Seifert W (ed): "Neurobiology of the Hippocampus." London: Academic Press, pp 335–373.

Oppenheim RW (1981): Neuronal cell death and some related regressive phenomena during neurogenesis: A selective historical review and progress report. In Cowan WM (ed): "Studies in Developmental Neurobiology." New York: Oxford University Press, pp 74–133.

Oyama S (1985): "the Ontogeny of Information." New York: Cambridge University Press.

Pennington SN, Boyd JW, Kalmus GW, Wilson RW (1983): The molecular mechanism of fetal alcohol syndrome (FAS). I. Ethanol-induced growth suppression. Neurotoxicol Teratol 5:259–262.

Pentney RJ (1982): Quantitative analysis of ethanol effects on Purkinje cell dendritic tree. Brain Res 249:397–401.

Pentney RJ, Cotter JR, Abel EL (1984a): Quantitative measures of mature neuronal morphology after in utero ethanol exposure. Neurotoxicol Teratol 6:59–65.

Pentney RJ, Cotter JR, Abel EL (1984b): Quantitative measures of dendritic networks after in utero ethanol exposure. Ann NY Acad Sci 435:471–474.

Pentney RJ, Quigley PJ (1987): Morphometric parameters of Purkinje dendritic networks after ethanol treatment during aging. Alcohol Clin Exp Res 11:536–540.

Phillips SC (1985): Age-dependent susceptibility of rat cerebellar Purkinje cells to ethanol exposure. Drug Alcohol Depend 16:273–277.

Phillips SC (1989): The threshold concentration of dietary ethanol necessary to produce toxic effects on hippocampal cells and synapses in the mouse. Exp Neurol 104:68–72.

Phillips SC, Cragg BG (1982): A change in susceptibility of rat cerebellar Purkinje cells to damage by alcohol during fetal, neonatal and adult life. Neuropathol Appl Neurobiol 8:441–454.

Phillips SC, Cragg BG (1984): Alcohol withdrawal causes a loss of cerebellar Purkinje cells in mice. J Stud Alcohol 45:475–480.

Pierce DR, Goodlett CR, West JR (1989): Differential neuronal loss following early postnatal alcohol exposure. Teratology 40:113–126.

Pierce DR, West JR (1986a): Alcohol-induced microencephaly during the third trimester equivalent: Relationship to dose and blood alcohol concentration. Alcohol 3:185–191.

Pierce DR, West JR (1986b): Blood alcohol concentration: A critical factor for producing fetal alcohol effects. Alcohol 3:269–272.

Pierog S, Chandavasu O, Wexler I (1977): Withdrawal symptoms in infants with the fetal alcohol syndrome. J Pediatr 90:630–633.

Riley EP, Barron S, Hannigan JH (1986): Response inhibition deficits following prenatal ethanol exposure: A comparison of the effects of hippocampal lesions in rats. In West JR (ed): "Alcohol and Brain Development." New York: Oxford University Press, pp 71–102.

Riley JN, Walker DW (1978): Morphological alterations in hippocampus after long-term alcohol consumption in mice. Science 201:646–648.

Samson HH (1986): Microcephaly and fetal alcohol syndrome: Human and animal studies. In West JR (ed): "Alcohol and Brain Development." New York: Oxford University Press, pp 167–183.

Samson HH, Diaz J (1982): Effects of neonatal ethanol exposure on brain development in rodents. In Abel EL (ed): "Fetal Alcohol Syndrome. Volume III, Animal Studies." Boca Raton: CRC Press, pp 131–150.

Samson HH, Grant KA, Coggan S, Sachs VM (1982): Ethanol induced microcephaly in the neonatal rat: Occurrence without withdrawal. Neurotoxicol Teratol 4:115–116.

Schapiro MB, Rosman NP, Kemper TL (1984): Effects of chronic ethanol exposure to alcohol on the developing brain. Neurotoxicol Teratol 6:351–356.

Schlessinger AR, Cowan WM, Swanson LW (1978): The time of origin of neurons in Ammon's horn and the associated retrohippocampal fields. Anat Embryol 154:153–173.

Segarnick DJ, Cordasco DM, Rotrosen J (1982): Biochemical and behavioral interactions between prostaglandin E_1 and alcohol. In Horrobin DF (ed): "Clinical Uses of Essential Fatty Acids." Montreal: Eden Press, Inc., pp 175–189.

Sellers EM, Kalant S, Kalow W (1980): Principles of drug administration, disposition and dosage. In Seeman P, Sellers EM, Roschlau WHE (eds): "Principles of Medical Pharmacology." Toronto: University of Toronto Press, pp 11–19.

Shaywitz SE, Cohen DJ, Shaywitz BA (1980): Behavior and learning difficulties in children of normal intelligence born to alcoholic mothers. J Pediatr 96:978–982.

Smith DE, Foundas A, Canale J (1986): Effect of perinatally administered ethanol on the development of the cerebellar granule cell. Exp Neurol 92:491–501.

Solomon PR (1979): Temporal versus spatial information processing theories of hippocampal function. Psych Bull 86:1272–1279.

Stanfield BB, O'Leary DDM, Fricke C (1982): Selective collateral elimination in early postnatal development restricts cortical distribution of rat pyramidal tract neurons. Nature 298:371–373.

Steinhausen H-C, Gobel D, Nestler V (1984): Psychopathology in the offspring of alcoholic parents. J Acad Child Psychiatr 23:465–471.

Stent GS (1985): Hermeneutics and the analysis of complex biological systems. In Depew DJ, Weber BH (eds): "Evolution at a Crossroads: The New Biology and the New Philosophy of Science." Cambridge: The MIT Press, pp 209–225.

Streissguth AP (1986): The behavioral teratology of alcohol: Performance, behavioral, and intellectual deficits in prenatally-exposed children. In West JR (ed): "Alcohol and Brain Development." New York: Oxford University Press, pp 3–44.

Streissguth AP, Herman CS, Smith DW (1978): Intelligence, behavior and dysmorphogenesis in the fetal alcohol syndrome: A report on 20 patients. J Pediatr 92:363–367.

Sun GY, Sun AY (1985): Ethanol and membrane lipids. Alcohol Clin Exp Res 9:164–180.

Swanson LW, Wyss JM, Cowan WM (1978): An autoradiographic study of the organization of intrahippocampal association pathways in the rat. J Comp Neurol 181:681–716.

Taraschi TF, Rubin E (1985): Biology of disease: Effects of ethanol on the chemical and structural properties of biologic membranes. Lab Invest 52:120–131.

Tavares MA, Paula-Barbosa MM (1982): Alcohol-induced granule cell loss in the cerebellar cortex of the adult rat. Exp Neurol 78:574–582.

Volk B (1984a): Neurohistological and neurobiological aspects of fetal alcohol syndrome in the rat. In Yanai J (ed): "Neurobehavioral Teratology." New York: Elsevier Science Publishers, pp 163–193.

Volk B (1984b): Cerebellar histogenesis and synaptic maturation following pre- and postnatal alcohol administration. Acta Neuropathol 63:57–65.

Volk B, Maletz J, Tiedemann M, Mall G, Klein C, Berlet HH (1981): Impaired maturation of Purkinje cells in the fetal alcohol syndrome of the rat. Acta Neuropathol 54:19–29.

Wahlsten D (1977): Heredity and brain structure. In Oliverio A (ed): "Genetics, Environment and Intelligence." North Holland: Elsevier/North Holland Biomedical Press, pp 93–115.

Wainwright P, Ward GR, Molnar JD (1985): Gamma-linolenic acid fails to prevent the effects of prenatal ethanol exposure on brain and behavioral development in B6D2F$_2$ mice. Alcohol Clin Exp Res 9:377–383.

Walker DW, Barnes DE, Zornetzer SF, Hunter BE, Kubanis P (1980): Neuronal loss in hippocampus induced by prolonged ethanol consumption in rats. Science 209:711–713.

Walker DW, Hunter BE, Abraham WC (1981): Neuroanatomical and functional deficits subsequent to chronic ethanol administration in animals. Alcohol Clin Exp Res 5:267–282.

Wallgren H, Barry H (1970): "Actions of Alcohol." Amsterdam: Elseirer.

Weinberg J (1985): Effects of ethanol and maternal nutritional status on fetal development. Alcohol Clin Exp Res 9:49–55.

West JR (1983): Distal infrapyramidal and longitudinal mossy fibers at a midtemporal hippocampal level. Brain Res Bull 10:137–146.

West JR (1984): Age dependent sprouting in the dentate gyrus demonstrated with anterograde HRP. Brain Res Bull 12:323–330.

West JR (1987): Fetal alcohol-induced brain damage and the problem of determining temporal vulnerability: A review. Alcohol Drug Res 7:423–441.

West JR, Dewey SL, Cassell MD (1984): Prenatal ethanol exposure alters the post-lesion reorganization (sprouting) of acetylcholinesterase staining in the dentate gyrus of adult rats. Dev Brain Res 12:83–95.

West JR, Goodlett CR, Bonthius DJ, Pierce DR (1989) : Manipulating peak blood alcohol concentrations in neonatal rats: Review of an animal model for alcohol-related developmental effects. Neurotoxicology 10:347–366.

West JR, Hamre KM, Cassell MD (1986): Effects of ethanol exposure during the third trimester equivalent on neuron number in rat hippocampus and dentate gyrus. Alcohol Clin Exp Res 10:190–197.

West JR, Hamre KM (1985): Effects of alcohol exposure during different periods of development: Changes in hippocampal mossy fibers. Dev Brain Res 17:280–284.

West JR, Hodges CA, Black AC Jr (1981): Prenatal ethanol exposure alters the organization of hippocampal mossy fibers in rats. Science 211:957–959.

West JR, Hodges-Savola CA (1983): Permanent hippocampal mossy fiber hyper-development following prenatal ethanol exposure. Neurotoxicol Teratol 5:139–150.

West JR, Lind MD, Demuth RM, Parker ES, Alkana RL, Cassell M, Black AC Jr (1982): Lesion-induced sprouting in the rat dentate gyrus is inhibited by repeated ethanol administration. Science 218:808–810.

West JR, Pierce DR (1984): The effect of in utero ethanol exposure on hippocampal mossy fibers: An HRP study. Dev Brain Res 15:275–279.

Wigal T, Amsel A (1990): Behavioral and neuroanatomical effects of prenatal, postnatal, or combined exposure to ethanol in weanling rats. Behav Neurosci 104:-116–126.

Yanai J, Waknin S (1985): Comparison of the effects of barbiturate and ethanol given to neonates on the cerebellar morphology. Acta Anat 123:145–147.

Zimmer J, Haug FMS (1978): Laminar differentiation of the hippocampus, fascia dentata and subiculum in developing rats, observed with the Timm sulphide silver method. J Comp Neurol 179:581–618.

Development of the Central Nervous System:
Effects of Alcohol and Opiates, pages 139–167
© 1992 Wiley-Liss, Inc.

7

Effects of In Utero Ethanol Exposure on the Development of Neurotransmitter Systems

MARY J. DRUSE

Department of Molecular and Cellular Biochemistry, Loyola University of Chicago, Stritch School of Medicine, Maywood, Illinois

INTRODUCTION

Mental retardation, hyperactivity, attention deficits, and behavioral problems comprise some of the most severe and commonly seen problems associated with the fetal alcohol syndrome (FAS) (reviewed by Clarren and Smith, 1978; Streissguth, 1983; Streissguth et al., 1988). In an attempt to determine the underlying causes of these central nervous system problems, considerable attention has been given to the effects of ethanol on the development of major CNS neurotransmitter systems in animal models of FAS. To date, the best studied systems include those associated with the neurotransmitters serotonin, dopamine, noradrenaline, glutamate, and acetylcholine. Less attention has been given to GABA, glycine, and histamine.

In this chapter, I will review studies of the effects of in utero ethanol exposure on developing neurotransmitter systems. To provide a frame of reference, I have provided information about the normal development of several neurotransmitter systems. In addition, several hypotheses are made regarding how in utero ethanol exposure might alter the development of a number of neurotransmitter systems through one or more common mechanism.

The research findings discussed here are grouped by the neurotransmitter studied. Table I summarizes the authors and feeding paradigms used in the studies reviewed. These studies were done using a variety of animal models, a wide range of ethanol doses, different timings of ethanol exposure, and different ages of assessment. It is somewhat difficult to compare the results because experimental outcome is dependent upon these variables, as well as on blood alcohol levels (Pierce and West, 1986), genetic susceptibility (Gilliam et al., 1988), choice of control animals, the presence or absence of circulating ethanol at the time of sacrifice, age of analysis, and regions analyzed. In many cases, regional changes were masked by whole brain analyses. In addition, circadian variations in several neuro-transmitter systems (reviewed by Wirz-Justice, 1987) are not always considered.

Despite the concerns mentioned, it is possible to draw general conclusions if studies of a given neurotransmitter system are grouped by common factors. Occasional differences with the majority consensus are presumably due to differences in one or more of the factors mentioned.

In the following tables and discussion, studies are grouped on the basis of timing, duration and dose of ethanol, and the use of either whole brain tissue or selected brain regions. An attempt has been made to follow the brain divisions specified by each author. Thus, a table may include data on a region (e.g., brain stem) as well as on some of its components (e.g., diencephalon, hypothalamus). In rare cases, a smaller component (e.g., caudate) is grouped with the larger associated region (e.g., striatum). Tables II–IX present this author's interpretation of data presented in the reports reviewed. Most reports do not indicate whether the first day of gestation is the day of conception or the next day. Nor do they indicate whether the first postnatal day is the day of birth or the following day. Consequently, I have used each author's own time reference; another author's time reference may differ by 24 hours. Percent differences between control and ethanol-treated animals are given as approximations (to the closest 5%) of data which the original author found significant. The reported units of measurement were based either on tissue weight, protein content, or an entire region. This author's calculated percent differences represent a comparison of values reported in the original study. Potentially important, nonsignificant data trends are generally excluded from tables and discussion. Some authors include control and pair-fed experimental animals as well as additional nutritional or drug-treatment groups. For the sake of simplicity and consistency, this review is limited to control and ethanol-treated rats. Ethanol treatment is categorized as a "low" dose if ethanol was administered at low concentration or in the drinking water. Pair-fed liquid diets are categorized as a "higher" dose.

SEROTONIN

The cell bodies of serotonin-containing neurons are found in the raphe nuclei, which are located in the brain stem. The raphe neurons send ascending and descending projections to many areas of the brain (B4–B9) as well as to the spinal cord (B1–B3). Neurons in the nuclei raphe dorsalis (B7 group) send projections to the neocortex, piriform cortex, neostriatum, and hippocampus, while neurons in the nucleus centralis superior (B8 group) send projections to the cerebral cortex and anterior hypothalamic area (reviewed by Green, 1989).

Studies of fetal/embryonic CNS development have shown that serotonergic nerves mature particularly early. In the rat, 5-HT synthesis can be detected on the 12th–13th day of gestation (G) in cells of the B4–B9 complex (Lauder and Krebs, 1978; Wallace and Lauder, 1983; Aitken and Tork, 1988). The peak of cell differentiation for serotonergic neurons occurs on

TABLE I. Summary of Ethanol Treatment[a]

Name	Rat/Mouse	Time	Ethanol
Boggan et al. (1979)	Mouse	G5—>G11	LD
Chan and Abel (1982)	Rat	G5—>0	LD
Cooper and Rudeen (1988)	Rat	P18	Chronic
Detering et al. (1980a)	Rat	G14—>0; 0—>21	LD
Detering et al (1980b)	Rat	G14—>0; 0—>21	LD
Detering et al. (1980c)	Rat	G14—>0; 0—>21	LD
Detering et al. (1980d)	Rat	G14—>0; 0—>21	LD
Detering et al. (1981)	Rat	G14—>0	LD
Druse and Paul (1989)	Rat	Chronic—>G—>0	LD
Druse et al. (1990)	Rat	Chronic—>G—>0	LD
Druse et al. (1991)	Rat	Chronic—>G—>0	
Druse et al. (in press)	Rat	Chronic—>G—>0	LD
Elis et al. (1976)	Mouse	G1—>0	GI
Elis et al. (1978)	Mouse	G1—>7, G8—>G14, G5—>0	GI
Espina et al. (1989)	Rat	G6—>G20	LD
Farr et al. (1988)	Rat	G—>0	LD
Farr et al. (1989)	Rat	G—>0	LD
Griezerstein and Aldrich (1983)	Rat	G(6,7,9,12,15 & 18)	GI
Hard et al. (1985a)	Rat	Chronic—>G—>0	W
Hard et al. (1985b)	Rat	Chronic—>G—>0	W
Kelley et al. (1986)	Rat	Chronic—>G—>0	LD
Krsiak et al. (1977)	Mouse	G1—>0 or 1 trimester	GI
Light et al. (1989)	Rat	P4—>8	GI
Lucchi et al. (1983)	Rat	G4—>0, G4—>P21, 0—>P21	W
Martin et al. (1989)	Rat	G—>0	LD
Mena et al. (1982)	Rat	G3—>P4	W
Mena et al. (1984)	Rat	G0—>P18, G0—>0	W
Morrissett et al. (1989)	Rat	G—>0	LD
Nelson et al. (1982)	Rat	G7, G13 or G14—>G20	W
Rathbun and Druse (1985)	Rat	Chronic—>G—>0	LD
Rawat (1977)	Rat	Chronic—>study	LD
Rawat (1980)	Rat	G—>P10	LD
Savage (personal communication)	Rat	G	LD
Serbus et al. (1986)	Rat	P4—>8	GI
Shoemaker et al. (1983)	Rat	G1—>10	LD
Slotkin et al. (1980)	Rat	G13—>G19	LD
Tajuddin and Druse (1989a)	Rat	Chronic—>G—>0	LD
Tajuddin and Druse (1989b)	Rat	Chronic—>G—>0	LD

[a]Complete references are provided in the reference section. Several abbreviations were used to define the times during which ethanol was administered. When the letter G precedes a number, it refers to a gestational day. G alone denotes all of gestation. P refers to postnatal ages. Day 0 indicates the day of parturition. Abbreviations: LD, liquid diet; GI, gastric intubation; W, water.

G15 or G16 (Lauder and Krebs, 1978). At about this time, the cells aggregate into subgroups, which can be correlated somewhat with the B4–B9 complex (Wallace and Lauder, 1983), and by G19 the distribution of 5-HT neurons resembles that found in the adult (Lidov and Molliver, 1982). Projections to the caudal diencephalon are found on G14, while those to the neocortex are found on G17 (Lauder et al., 1983; Wallace and Lauder, 1983). Synaptic contacts are detected by G20 (reviewed by Lidov and Molliver, 1982) and $5-HT_1$ receptors have been reported in rats on postnatal day 1 (P1) (Whitaker-Azmitia et al., 1987). $5-HT_2$ receptors can be detected at birth and peak at around 5 weeks (Bruinink et al., 1983a). The diurnal variations in $5-HT_2$ sites appear at about 40 days (Bruinink et al., 1983b).

Recent work has emphasized the importance of 5-HT in the normal development of both the pre- and postsynaptic components of the serotonergic system and the close interrelationship of the development and maturation of the serotonergic neurons and their postsynaptic target areas. Elegant studies of cultured snail Helisoma ganglion cells demonstrate that exogenous 5-HT has the potential to cause cessation of neurite outgrowth and elongation from growth cones (Haydon et al., 1984, 1987; McCobb et al., 1988). In early fetal vertebrate development, serotonin appears to act on its own neurons via a presynaptic autoreceptor of the $5-HT_1$ class (tentatively identified as the $5HT_{1A}$ receptor) (Whitaker-Azmitia and Azmitia, 1986; Whitaker-Azmitia et al., 1987). During this early developmental period, 5-HT inhibits neurite outgrowth to 5-HT target areas and promotes collateral connections between serotonergic neurons (Whitaker-Azmitia et al., 1987). 5-HT also exerts an epigenetic, maturational influence on 5-HT target tissues (Chumasov et al., 1980; Lauder and Krebs, 1978, 1984; Lauder et al., 1983, 1985; Chubakov et al., 1986). 5-HT causes the target tissues to cease cell division and to begin differentiation. Through cerebrospinal fluid-derived 5-HT, the development and maturation of non-5-HT target tissue may also be influenced (Lauder and Krebs, 1984). In addition, a factor from the postsynaptic 5-HT targets can enhance the maturation of the presynaptic serotonergic neurons (Whitaker-Azmitia and Azmitia, 1986; Azmitia and deKloet, 1987; Zhou et all, 1987). This soluble neurotrophic factor is increased in 5-HT target areas following denervation (Zhou et al., 1987).

The importance of the neurotrophic and epigenetic factors mentioned in development is demonstrated by studies in which pregnant animals were treated either with a 5-HT agonist (5-methoxytryptamine, 5-MT) or a tryptophan hydroxylase inhibitor (parachlorophenylalanine, PCPA). Removal of the 5-HT signal, via PCPA treatment, results in the depletion of 5-HT levels in the cell bodies and axons of embryonic raphe nuclei of the B4–B9 complex, delayed differentiation of the postsynaptic target areas of 5-HT neurons (Lauder and Krebs, 1978; Lauder et al., 1985), and a delay in the normal early postnatal decline of $5-HT_1$ receptors in the forebrain and brain stem (Whitaker-Azmitia et al., 1987). In contrast, prenatal treatment with 5-MT appears to accelerate the early postnatal $5-HT_1$ receptor decline (Whitaker-Azmitia et al., 1987).

The prenatal development of several components of the serotonergic system and the potential sensitivity of this system to maternal stresses have made this system interesting to examine in animal models of FAS. Studies of the effects of in utero ethanol exposure on the developing serotonergic system have examined several components: the steady-state levels of serotonin (5-HT), its precursor 5-hydroxytryptophan (5-HTP) and metabolite 5-hydroxyindoleacetic acid (5-HIAA); the activity of enzymes involved with the synthesis or degradation of 5-HT; the presynaptic uptake of serotonin; and serotonin receptors. Although postnatal development has been a primary focus, recent studies have examined fetal/embryonic development of the serotonergic system as well.

Differences in the concentration of whole brain serotonin (5-HT) or its acid metabolite 5-HIAA (Table II) are not detected in offspring of rats that received ethanol in a low dose (i.e., in drinking water) or for a short and relatively early period of time (i.e., G5–G11) (Boggan et al., 1979). However, when rodent mothers are given a higher ethanol dose or a moderate ethanol dose for a longer period of time, whole brain serotonin is markedly decreased in brains of older animals. In fact, Elis et al. (1976, 1978) and Krsiak et al. (1977) found more than a 50% decrease in 5-HT levels in the brains of 3- and 6-month-old offspring of rats whose mothers received 1 g ethanol/kg, via gastric intubation, for one or more trimesters of gestation (Table II).

The 5-HT deficiency is apparently localized to selected brain regions. Studies from our laboratory have shown that the 19- and 35-day-old offspring of rats, fed a 6.6% (v/v) ethanol-containing liquid diet on a chronic basis prior to parturition, have a 20–50% deficiency of 5-HT and 5-HIAA in the cortex, a 50% deficiency in the motor cortex, and a 20–40% deficiency in the somatosensory cortex (Rathbun and Druse, 1985, Druse et al., in press). 5-HT and 5-HIAA were also reduced in the cerebellum. In contrast, normal levels (a nonsignificant decrease) of 5-HT were found in the hypothalamus, corpus striatum, and hippocampus (Rathbun and Druse, 1985).

Recent data from our laboratory indicates that the cortical deficiency of 5-HT and 5-HIAA is also present as early as P5 and that the concentration of 5-HIAA is reduced by 40% in ethanol-exposed rats on G19. It is particularly interesting that on G15, G19, and P5 there is a marked decrease of 5-HT and 5-HIAA in the brain stem (Druse et al., in press) where the raphe nuclei are located. This observation is significant in light of reports that embryonic 5-HT is essential for the normal development of 5-HT-containing neurons and their target areas, as well as for normal development of other CNS areas (Lauder and Krebs, 1978, 1984; Lauder et al., 1983, 1985; Whitaker-Azmitia et al., 1987). Lack of such a key signal for differentiation or maturation at this critical period could result in a failure of serotonergic terminals to reach their target areas at the appropriate time (hence leading to cell death). Lack of 5-HT in the fetal brain could also contribute to abnormal development of nonserotonergic neurons (Lauder and Krebs, 1984).

TABLE II. Ethanol Effects on the Development of Components of
the Serotonergic System in Whole Brain[a]

Low ethanol dose or short ethanol exposure	
5-HT	
Boggan et al. (1979)	
G19–60 days	NC
Mena et al. (1982)	
G21, 1 day	NC
Nelson et al. (1982)	
0 days	NC–40%↓
4 days	25%↑
Higher ethanol dose or longer period of ethanol exposure	
5-HT and/or 5-HIAA	
Rawat (1977)	
G17–19 days	NC
Shoemaker et al. (1983)	
0 days	NC
Rawat (1977)	
5–10 days	NC
Elis et al. (1976, 1978)	
3 and 5 months	60%↓
Krsiak et al. (1977)	
3 months	60%↓
5-HT uptake	
Slotkin et al. (1980)	
2 days	15%↓
4–19 days	NC

[a]Ethanol administered in drinking water is described as a low dose. Ethanol administration via liquid diets is considered as a higher physiological dose than that in the drinking water. Please refer to the introduction to the text for additional information regarding this author's interpretation of reported data.
Abbreviations: 5-HT, 5-hydroxytryptamine (serotonin); 5-HIAA, 5-hydroxyindoleacetic acid; G, gestation; NC, no change.

One might expect that the decreased concentration of serotonin could be due either to decreased synthesis or increased degradation of serotonin. The latter explanation seems unlikely in light of decreased levels of 5-HIAA, a product of 5-HT metabolism, in the same brain regions where there is a 5-HT deficiency. Thus, it seems that synthesis of both 5-HT and 5-HIAA is decreased in selected brain regions from offspring exposed to ethanol in utero. Consistent with this conclusion is the observation that synthesis of 5-HTP, a precursor of 5-HT and 5-HIAA, is decreased in the whole brain and limbic system (Hard et al., 1985a, b).

Additional studies indicate that the 5-HT deficiency cannot be attributed to a basic metabolic effect. Rather, it appears that the offspring of ethanol-fed rats have fewer serotonergic projections and, hence, a decreased concentration of substances which are normally found at the serotonergic nerve terminals. Consistent with this hypothesis is the evidence that K^+-stimulated 5-HT release is decreased in young, ethanol-exposed offspring (Boggan et al., 1979) and that there is a 15–30% decrease in 5-HT uptake sites in the motor cortex of 19- and 35-day-old offspring of rats that were fed an ethanol-containing liquid diet on a chronic basis prior to parturition (Druse and Paul, 1989) (Table III). (Both 5-HT release and reuptake are localized to serotonergic projections and thus serve as markers for serotonin-containing terminals.) The deficiency of 5-HT uptake sites is region-specific and not found in the somatosensory cortex (Druse and Paul, 1989) or in analyses of whole brain 5-HT uptake sites in rats 4 days and older (Slotkin et al., 1980).

Recently, our laboratory demonstrated a 10–40% reduction of total 5-HT_1 binding sites on membranes from motor, somatosensory, and whole cortex in the 19- and 37-day-old offspring of rats pair-fed an ethanol-containing liquid diet on a chronic basis prior to parturition (Tajuddin and Druse, 1989a). Additional studies suggest that 5-HT_{1A}, but not 5-HT_{1B}, sites are decreased in postnatal rats (Druse et al., in press; Savage et al., unpublished data). Because 5-HT_1 binding sites represent a mixture of the 1A, 1B, and 1C subtypes, each of which is located both pre- and postsynaptically (Blurton and Wood, 1986; Whitaker-Azmitia, et al. 1987), presynaptic lesioning studies are needed to determine whether the 5-HT_1 and 5-HT_{1A} deficits are located pre- or postsynaptically.

Studies of fetal and neonatal rats (Druse et al., in press) indicate that the young (P5 and G19) offspring of rats exposed to ethanol in utero have a deficiency of 5-HT_{1A} receptors in cortex. This may be particularly important because fetal 5-HT_{1A} receptors have been associated with an autoreceptor function related to collateral formation between neighboring serotonergic neurons. A deficiency of fetal 5-HT_{1A} receptors could thus contribute to the abnormal development of serotonergic projections.

It is interesting to note that 5-HT_2 receptors, which are located postsynaptically on neurons innervated by serotonergic neurons (Leysen et al., 1983), are not affected by in utero ethanol exposure (Table III) (Tajuddin and Druse, 1989b). Thus, it would appear that the abnormalities in the serotonergic system, induced by in utero ethanol exposure, may be limited to the serotonin-containing neurons themselves, and not necessarily found in the targets innervated by serotonergic neurons. This observation is somewhat surprising because chemical denervation of serotonin-containing neurons in adult animals produces a supersensitivity to serotonin in the terminal field (Mueller et al., 1985). However, the developing rat may not respond to a long term 20–50% deficiency of 5-HT input in the same way that mature animals respond to an abrupt loss of 5-HT input.

In summary, in utero exposure to a lower ethanol dose produces little effect on whole brain serotonin. In contrast, exposure to a higher ethanol dose results in a deficiency of 5-HT and 5-HIAA, that is particularly evident in cortical regions of postnatal rats. These postnatal rats also have a

TABLE III. Ethanol Effects on the Development of Components of the Serotonergic System in Brain Regions[a]

	Cortex and cortical regions		
	Whole cortex	Motor cortex	Somatosensory cortex
Low ethanol dose Nelson et al. (1982)			
21 days	5-HT: NC		
Higher ethanol dose Druse et al. (in press)			
G19	5-HT: NC 5-HIAA: 40%↓		
5 days	5-HT: 40%↓ 5-HIAA: 30%↓		
Rathbun and Druse (1985)			
19 and 35 days	5-HT: 50%↓ 5-HIAA:20–40%↓		
Druse et al. (in press)			
19 and 35 days		5-HT: 50%↓ 5-HIAA:50%↓	5-HT: 20–40%↓ 5-HIAA:20–40%↓
5-HT uptake (higher ethanol dose) Druse and Paul (1989)			
19 and 35 days		Uptake: 15–30%↓	Uptake: NC
5-HT receptors (higher ethanol dose) Tajuddin and Druse (1989a, b)			
19 and 35 days		5-HT$_1$:25%↓ 5-HT$_2$:NC	5-HT$_1$:25%↓ 5-HT$_2$: NC
Chan and Abel (1982)			
4–5 months	Total 5-HT: NC		
Druse et al. (in press)			
G19	5-HT$_{1A}$: 40%↓		
5 days	5-HT$_{1A}$: 25%↓		
19 days	5-HT$_{1A}$: > 25%↓		

TABLE III. Ethanol Effects on the Development of Components of the Serotonergic System in Brain Regions[a] (Continued)

		Noncortical regions				
		BS	CB	HT	CS	HC
5-HT and 5-HIAA						
Low ethanol dose						
Nelson et al. (1982)						
21 days	5-HT:	NC	NC	NC		
Higher ethanol dose						
Druse et al. (in press)						
G19	5-HT:	65%↓	20–30%↓			
	5-HIAA:	60%↓	20–30%↓			
5 days	5-HT:	40%↓	20–30%↓			
	5-HIAA:	30%↓				
Rathbun and Druse (1985)						
19 or 35 days	5-HT:	20%↓	20–30%↓	NC	NC	NC
19 or 35 days	5-HIAA:	20%↓	20–40%↓			
Receptors						
Chan and Abel (1982)						
4–5 months	5-HT:			NC	NC	

Abbreviations: 5-HT, 5 hydroxytryptamine (serotonin); 5-HIAA, 5 hydroxyindole acetic acid; G, gestation; NC, no change. Brain regions: CB, cerebellum; HT, hypothalamus; CS, corpus striatum; HC, hippocampus; BS, brain stem.
[a]Ethanol administered in drinking water is described as a low dose. Ethanol administration via liquid diets is considered a higher dose than that in drinking water. Please refer to the introduction to the text for additional information regarding this author's interpretation of reported data.

deficit of 5-HT uptake and 5-HT_1 binding sites. Apparently, the 5-HT_2 receptors, which are found on the neurons innervated by 5-HT-containing neurons, are unaffected by in utero ethanol exposure. Thus, the developing rat serotonergic system seems to be highly sensitive to in utero ethanol exposure. The deficiency of 5-HT or 5-HIAA is apparent very early in the development of both the brain stem (G15) and cortex (G19). A cortical 5-HT_{1A} receptor deficit is also found in neonatal rats.

DOPAMINE

The three major groups of dopamine-containing neurons include the nigrostriatal, mesocortical, and tuberohypophyseal neurons. The corpus striatum is densely innervated by neurons which originate in the substantia nigra. Less dense innervation is provided to the forebrain by neurons whose cell bodies are found medial to the substantia nigra. The areas so innervated include the frontal cortex, the cingulate cortex, the olfactory tubercle, the septal nuclei and the nucleus accumbens. The third group of dopamine-containing cell bodies are in the hypothalamus and these neurons innervate a portion of the pituitary and median eminence (reviewed by Weiner and Molinoff, 1989).

Dopamine is ultimately derived from the amino acid tyrosine. The enzyme tyrosine hydroxylase converts tyrosine to 3,4-dihdroxyphenylalanine (DOPA). DOPA is then converted to dopamine by the action of aromatic amino acid decarboxylase (AADC). In noradrenergic neurons, dopamine is converted to norepinephrine by dopamine β-hydroxylase.

The initial development of dopamine-containing cells in rat brain begins late in gestation. Dopamine-containing cells are found in the ventral prosencephalon on G13 and in the ventral mesencephalon on G14 (Voorn et al., 1988). Afferents to the striatum, anterior frontal cortex, and lateral neocortex are detected by G15–G17 (Verney et al., 1982; Kalsbeek et al., 1988; Voorn et al., 1988). By G21, the primordia of dopaminergic cell groups are found in the substantia nigra pars compacta and pars reticulata (Voorn et al., 1988). Dopaminergic fibers are found in the lateral frontal, prefrontal, and parietal cortex after birth (Verney et al., 1982; Kalsbeek et al., 1988).

Striatal dopamine content and dopamine uptake increase postnatally in rats until near adult levels are reached at 3–4 weeks of age (Coyle and Campochiaro, 1976; Noison and Thomas, 1988). Striatal dopamine D_1 receptors are first detected in late gestation (Bruinink et al., 1983a; Noison and Thomas, 1988) and rise to a peak at around 21 days postnatal (Murrin and Zeng, 1986; Zeng et al., 1988). Dopamine D_2 receptors also peak at approximately P21 (Zeng et al., 1988). The development of D_1 receptors does not depend on proliferation of dopaminergic nerve endings (Giorgi et al., 1987); in fact, it precedes terminal development (Murrin and Zeng, 1989).

The general consensus indicates that neither a low nor a high dose of ethanol during gestation produces a significant change in whole brain dopamine levels or dopamine uptake in young to 3-month-old rodents (Table IV) (Elis et al., 1976, 1978; Krsiak et al., 1977; Detering et al., 1980a; Slotkin et al., 1980; Mena et al., 1982, 1984; Nelson et al., 1982; Shoemaker et al., 1983). The findings in a study by Lucchi et al. (1983) disagree with the above studies. Lucchi et al. reported that dopamine D_2 receptors are decreased by 25% in 63-day-old rats exposed to a low ethanol dose (Lucchi et al., 1983).

Although there are conflicting findings on the effect of in utero ethanol exposure on whole brain dopamine content, it appears that exposure to a higher ethanol dose results in a dopamine or dopamine receptor deficiency in the hypothalamus and striatum, and possibly in the frontal cortex, in rats aged P18–P35 (Table V). At about 3 weeks of age, rats exposed to ethanol in utero had a significant deficiency (25–35%) of hypothalamic dopamine, a 25–45% deficiency of striatal dopamine (Detering et al., 1980a; Cooper and Rudeen, 1988), and more than a 20% decrease in striatal D_1 receptors (Druse et al., 1990). In contrast, striatal D_2 receptors were not significantly altered (Druse et al., 1990). Cortical dopamine and D_1 recep-

TABLE IV. Effects of In Utero Ethanol Exposure on
Dopamine Content and Uptake: Whole Brain Analyses[a]

Dopamine	
Low ethanol dose or short period of exposure	
Mena et al. (1982)	
G1, 1, and 4 days	NC
Nelson et al. (1982)	
0 days	NC–50%↓
Elis et al. (1976, 1978)	
3 months	NC
Krsiak et al. (1977)	
3 months	NC
High ethanol dose	
Detering et al. (1980a)	
G17, G19, 0 days	NC
Shoemaker et al. (1983)	
0 days	NC
Detering et al. (1980a)	
7, 14, and 21 days	NC
Dopamine uptake (higher ethanol dose)	
Slotkin et al. (1980)	
2–17 days	NC

Abbreviations: G, gestation; NC, no change.
[a]Please refer to the introduction to the text for additional information regarding this author's interpretation of reported data. Low dose is ethanol administered in drinking water. A higher dose is ethanol administered via liquid diets.

tors were also transiently affected by early exposure to ethanol (Rathbun and Druse, 1985; Druse et al., 1990).

Our laboratory's recent observation of a dopamine deficiency in the brain stem and cortex of 5-day-old ethanol-exposed rats (Druse et al., 1991) could be quite important. A marked dopamine deficiency at 5 days of age indicates that the early development of the dopaminergic system is markedly impaired by in utero ethanol exposure. Specifically, it appears that the development of the dopamine-containing cell bodies, generally located in brain stem structures, is impaired by ethanol exposure. A permanent reduction in the number of dopamine-containing neurons could explain alterations in dopaminergic projections to the hypothalamus, striatum, and cortex. Furthermore, since dopamine appears to play the role of a growth regulator in neuronal differentiation via its action on the embryonic D_1 receptor (Lankford et al., 1987, 1988) and on neurite elongation (McCobb et al., 1988), an early dopamine deficiency could contribute to the abnormal dopaminergic development. From brain region studies it appears that portions of the major dopaminergic projection systems (projection and/or cell body) are affected by in utero exposure to ethanol.

TABLE V. Ethanol Effects on the Developing Dopaminergic System[a]

Dopamine content	Brain regions				
	CX	CS	DI	BS	HT
Low ethanol dose					
Mena et al. (1984)					
15 days	NC	NC	NC		
Higher ethanol dose					
Druse et al. (1990)					
5 days	30%↓			40%↓	
Rathbun and Druse (1985)					
19 days	NC	NC		NC	NC
Druse et al. (1990)					
19 days		45%↓			25%↓
Detering et al. (1980a)					
21 days		25%↓			35%↓
Cooper and Rudeen (1988)					
18 days	NC				30%↓
Rathbun and Druse (1985)					
35 days	80%↓	NC		NC	NC
Druse et al. (1990)					
35 days		NC			
Low ethanol dose					
Mena et al. (1984)					
15 days				NC	
Dopamine receptors					
Lower ethanol dose					
Lucchi et al. (1983)					
63 days D_2		25%↓			
Higher ethanol dose					
Druse et al. (1990)					
19 days D_1	NC	20%↓			
35 days D_1	40%↓	20%↓			
Druse et al. (1990)					
19 and 35 days D_2		NC			
Dopamine uptake					
Higher ethanol dose					
Druse et al. (1990)	NC	25%↓			

Abbreviations: G, gestation; NC, no change; brain regions: CX, cortex; CS, corpus striatum; DI, diencephalon; BS, brain stem; HT, hypothalamus.

[a]Ethanol in drinking water is described as a low dose. Ethanol administered via liquid diets is described as a higher dose. Please refer to the introduction to the text for additional information regarding this author's interpretation of reported data.

**TABLE VI. Effects of Ethanol on Norepinephrine in
Developing Brain Whole Brain Norepinephrine Content[a]**

Low ethanol dose or short period of exposure	
Mena et al. (1982)	
G21, 1 day	10–25%↑
4 days	NC
Nelson et al. (1982)	
0 days	NC–25%↓
Elis et al. (1976, 1978)	
3 months	NC
Krsiak et al. (1977)	
3 months	NC
Higher ethanol dose or long period of exposure	
Rawat (1977)	
G17–G19	NC
Detering et al. (1980a)	
G19, 0, 7 days	30–35%↓
Shoemaker et al. (1980)	
0 days	10%↓
Rawat (1977)	
5–10 days	NC
Detering et al. (1980a)	
14 days	NC
21 days	20%↓

Abbreviations: G, gestation; NC, no change.
[a]Ethanol in drinking water is described as a low dose. Ethanol administered via liquid diets is described as a higher dose. Please refer to the introduction to the text for additional information regarding this author's interpretation of reported data.

There is additional evidence that in utero ethanol exposure impairs the development of striatal dopamine-containing neurons and possibly the targets of the dopaminergic neurons. Evidence of a deficiency of presynaptic components of striatal dopaminergic projections is provided by the studies described above and evidence of decreased striatal DOPA synthesis (Hard et al., 1985a, b) and dopamine uptake at 35 days (Druse et al., 1990).

In summary, in utero exposure to a low ethanol dose appears to have little effect on whole brain dopamine content in postnatal rats. In contrast, either dopamine content, dopamine uptake, or dopamine receptors are decreased in the striatum, hypothalamus, or frontal cortex of postnatal rats. Consequently, it appears that in utero exposure to a higher ethanol dose adversely affects the development of certain components of the dopaminergic system.

NOREPINEPHRINE

The noradrenergic system is another CNS projection system, which has cell bodies in the midbrain, pons, and medulla. Projections are sent from

TABLE VII. Effects of Ethanol on Norepinephrine in Brain Regions of
Developing Rats[a]

Low ethanol dose	L	CS	CX/H	DI	BS
Mena et al. (1984)					
15 days	NC–20%↑	NC	30%↑	25%↑	10–20↑
Nelson et al. (1982)					
21 days			NC		NC
Higher ethanol dose	SA	CX/H	DI	CB	HT
Cooper and Rudeen (1988)					
18 days	25%↓	NC	NC	NC	NC
	Th	CS	BS		
Detering et al. (1980a, 1981)					
21 days	NC	25%↓	40–60%↓		
26 weeks			20–25%↓		

Abbreviations: NC, no change. Brain regions: L, limbic system; CS, corpus striatum; CX, cortex; H, cerebral hemisphere; DI, diencephalon; BS, brain stem; SA, septal area; CB, cerebellum; HT, hypothalamus; Th, thalamus.
[a]Ethanol in drinking water is described as a low dose. Ethanol administered via liquid diets is described as a higher dose. Please refer to the introduction to the text for additional information regarding this author's interpretation of reported data.

the locus coeruleus to the spinal cord, cerebellum, cerebral cortex, and hippocampus. Additional populations of neurons project to the hypothalamus and brain stem (reviewed by Weiner and Molinoff, 1989). Several reports indicate that norepinephrine (NE) may modulate the development of neurons and glia during embryonic or fetal development (e.g., Felten et al., 1982; Chumasov et al., 1984; reviewed by Lauder and Krebs, 1984).

In the rat, locus coeruleus neurons cease dividing by G11–G13 (Lauder and Bloom, 1974). NE synthesis can be detected by G13. Superficial cortical fibers and cortical NE can be found by G13–G14 (Elias et al., 1982). Noradrenergic innervation of the cortex is present in all regions by birth; the adult innervation pattern and density are established by P6–P7 (Lidov et al., 1978; Levitt and Moore, 1979). Nonetheless, levels of NE and tyrosine hydroxylase increase until 42–52 days (Johnston and Coyle, 1980; Storm and Fechter, 1985), although the NE peak in cerebellum occurs 1–2 weeks earlier (Storm and Fechter, 1985).

The results of studies of early exposure to a low dose of ethanol on whole brain or brain region NE in neonatal or older rats have been inconsistent (Tables VI and VII) (Elis et al., 1976, 1978; Krsiak et al., 1977; Mena et al., 1982, 1984; Nelson et al., 1982). Although Rawat (1977) demonstrated no change in whole brain NE content in rats exposed to the higher ethanol dose, other comparable studies found a deficiency of brain NE (Detering et al., 1980a, b; 1981; Shoemaker et al., 1983). Those brain areas particularly affected by in utero ethanol exposure include the septal area (Cooper and Rudeen, 1988), the hypothalamus, and the striatum (Detering et al., 1980a, 1981). In fact, hypothalamic NE remained decreased for as long as 26 weeks (Detering et al., 1981). Evidence of decreased NE content and turnover in the hypothalamus is reportedly indicative of impaired development of noradrenergic neurons (Detering et al., 1980c). Consequently, it appears that development of the noradrenergic system in the striatum, septal area, and particularly in the hypothalamus of postnatal rats is significantly affected by in utero exposure to a higher ethanol dose.

ACETYLCHOLINE

Acetylcholine is formed from choline and acetyl coenzyme A in a reaction catalyzed by the enzyme choline acetyltransferase (ChAT). Although ChAT activity is localized in neurons where acetylcholine synthesis occurs, the enzyme involved with acetylcholine (ACh) degradation, acetyl-cholinesterase (AChE), is found both in cholinergic neurons and in cholinoceptive sites. Cholinergic neurons also have a high affinity choline uptake system (reviewed by Taylor and Brown, 1989).

In rodents, the levels of several components of the cholinergic system are low during the first postnatal week. For example, striatal ChAT activity is low in the newborn rat (Coyle and Campochiaro, 1976) and is first detected in mouse forebrain on P6 (Hohmann and Ebner, 1985). In addition, neonatal striatal ACh is 23% of that in the adult rat and there is little striatal high affinity choline uptake until P10–P15 (Coyle and Yamamura, 1976). However, the cholinergic system develops rapidly in the rat CNS during the first few postnatal weeks. Striatal ChAT activity, ACh content, and high affinity choline uptake reach near-adult levels by 0–4 weeks. Adult cerebellar ChAT is found by 7 weeks (Coyle and Campochiaro, 1976; Coyle and Yamamura, 1976; Johnston and Coyle, 1980; Hohmann and Ebner, 1985; Clos et al., 1989; Represa et al., 1989). Binding sites for quinuclidinyl benzilate (QNB), which labels muscarinic cholinergic receptors, reach peak levels in the hippocampal CA1 and CA3 regions by 2 weeks, and in the fascia dentata and cerebellum by 3 weeks (Mallol et al., 1984; Represa et. al., 1989).

There are limited reports of the effects of ethanol on the developing cholinergic system (Table VIII). These studies indicate that the development of select brain cholinergic components is transiently affected by in utero ethanol exposure. Although whole brain ACh is not significantly changed in young (G17–P10) ethanol-exposed rats (Rawat, 1977), there is a transient increase in cortical muscarinic receptors. The increase in cortical QNB receptors is found at 8 days, but not at 20 days (Serbus et al., 1986) or at 4–5 months (Chan and Abel, 1982).

Most studies of the effects of in utero ethanol exposure on neurotransmitters are limited either to male animals or to mixed sexes. However, one study that examined ethanol effects on male and female rats found that cortical activity of AChE and ChAT was unchanged in both male and female rats at 20 days of age (Light et al., 1989). In contrast, the normal

TABLE VIII. Effects of Ethanol on the Development
of the Cholinergic System

	CX	CS	Th/HT
Brain acetylcholine			
Rawat (1977)			
G17, G20, 5, and 10 days	25–35%↓		
Brain region acetylcholine receptors (QNB)			
Chan and Abel (1982)			
4–5 months	NC	NC	NC
Serbus et al. (1986)			
8 days	40%↑		
20 days	NC		
Brain region acetylcholine enzymes			
Light (1989)			
AChE: 20 days	NC	loss of gender-based difference	
ChAT: 20 days	NC	NC	

Abbreviations: G, gestation; NC, no change. AChE, acetylcholine esterase; ChAT, choline acetyltransferase; QNB, quinuclidinyl benzilate; CX, cortex; CS, corpus striatum; Th, thalamus; HT, hypothalamus.
[a]Ethanol in drinking water is described as a low dose. Ethanol administered via liquid diets is described as a higher dose. Please refer to the introduction to the text for additional information regarding this author's interpretation of reported data.

gender difference in striatal AChE activity in 20-day-old rats is lost in the ethanol-exposed group.

GLUTAMATE

Glutamate is an acidic amino acid that has a CNS concentration hundreds to thousands of times higher than that of any of the monoamines. Although glutamate is found in many brain areas, the most widely accepted glutamate pathways are descending pathways, which originate in hippocampal pyramidal and cortical cells (reviewed by McGeer and McGeer, 1989).

In comparison with the monoamines, there are presently only a limited number of studies that have examined the effects of ethanol exposure on glutamate concentration in the CNS. Although studies of glutamate concentration have produced conflicting findings (Table IX), the results of analysis of glutamate receptors are relatively consistent. Early exposure to ethanol results in a transient decrease of [3H]-glutamate binding sites in whole brain and in the hippocampus (Kelly et al., 1986; Farr et al., 1988). However, cortical [3H]-glutamate binding sites are not decreased (Kelly et

TABLE IX. Effects of Ethanol on CNS Glutamate
and Glutamate Receptors[a]

Glutamate concentration in brain	
Griezerstein (1983)	
G19	15%↓
Rawat (1977)	
G19–10 days	20–50%↑
Glutamate receptors	
Brain [³H]-glutamate binding sites	
Kelly (1986)	
14 days	NC
17 days	50%↓
20 and 26 days	NC
Cortical glutamate binding sites	
Kelly (1986)	
20 days	40%↑
Hippocampal glutamate binding sites	
Farr (1988)	
5 days	50%↓
NMDA sites	
Savage (1989)	
45 days	Decreased NMDA binding sites in the dentate gyrus, HC CA1, and subiculum of dorsal HC formation; NC in ventral HC, CB, lateral entorhinal CX, and posterior neoCX
Morrissett (1989)	
45 days	Decreased electrophysiological response of HC CA1 to NMDA
Martin (1989)	
45 days	Abnormal response to NMDA in HC CA1
Vinylidine kainic acid sites	
Farr (1989)	
45 days	Decreased vinylidine kainic acid sites in entorhinal CX, ventral HC CA3, and stratum lucidum; NC in dorsal HC CA3, stratum lucidum, and CB

Abbreviations: G, gestation; NC, no change; NMDA, N-methyl-D-aspartate; HC, hippocampus; CB, cerebellum; CX, cortex.

[a]Ethanol in drinking water is described as a low dose. Ethanol administered via liquid diets is described as a higher dose. Please refer to the introduction to the text for additional information regarding this author's interpretation of reported data.

al., 1986). Savage and colleagues have shown regional specificity of the hippocampal glutamate binding site abnormalities. They have demonstrated that in utero ethanol exposure results in a decreased number of the N-methyl-D-aspartate (NMDA) subtype of glutamate receptors in the dentate gyrus, hippocampal CA1 region, and subiculum of the dorsal hippocampal formation, and an abnormal response of the hippocampal CA1 region to NMDA (Farr et al., 1988; Savage, personal communication; Martin et al., 1989; Morrisett et al., 1989). In contrast, they found that the NMDA binding sites are not significantly changed in similar regions of the ventral hippocampal formation, nor in the cerebellum, lateral entorhinal cortex, or posterior neocortex (Savage, personal communication). In addition to abnormalities in NMDA-sensitive glutamate receptors, Savage and colleagues have found a significant deficiency of the kainate-sensitive receptor subtype of glutamate receptors in the entorhinal cortex and in the ventral hippocampal CA3 stratum lucidum of 45-day-old offspring of rats that consumed a 3.35% ethanol-containing liquid diet during pregnancy (Farr et al., 1989). No significant differences are found in vinylidene kainic acid sites in the same regions from offspring of rats that consumed a diet containing 6.7% (v/v) ethanol.

OTHER NEUROTRANSMITTERS

At this time there is a paucity of studies on the effects of early ethanol exposure on other neurotransmitter systems. Those neurotransmitters which have been studied include gamma-aminobutyric acid (GABA), glycine, and histamine (Table X). It has been reported that early ethanol exposure has little effect on whole brain GABA concentration (Mena et al., 1982; Espina et al., 1989) or on the concentration of GABA in the striatum and amygdaloid cortex (Moloney and Leonard, 1983). However, both glycine and histamine appear sensitive to the effects of early ethanol exposure. Specifically, there is a 30% deficiency of brain glycine in ethanol-exposed rats on G19 (Griezerstein and Aldrich, 1983). In addition, Rawat (1980) reports no significant differences in brain histamine in rats from G17–P120. In contrast, there appears to be a 40–80% deficiency of cerebellar histamine receptors (Serbus et al., 1986).

SUMMARY

The development of several neurotransmitter systems is markedly impaired by in utero ethanol exposure. The affected systems are those that use 5-HT, dopamine, NE, glutamate, ACh, and histamine as neurotransmitters. There are interesting similarities in the effects of in utero ethanol exposure on the developing monoamine systems in postnatal animals. Administration of an amount of ethanol expected to produce low blood alcohol levels had little effect on whole brain levels of NE, dopamine, or 5-HT. In contrast, administration of a higher ethanol dose (e.g., that obtained from ethanol-containing liquid diets) or a moderate ethanol dose for a longer time period produced a significant CNS deficiency of the three neurotransmitters. 5-HT and dopamine synthesis and uptake were also decreased. In

TABLE X. Effects of Ethanol on Other Developing
Neurotransmitter Systems

Glycine		
	Brain	
Griezerstein and Aldrich (1983)		
G19	30%↓	
Histamine		
	Brain	
Rawat (1980)		
G17, 10, and 120 days	NC	
Histamine receptors		
	Cerebellum	
Serbus et al. (1986)		
8 and 20 days	40–80%↓	
GABA		
	Brain	
Rawat (1977)		
G17, G19, 5, and 10 days	20-250%↑	
Mena et al. (1982)		
G21, 1, and 4 days	NC	
Espina et al. (1989)		
7–28 days	NC	
Brain region GABA		
	Amygdaloid cortex	Corpus striatum
Moloney and Leonard (1983)		
21 days	Near normal	Near normal

Abbreviations: G, gestation; NC, no change; GABA, gamma-aminobutyric acid.
[a]Please refer to the introduction to the text for additional information regarding this author's interpretation of reported data. Low dose is ethanol administered in drinking water. A higher dose is ethanol administered via liquid diets.

addition, there were low levels of NE turnover. Regional studies localized monoamine deficiencies to brain areas that normally contain either the terminals of the major projections or the neuronal cell bodies.

In the cases of 5-HT and dopamine, the neurotransmitter deficiencies were found in embryonic/neonatal rats as well as in the older rats mentioned above. Given the reported role of these two neurotransmitters as embryonic trophic factors involved with the development of their own systems (5-HT and dopamine effects) and other neurotransmitter systems (5-HT effects) (Lauder and Krebs, 1978, 1984; Chumasov et al., 1980; Lauder et al., 1983, 1985; Haydon et al., 1984, 1987; Chubakov et al., 1986; Lankford et al., 1987, 1988; Whitaker-Azmitia and Azmitia, 1986; Whitaker-Azmitia et al., 1987), an early deficit may contribute to the abnormal development of one or more neurotransmitter systems. Future analysis of embryonic and neonatal NE levels are needed to determine if a third neurotransmitter trophic factor (Felten et al., 1982; Chumasov et al., 1984; and reviewed by Lauder and Krebs, 1984) is also deficient in embryonic animals exposed to ethanol in utero.

Besides adversely affecting the development of the catecholamine and indoleamine systems, in utero ethanol exposure alters the development of the neurons containing glutamate, ACh, and histamine. Of the neurotransmitter systems reviewed here, the only one for which development is reportedly minimally affected by ethanol is that containing GABA, and comprehensive studies of GABA have not yet been performed.

Although the precise mechanism(s) by which in utero ethanol exposure is able to adversely affect the development of several neurotransmitter systems is unknown, there are several potential explanations.

1. The development of some of the embryonic cell bodies containing the affected neurotransmitters may be damaged or destroyed as a consequence of in utero ethanol exposure. Consistent with this hypothesis, ethanol appears to be toxic to developing astrocytes (Kennedy and Mukerji, 1986a, b) and neurites (Dow and Riopelle, 1985). Alternatively, transient anoxia (e.g., produced by ethanol-induced placental constriction) (Altura et al., 1983; Savoy-Moore et al., 1989) could permanently damage developing neural cells. Destruction of a portion of the developing cell bodies would ultimately result in fewer cell bodies and hence, fewer projections from these cell bodies. Thus, there would be a reduction in components associated with terminals of these projections, such as neurotransmitter, uptake sites, synthetic enzymes, and presynaptic receptors. Such observations have been made in studies of the serotonergic and dopaminergic systems and, to a lesser extent, with the noradrenergic system.

2. Ethanol, an ethanol metabolite, or ethanol-induced alterations in the levels of another factor (e.g., hormone or second messenger) may result in abnormal levels of one or more embryonic neurotrophic factors. Relevant to this hypothesis, the levels of the neurotransmitter-neurotrophic factors, 5-HT and dopamine, are decreased in embryonic/neonatal brain (Druse et al., in press). Furthermore, our recent studies showed that the number of cortical 5-HT_{1A} receptors are low in rat neonates. Because fetal serotonin is involved with the development of serotonergic neurons and their targets as well as normal CNS development (Lauder and Krebs, 1978, 1984; Lauder et al., 1983; Whitaker-Azmitia and Azmitia, 1986; Whitaker-Azmitia et al., 1987), an embryonic deficiency of 5-HT and/or 5-HT_{1A} receptors may adversely affect the development of several neurotransmitter systems. Likewise, an embryonic deficiency of dopamine may adversely affect dopaminergic development. Additional embryonic neurotransmitter-neurotrophic factors may also be affected by in utero ethanol exposure.

3. Considering that the affected neurotransmitter systems are largely projection systems, it is possible that ethanol interferes with the ability of neurons to project to target areas. This could happen if in utero ethanol exposure either directly or indirectly interferes with the epigenetic regulation of molecules involved with the guidance of projections to the target

areas. Such factors could include chemotactic factors, cellular adhesion molecules (CAMs) on neurons or glia, and components of the extracellular matrix (substrate adhesion molecules, SAMs). These adhesion and guidance molecules are essential to normal fetal/embryonic neural development (Edelman and Crossin, 1988). An alteration in the levels of these molecules could also interfere with an earlier step—neuronal migration. Anatomical studies suggest that neuronal migration is delayed by in utero ethanol exposure (Miller, 1986). In addition, the pattern of neurite outgrowth and functional characteristics of neurons depend on the substrate on which the neurons grow (Chiquet and Acklin, 1986; Chiquet and Nicholls, 1987; Ross et al., 1988). Thus, interference with the normal pattern of expression of genes coding for one or more guidance or adhesion molecules could seriously impair normal CNS development. An abnormality in one SAM or CAM could impact on many neurotransmitter systems. Abnormal expression of the genes for several SAMs and/or CAMs might well have devastating effects on CNS development.

Of these three possible mechanisms, the first involves a potential neurotoxicity of ethanol or related compound, while the latter two imply that ethanol may directly or indirectly interfere with the expression of one or more genes. Interference with normal gene expression might happen in several ways. 1) Ethanol may alter levels of the second messengers $3',5'$-cyclic AMP (cAMP) or diacylgylcerol, which are both involved with the regulation of gene transcription via their action on transcription factors (Montminy et al., 1986; Angel et al., 1987). An alteration in their levels could affect the transcription of certain responsive genes. One such cAMP-regulated gene is tyrosine hydroxylase (Lewis et al., 1983), the rate limiting enzyme in the synthesis of two of the affected neurotransmitters—dopamine and NE. An ethanol-induced alteration in the levels of second messengers in fetal brain is plausible because of evidence of altered responsiveness of adenylate cyclase to prostaglandin PGE_2 in embryonic chick brain (Pennington, 1988; see also Chapter 9). Furthermore, there are alterations in cAMP and the binding of cAMP by the regulatory subunit (R_{II}) of protein kinase (Beeker et al., 1988). In addition, chronic ethanol exposure causes a decrease in the stimulation of cAMP formation and phosphoinositide turnover (which yields diacylglycerol) in mature animals (Lucchi et al., 1983a, b; Gordon et al., 1986; Hoffman et al., 1986). 2) Ethanol exposure has been shown to alter the levels of both glucocorticoids and thyroid hormones (reviewed by Weinberg et al; 1986; Hannigan et al., 1989; Weinberg, 1989). Altered levels of either of these hormones could directly alter the expression of cortisol- or thyroid hormone-specific genes. 3) It is possible that ethanol is converted to another compound, for which there is a specific nuclear binding site, involved in the regulation of gene transcription. At present, the latter scenerio is purely speculative.

Other factors may also contribute to the abnormalities found in several neurotransmitter systems in animal models of FAS. For example, chronic ethanol exposure is known to result in decreased voltage-dependent calcium uptake by synaptosomes (Harris and Hood, 1980; Leslie et al., 1983). Both calcium and AMP reportedly regulate the outgrowth of neurites from specific neurons (Mattson and Kater, 1987; Mattson et al., 1988). In addition, undernourishment of the CNS could produce numerous generalized CNS abnormalities. Although most researchers pair-feed animals, placental transfer of nutrients may be altered by ethanol exposure (examples in Fisher et al., 1981, 1985; Henderson et al., 1981). Finally, several laboratories hypothesize that the levels of certain prostaglandins may be increased by in utero ethanol exposure (Pennington et al., 1981, 1985; Randall et al., 1987). Since prostaglandins are hormonal mediators in many cell types, altered levels of these compounds could impact on several neurotransmitter systems.

If there were a single hormone or factor which was generally necessary for the differentiation, migration, or maturation of many or all neurons, then a single mechanism could be proposed. Such an important factor could be involved with the epigenetic regulation of multiple genes in different neurons and brain areas. Thus, the varied effects of ethanol on multiple neurotransmitter systems in one or more brain regions may be explained by the timing of the development of such regions or systems. Alternatively, it is possible that ethanol interferes with the expression of a number of genes, the products of which affect several neurotransmitter systems.

However, it is also possible that ethanol and/or an ethanol metabolite may have multiple actions, including neurotoxicity, altered epigenetic regulation of CAMs or SAMs, altered synthesis of hormones, prostaglandins, neurotransmitter-neurotrophic factors, and chemotactic factors. The future beckons us to elucidate the primary mechanisms underlying the devastating effects of ethanol on the developing CNS, and to determine whether pharmacological manipulations of key hormones, neurotransmitters, or second messengers can protect against or reverse the adverse effects of ethanol on the developing CNS.

REFERENCES

Aitken AR, Tork I (1988): Early development of serotonin-containing neurons and pathways as seen in wholemount preparations of the fetal rat brain. J Comp Neurol 274:32–47.

Altura BM, Altura BT, Carella A, Chatterjee M, Halvey S, Tejani N (1983): Alcohol produces spasms of human umbilical blood vessels: Relationship to fetal alcohol syndrome (FAS). Eur J Pharmacol 86:311–312.

Angel P, Imagawa M, Chiu R, Stein B, Imbra RJ, Rahmsdorf HJ, Jonst C, Herrlich P, Karin M (1987): Phorbol ester-inducible genes contain a common cis element recognized by a TPA-modulated trans-acting factor. Cell 49:729–739.

Azmitia EC, DeKloet ER (1987): ACTH neuropeptide stimulation of serotonergic neuronal maturation in tissue culture: Modulation by hippocampal cells. Prog Brain Res 72:311–318.

Beeker K, Deane D, Elton C, Pennington S (1988): Ethanol-induced growth inhibition in embryonic chick brain is associated with changes in cytoplasmic cyclic-AMP-dependent protein kinase regulatory subunit. Alcohol Alcohol 23:477–482.

Blurton PA, Wood MD (1986): Identification of multiple binding sites for [³H]-5-hydroxytryptamine in the rat CNS. J Neurochem 46:1392–1398.

Boggan WO, Randall CL, Wilson-Burrows C, Parker LS (1979): Effect of prenatal ethanol on brain serotonergic systems. Trans Am Soc Neurochem 10:186.

Bruinink A, Lichtensteiger W, Schlumpf M (1983a): Pre- and postnatal ontogeny and characterization of dopaminergic D₂, serotonergic S₂, and spirodecanone binding sites in rat forebrain. J Neurochem 40:1227–1236.

Bruinink A, Lichtensteiger W, Schlumpf M (1983b): Ontogeny of diurnal rhythms of central dopamine, serotonin and spirodecanone binding sites and of motor activity in the rat. Life Sci 33:31–38.

Chan AWK, Able EL (1982): Absence of long-lasting effects on brain receptors for neurotransmitters in rats prenatally exposed to alcohol. Res Commun Subst Abuse 3:219–224.

Chiquet M, Acklin SE (1986): Attachment to Con A or extracellular matrix initiates rapid sprouting by cultured leech neurons. Proc Natl Acad Sci USA 83:6188–6192.

Chiquet M, Nicholls JG (1987): Neurite outgrowth and synapse formation by identified leech neurons. J Exp Biol 132:191–206.

Chubakov AR, Gromova EA, Konovalov GV, Sarkisova EF, Chumasov EI (1986): The effects of serotonin on the morpho-functional development of rat cerebral neocortex in tissue culture. Brain Res 369:285–297.

Chumasov EI, Chubakov AR, Konovalov GV, Gromova EA (1980): Effect of serotonin on growth and differentiation of hippocampal cells in culture. Neurosci Behav Physiol 10:125–131.

Chumasov EI, Chubakov AR, Konovalov GV, Gromova EA (1984): Effect of noradrenaline on growth and differentiation of explanted rat hippocampal cells Neurosci Behav Physiol 11.7–14.

Clarren SK, Smith DW (1978): The fetal alcohol syndrome. N Engl J Med 298:1063–1067.

Clos J, Ghandour S, Eberhart R, Vincendon G, Gombos G (1989): The cholinergic system in developing cerebellum: Comparative study of normal, hypothyroid and underfed rats. Dev. Neurosci. 11:188–204.

Cooper JD, Rudeen PK (1988): Alterations in regional catecholamine content and turnover in the male rat brain in response to in utero ethanol exposure. Alcohol Clin Exp Res 12:282–285.

Coyle JT, Campochiaro P (1976): Ontogenesis of dopaminergic-cholinergic interactions in the rat striatum: A neurochemical study. J Neurochem 27:673–678.

Coyle JT, Yamamura HI (1976): Neurochemical aspects of the ontogenesis of cholinergic neurons in the rat brain. Brain Res 118:429–440.

Detering N, Collins R, Hawkins RL, Ozand PT, Karahasan AM (1980a): The effects of ethanol on developing catecholamine neurons. Adv Exp Med Biol 132:721–727.

Detering N, Collins RM, Hawkins RL, Ozand PT, Karahasan A (1980b): Comparative effects of ethanol and malnutrition on the development of catecholamine neurons: Changes in neurotransmitter levels. J Neurochem 34:1587–1593.

Detering N, Collins RM, Hawkins RL, Ozand PT, Karahasan A (1980c): Comparative effects of ethanol and malnutrition on the development of catecholamine neurons: Changes in norepinephrine turnover. J Neurochem 34:1788–1791.

Detering N, Collins RM, Hawkins RL, Ozand PT, Karahasan A (1981): Comparative effects of ethanol and malnutrition on the development of catecholamine neurons: A long lasting effect in the hypothalamus. J Neurochem 36:2094–2096.

Detering N, Edwards E, Ozand P, Karahasan A (1980d): Comparative effects of ethanol and malnutrition on the development of catecholamine neurons: Changes in specific activities of enzymes. J Neurochem 34:297–304.

Dow KE, Riopelle RJ (1985): Ethanol neurotoxicity: Effects on neurite formation and neurotrophic factor production in vitro. Science 228:591–593.

Druse MJ, Paul LH (1989): Effects of in utero ethanol exposure on serotonin uptake in cortical regions. Alcohol 5:455–459.

Druse MJ, Tajuddin N, Kuo AP, Connerty M (1990): Effects of in utero ethanol exposure on the developing dopaminergic system in rats. J Neurosci Res 27:233–240.

Druse MJ, Kuo A, Tajuddin N (in press): Effects of in utero ethanol exposure on the developing serotonergic system. Alcoholism: Clin Exp Res.

Edelman GM, Crossin KL (1988): The molecular regulation of neural morphogenesis. In Easter SS, Barald KF, Carlson BM (eds): "From Message to Mind." Sunderland, Ma: Sinauer Assoc., Inc., pp 4–22.

Elias M, Deacon T, Caviness VS (1982): The development of neocortical noradrenergic innervation in the mouse: A quantitative radioenzymatic analysis. Dev Brain Res 3:652–656.

Elis J, Krsiak M, Poschlova N (1978): Effect of alcohol given at different periods of gestation on brain serotonin in offspring. Act Nerv Super (Praha) 20:287–288.

Elis J, Krsiak M, Poschlova N, Masek K (1976): The effect of alcohol administration during pregnancy on the concentration of noradrenaline, dopamine and 5-hydroxytryptamine in the brain of offspring of mice. Act Nerv Super (Praha) 18:220–221.

Espina N, Hannigan JH, Martin DL (1989): Neuroactive amino acid levels following prenatal exposure to ethanol. Alcoholism: Clin Exp Res 13:319.

Farr KL, Montano CY, Paxton LL, Savage DD (1988): Prenatal ethanol exposure decreases hippocampal ^{3}H-glutamate binding in 45-day-old rats. Alcohol 5:125–133.

Farr KL, Montano CY, Paxton LL, Savage DD (1989): Prenatal ethanol exposure decreases hippocampal ^{3}H-vinylidene kainic acid binding in 45-day-old rats. Neurotoxicol Teratol 10:563–568.

Felton DL, Hallman H, Jonsson G (1982): Evidence for a neurotrophic role of noradrenaline neurons in the postnatal development of rat cerebral cortex. J Neurocytol 11:119–135.

Fisher SE, Atkinson M, Van Thiel DH, Rosenblum E, Holzman DR (1981): Selective fetal malnutrition: Effect of ethanol and acetaldehyde upon in vitro uptake of alpha-aminoisobutyric acid by human placenta. Life Sci 29:1283–1288.

Fisher SM, Inselman LS, Duffy L, Atkinson M, Spencer H, Chang B (1985): Ethanol and fetal nutrition: Effect of chronic ethanol exposure on rat placental growth and membrane-associated folic acid receptor binding activity. J Pediatr Gastroenterol Nutr 4:645–649.

Gilliam DM, Kotch LE, Dudek BC, Riley EP (1988): Ethanol teratogenesis in mice selected for differences in alcohol sensitivity. Alcohol 5:513–519.

Giorgi O, DeMontis G, Porceddu ML, Mele S, Calderini G, Toffano G, Biggio G (1987): Developmental and age-related changes in D_1-dopamine receptors and dopamine content in the rat striatum. Dev Brain Res 35:283–290.

Gordon AS, Collier K, Diamond I (1986): Ethanol regulation of adenosine receptor-stimulated cAMP levels in a clonal neural cell line: An in vitro model of cellular tolerance to ethanol. Proc Natl Acad Sci USA 83:2105–2108.

Green JP (1989): Histamine and serotonin. In Siegel G, Agranoff B, Albers RW, Molinoff P (eds): "Basic Neurochemistry, 4th Edition." New York: Raven Press, pp 253–269.

Griezerstein HB, Aldrich LK (1983): Ethanol and diazepam effects on intrauterine growth of the rat. Dev Pharmacol Ther 6:409–418.

Hannigan J, Bellasario R, Nalwalk J (1989): Reduced serum thyroxine (T_4) in young rats exposed to ethanol in utero. Alcohol 13:324.

Hard E, Engel J, Larsson K, Liljequist S, Musi B (1985a): Effects of maternal ethanol consumption in the offspring sensory-motor development, ultrasonic vocalization, audiogenic immobility reaction and brain monoamine synthesis. Acta Pharmacol Toxicol 56:354–363.

Hard E, Musi B, Dahlgren IL, Engel J, Larsson K, Liljequist S, Lindh AS (1985b): Impaired maternal behaviour and altered central serotonergic activity in the adult offspring of chronically ethanol treated dams. Acta Pharmacol Toxicol 56:347–353.

Harris RA, Hood WF (1980): Inhibition of synapto-calcium uptake by ethanol. J Pharmacol Exp Ther 213:562–568.

Haydon PG, McCobb DP, Kater SB (1984): Serotonin selectively inhibits growth cone motility and synaptogenesis of specific identified neurons. Science 236:561–564.

Haydon PG, McCobb DP, Kater SB (1987): The regulation of neurite outgrowth, growth cone motility, and electrical synaptogenesis by serotonin. J Neurobiol 18:197–215.

Henderson GI, Turner D, Patwardhan RV, Lumeng L, Hoyumpa AM, Schenker S (1981): Inhibition of placental valine uptake following acute and chronic maternal ethanol consumption. J Pharmacol Exp Ther 216:465–472.

Hoffman PL, Moses F, Luther GR, Tabakoff B (1986): Acute and chronic effects of ethanol on receptor mediated phosphatidylinositol 4,5-bisphosphate breakdown in mouse brain. Mol Pharmacol 30:13–18.

Hohmann CF, Ebner FF (1985): Development of cholinergic markers in mouse forebrain. I. choline acetyltransferase enzyme activity and acetylcholinesterase histochemistry. Dev Brain Res 23:225–241.

Johnston MV, Coyle JT (1980): Ontogeny of neurochemical markers for noradrenergic, GABAergic and cholinergic neurons in neocortex lesioned with methylazoxymethanol acetate. J Neurochem 34:1429–1441.

Kalsbeek A, Voorn P, Buijs RM, Pool CW, Uylings HBM (1988): Development of the dopaminergic innervation in the prefrontal cortex of the rat. Comp Neurol 269:58–72.

Kelly GM, Druse MJ, Tonetti DA, Oden BG (1986): Maternal ethanol consumption: Binding of L-glutamate to synaptic membranes from whole brain, cortices, and cerebella of offspring. Exp Neurol 91:219–228.

Kennedy LA, Mukerji S (1986a): Ethanol neurotoxicity. 1. Direct effect on replicating astrocytes. Neurobehav Toxicol Teratol 8:11–15.

Kennedy LA, Mukerji S (1986b): Ethanol neurotoxicity. 2. Direct effects on differentiating astrocytes. Neurobehav Toxicol Teratol 8:17–21.

Krsiak M, Elis J, Poschlova N, Masek K (1977): Increased aggressiveness and lower brain serotonin levels in the offspring of mice given alcohol during gestation. J Stud Alcohol 38:1696–1704.

Lankford K, DeMello FG, Klein WL (1987): A transient embryonic dopamine receptor inhibits growth cone motility and neurite outgrowth in a subset of avian retina neurons. Neurochem Lett 75:169–174.

Lankford KL, DeMello FG, Klein WL (1988): D_1-type dopamine receptors inhibit growth cone motility in cultured retina neurons: Evidence that neurotransmitters act as morphogenic growth regulators in the developing central nervous system. Proc Natl Acad Sci USA 85:2839–2843.

Lauder JM, Bloom FE (1974): Ontogeny of monoamine neurons in the locus coeruleus. Raphe nuclei and substantia nigra of the rat. I. Cell differentiation. J Comp Neurol 155:469–481.

Lauder JM, Krebs H (1978): Serotonin as a differentiation signal in early neurogenesis. Dev Neurosci 1:15–30.

Lauder JM, Krebs H (1984): Neurotransmitters in development as possible substrates for drugs of use and abuse. In Yanai J (ed): "Neurobehavioral Teratology." Amsterdam: Elsevier Science Publishers BV, pp 289–314.

Lauder JM, Towle AC, Patrick K, Henderson P, Krebs H (1985): Decreased serotonin content of embryonic raphe neurons following maternal administration of p-chlorophenylalanine: A quantitative immunocytochemical study. Dev Brain Res 20:107–114.

Lauder JM, Wallace JA, Wilkie MB, DiNome A, Krebs H (1983): Roles for serotonin in neurogenesis. Monogr Neural Sci 9:3–10.

Leslie SW, Barr E, Chandler J, Farrar RP (1983): Inhibition of fast- and slow-phase depolarization-dependent synaptosomal calcium uptake by ethanol. J Pharmacol Exp Ther 225:571–575.

Levitt P, Moore RY (1979): Development of the noradrenergic innervation of neocortex. Brain Res 162:243–259.

Lewis EJ, Tank AW, Werner N, Chikaraishi DM (1983): Regulation of tyrosine hydroxylase mRNA by glucocorticoid and cyclic AMP in a rat pheochromocytoma cell line. J Biol Chem 258:14632–14637.

Leysen JE, van Gompel P, Verwimp M, Niemegeers CJE (1983): Role and localization of serotonin₂ (S₂)-receptor-binding sites: Effects of neuronal lesions. In Mandel P, DeFeudis FV (eds): "CNS Receptors - From Molecular Pharmacology to Behavior." New York: Raven Press, pp 373–383.

Lidov HGW, Molliver ME (1982): Immunohistochemical study of the development of serotonergic neurons in the rat CNS. Brain Res Bull 9:559–604.

Lidov HGW, Molliver ME, Zecevic NR (1978): Characterization of the monoaminergic innervation of immature rat neocortex: A histofluorescence analysis. J Comp Neurol 181:663–679.

Light KE, Serbus DC, Santiago M (1989): Exposure of rats to ethanol from postnatal days 4 to 8: Alterations of cholinergic neurochemistry in the cerebral cortex and corpus striatum at day 20. Alcoholism: Clin Exp Res 13:29–35.

Lucchi L, Covelli V, Petkov VV, Spano P-F, Trabucchi M (1983): Effects of ethanol, given during pregnancy on the offspring dopaminergic system. Pharmacol Biochem Behav 19:567–570.

Mallol J, Sarraga MC, Bartolome M, Ghandour MS, Gombos G (1984): Muscarinic receptor during postnatal development of rat cerebellum: An index of cholinergic synapse formation? J Neurochem 42:1641–1649.

Martin D, Morrisett RA, Savage DD, Wilson WA, Swarzwelder HS (1989): Prenatal ethanol exposure enhances Mg^{++} regulation of depolarizing responses to NMDA in rat hippocampal CA_1 pyramidal cells. Alcoholism: Clin Exp Res 13:-323.

Mattson MP, Kater SB (1987): Calcium regulation of neurite elongation and growth cone motility. J Neurosci 7:4034–4043.

Mattson MP, Taylor-Hunter A, Kater SB (1988): Neurite outgrowth in individual neurons of a neuronal population is differentially regulated by calcium and cyclic AMP. J Neurosci 8:1704–1711.

McCobb DP, Haydon PG, Kater SB (1988): Dopamine and serotonin inhibition of neurite elongation of different identified neurons. J Neurosci Res 19:19–26.

McGeer PL, McGeer EG (1989): Amino acid neurotransmitters. In Siegel G, Agranoff B, Albers RW, Molinoff PI (eds): "Basic Neurochemistry, 4th Edition." New York: Raven Press, pp 311–332.

Mena MA, Del Rio RM, Herrera E (1984): The effect of long-term ethanol maternal ingestion and withdrawal on brain regional monoamine and amino acid precursors in 15-day-old rats. Gen Pharmacol 15:151–154.

Mena MA, Salinas M, Martin Del Rio R, Herrera E (1982): Effects of maternal ethanol ingestion on cerebral neurotransmitters and cyclic-AMP in rat offspring. Gen Pharmacol 13:241–248.

Miller MW (1986): Effects of alcohol on the generation and migration of cerebral cortical neurons. Science 233:1308–1311.

Moloney B, Leonard BE (1983): Pre-natal and post-natal effects of alcohol in the rat II. Changes in gamma-aminobutyric acid concentration and adenosine triphosphatase activity in the brain. Alcoholism: Clin Exp Res 19:137–140.

Montminy MR, Sevarino KA, Wagner JA, Mandel G, Goodman GH (1986): Identification of a cyclic-AMP-responsive element within the rat somatostatin gene. Proc Natl Acad Sci USA 83:6682–6686.

Morrisett RA, Martin D, Savage DD, Wilson WA, Swartzwelder HS (1989): Prenatal ethanol exposure decreases sensitivity of adult rat hippocampus to N-methyl-D-aspartate. Alcohol 13:323.

Mueller RA, Towle A, Breese GR (1985): Serotonin turnover and supersensitivity after neonatal 5,7-dihydroxytryptamine. Pharmacol Biochem Behav 22:221–225.

Murrin LC, Zeng W (1986): Postnatal ontogeny of dopamine D_2 receptors in rat striatum. Biochem Pharmacol 35:1159–1162.

Murrin LC, Zeng W (1989): Dopamine D_1 receptor development in the rat striatum: Early localization in striosomes. Brain Res 480:170–177.

Nelson BK, Brightwell WS, Setzer JV, O'Donohue TL (1982): Prenatal interactions between ethanol and the industrial solvent 2-ethoxyethanol in rats: Neurochemical effects in the offspring. Neurobehav Toxicol Teratol 4:395–401.

Noisin EL, Thomas WE (1988): Ontogeny of dopaminergic function in the rat midbrain tegmentum, corpus striatum and frontal cortex. Dev Brain Res 41:241–252.

Pennington S (1988): Ethanol-induced growth inhibition: The role of cyclic AMP protein kinase. Alcoholism: Clin Exp Res 12:125–129.

Pennington S, Allen Z, Runion J, Farmer P, Rouland L, Kalmus G (1985): Prostaglandin synthesis inhibitors block alcohol-induced fetal hypoplasia. Alcoholism: Clin Exp Res 9:433–437.

Pennington SN, Rumbley RA, Woody DG (1981): Fetal 15-hydroxyprostaglandin dehydrogenase is altered by maternal ethanol exposure. Biol Neonate 40:246–251.

Pierce DR, West JR (1986): Blood alcohol concentration: A critical factor for producing fetal alcohol effects. Alcohol 3:269–272.

Randall CL, Anton RF, Becker HC (1987): Alcohol, pregnancy and prostaglandins. Alcoholism: Clin Exp Res 11:32–36.

Rathbun W, Druse MJ (1985): Dopamine, serotonin and acid metabolites in brain regions from the developing offspring of ethanol treated rats. J Neurochem 44:57–62.

Rawat AK (1977): Developmental changes in the brain levels of neurotransmitters as influenced by maternal ethanol consumption. J Neurochem 28:1175–1182.

Rawat AK (1980): Development of histaminergic pathways in brain as influenced by maternal alcoholism. Res Commun Chem Pathol Pharmacol 27:91–103.

Represa A, Chanez C, Flexor MA, Ben-Ari Y (1989): Development of the cholinergic system in control and intra-uterine growth retarded rat brain. Dev Brain Res 47:71–79.

Ross WN, Arechiga H, Nicholls JG (1988): Influence of substrate on the distribution of calcium channels in identified leech neurons in culture. Proc Natl Acad Sci USA 85:4075–4078.

Savoy-Moore RT, Dombrowski MP, Cheng A, Abel EA, Sokol RJ (1989): Low dose alcohol contracts the human umbilical artery in vitro. Alcoholism: Clin Exp Res 13:40–42.

Serbus DC, Stull RE, Light KE (1986): Neonatal ethanol exposure to rat pups: Resultant alterations of cortical muscarinic and cerebellar H_1-histaminergic receptor binding dynamics. Neurotoxicology 7:257–278.

Shoemaker WJ, Baetge G, Azad R, Sapin V, Bloom FE (1983): Effect of prenatal alcohol exposure on amine and peptide neurotransmitter systems. Monogr Neural Sci 9:130–139.

Slotkin TW, Schanberg SM, Kuhn CM (1980): Synaptic development in brains of rats exposed perinatally to ethanol. Experientia 36:1005–1007.

Storm JE, Fechter LD (1985): Alteration in the postnatal ontogeny of cerebellar norepinephrine content following chronic prenatal carbon monoxide. J Neurochem 45:965–969.

Streissguth AP (1983): Alcohol and pregnancy: An overview and an update. Subst Alcohol Actions Misuse 4:149–173.

Streissguth AP, Sampson PD, Barr HM, Clarren SK, Martin DC (1988): Studying alcohol teratogenesis from the perspective of the fetal alcohol syndrome: Methodological and statistical issues. Ann NY Acad Sci 477:63–86.

Tajuddin N, Druse MJ (1989a): Chronic maternal ethanol consumption results in decreased serotonergic 5-HT$_1$ sites in cerebral cortical regions from offspring. Alcohol 5:465–470.

Tajuddin N, Druse MJ (1989b): Effects of in utero ethanol exposure on cortical 5-HT$_2$ binding sites. Alcohol 5:461–464.

Taylor P, Brown JH (1989): Acetylcholine. In Siegel G, Agranoff B, Albers RW, Molinoff P (eds): "Basic Neurochemistry. 4th Edition." New York: Raven Press, pp 203–231.

Verney C, Berger B, Adrien J, Vigny A, Gay M(1982): Development of the dopaminergic innervation of the rat cerebral cortex. A light microscopic immunocytochemical study using anti-tyrosine hydroxylase antibodies. Dev Brain Res 5:41–52.

Voorn P, Kalsbeek A, Jorritsma-Byham B, Groenewegen HJ (1988): The pre- and postnatal development of the dopaminergic cell groups in the ventral mesencephalon and the dopaminergic innervation of the striatum of the rat. Neuroscience 25:857–887.

Wallace JA, Lauder JM (1983): Development of the serotonergic system in the rat embryo: An immunochemical study. Brain Res Bull 10:459–479.

Weinberg J (1989): Prenatal ethanol exposure alters adrenocortical development of offspring. Alcoholism: Clin Exp Res 13:73–83.

Weinberg J, Nelson LR, Taylor AN (1986): Hormonal effects of fetal alcohol exposure. In West J (ed): "Alcohol and Brain Development." New York: Oxford University Press, pp 310–342.

Weiner N, Molinoff PB (1989): Catecholamines. In Siegel G, Agranoff B, Albers RW, Molinoff P (eds): "Basic Neurochemistry. 4th Edition." New York: Raven Press, pp 233–252.

Whitaker-Azmitia PM, Azmitia EC (1986): Autoregulation of fetal serotonergic neuronal development: Role of high affinity serotonin receptors. Neurosci Lett 67:307–312.

Whitaker-Azmitia PM, Lauder JM, Shenner A, Azmitia EC (1987): Postnatal changes in serotonin$_1$ receptors following prenatal alterations in serotonin levels: Further evidence for functional fetal serotonin$_1$ receptors. Dev Brain Res 33:285–289.

Wirz-Justice A (1987): Circadian rhythms in mammalian neurotransmitter receptors. Prog Neurobiol 29:219–259.

Zeng W, Hyttel J, Murrin LC (1988): Ontogeny of dopamine D$_1$ receptors in rat striatum. J Neurochem 50:862–867.

Zhou FC, Auerback S, Azmitia E (1987): Denervation of serotonergic fibers in the hippocampus induced a trophic factor which enhances the maturation of transplanted serotonergic neurons but not norepinephrine neurons. J Neurosci Res 17:235–246.

Development of the Central Nervous System:
Effects of Alcohol and Opiates, pages 169–188
© 1992 Wiley-Liss, Inc.

8

Effects of Fetal Ethanol Exposure on Androgen-Sensitive Neural Differentiation

P. KEVIN RUDEEN

*Department of Anatomy and Neurobiology, University of Missouri
School of Medicine, Columbia, Missouri*

INTRODUCTION

A number of clinical reports have identified distinctive patterns of congenital abnormalities in the offspring of alcoholic mothers referred to as the fetal alcohol syndrome (FAS). FAS was described as a collection of anomalies first recognized clinically in the United States in 1973 (Jones and Smith, 1973; Jones et al., 1973). The most predominant characteristics of FAS include prenatal and/or postnatal growth retardation, neurological abnormalities, intellectual impairment, craniofacial malformations, and anomalous genitalia (Jones and Smith, 1973; Palmer et al., 1974; Hanson et al., 1976; Clarren et al., 1978; Tillner and Majewski, 1978; Clarren, 1981; Ernhart et al., 1987). The worldwide incidence of diagnosed FAS is approximately 1.9 per 1,000 live births (Sokol and Abel, 1988). It is likely that alcohol-related birth defects (ARBD), abnormal features present in individuals whose mothers have a history of alcohol abuse during pregnancy (Abel, 1984), represent an even more widespread health problem than FAS since it has been estimated that up to 5% of all congenital anomalies may be related to maternal alcohol consumption (Sokol, 1981). The focus of the present research review concerns the more subtle effects of in utero ethanol exposure and a hormonal mechanism by which ethanol exposure during a critical period of brain development results in the alteration of brain sexual differentiation. Alterations in this developmental process appear to be related to neurobehavioral abnormalities present in the adult.

Alcohol Use During Pregnancy

Ethanol was utilized clinically to prevent or stop premature onset of labor because of its inhibitory effects on uterine contractions (Fuchs et al., 1967; Caritis et al., 1979). The clinical application of the use of ethanol in the pregnant mother prompted investigation into the ability of ethanol to traverse the placenta and interact with the fetus. Studies have found that when ethanol was given to the mother, it readily traversed the placenta and was ubiquitously distributed through the fetal tissues (Dilts, 1970; Idanpaan-Heikkila et al., 1971; Mann et al., 1975). Interestingly, the levels of alcohol in the fetus were slower to rise than in the mother, and remained slightly higher than in the maternal tissues (Jung et al., 1980). This suggests that there is a slower partition of ethanol to the fetus from the mother and a reduced ability of the fetus to metabolize and/or to eliminate ethanol. Experimental observations confirmed the reduced ability of the fetus to metabolize alcohol (Idanpaan-Heikkila et al., 1972; Gartner and Ryden, 1972), and demonstrated low alcohol and acetaldehyde dehydrogenase activities in both the human and rat fetus (Kesaniemi, 1974). It has been suggested that ethanol elimination in the fetus is due primarily to the elimination of ethanol in the mother. This maternal-fetal relationship is detrimental to the fetus because of the reduced ability of the human fetal liver to metabolize both ethanol and acetaldehyde.

Alcohol-Induced Defects of the Central Nervous System

The maternal-fetal unit provides a situation whereby elevated levels of both ethanol and acetaldehyde in the fetus are prolonged following maternal ethanol administration. The harmful effects of ethanol on the development of the central nervous system and on different organ systems vary according to the period of time during development that ethanol is present, and the length of time ethanol exposure occurs (Clarren et al., 1988). For this reason, important implications exist for studies attempting to compare the effects of a given dosage of alcohol during different periods of time of development (Kelley et al., 1987). Damage to the central nervous system has been recognized as one of the most serious consequences of ethanol consumption during pregnancy since the developing central nervous system is particularly vulnerable to prenatal ethanol exposure (Sulik et al., 1981). Animal models of fetal alcohol effects have reported anatomical changes in several areas of the brain including the hippocampus (Abel et al., 1983; Barnes and Walker, 1981; West and Hodges, 1983), cerebral cortex (Miller, 1986, 1988; Kotkoskie and Norton, 1989), cerebellum (Volk et al., 1981; Bonthius and West, 1990), and olfactory bulb (Nyquist-Battie and Gochee, 1985). Morphological and functional effects of ethanol exposure during development have been demonstrated experimentally in rats even in the absence of outward physical abnormalities (Barnes and Walker, 1981; West et al., 1981).

A number of mechanisms have been proposed that provide possible explanations for the effects of ethanol exposure on the development of the central nervous system (Rudeen and Creighton, 1989). The putative mechanisms basic to the effects of ethanol on the development of the brain can be grouped into two general areas: 1) effects on neuronal birth, migration, and differentiation, and 2) effects on metabolic processes of cells or cellular products. This report will focus on a specific mechanism included in the latter general area. The effects of ethanol on metabolic processes of cells or cellular products can be subdivided into several categories including (but not limited to): a) protein synthesis, b) prostaglandin metabolism, c) free-radical oxygen generation, and d) endocrine effects. The endocrine effects on the development of the central nervous system have been extensively investigated. Several different hormones, including corticosteroids (Scheff et al., 1987), thyroid hormones (Crockett and Kiernan, 1973; Davis and Martin, 1982; Gottesfeld et al., 1987; Gottesfeld and Silverman, 1990; Hannigan et al., 1990), and gonadal hormones (Loy and Milner, 1980; Milner and Loy, 1982) have been shown to influence a variety of developmental factors, including neuronal synaptogenesis and lesion-induced axon sprouting. An example of a sex steroid-dependent process is the neuronal sprouting response of septal afferents to the hippocampal formation. Removal of the testes of neonates permits sprouting equivalent to that in untreated females, and neonatal testosterone treatment of females results in a reduced sprouting response, equivalent to that in intact males (Loy and Milner, 1980; Milner and Loy, 1982). However, limited information is available on the effects of ethanol exposure on the endocrine-related developmental processes in the central nervous system (Kornguth et al., 1979; Kakihana et al., 1980).

CENTRAL NERVOUS SYSTEM SEXUAL DIFFERENTIATION

It is now well recognized that the central nervous systems of male and female mammals differ both structurally and functionally (see review by Serio et al., 1984). Testicular androgens from the perinatal testes serve as an inducer for neural differentiation. The development of noncyclic neuroendocrine patterns, referred to as brain masculinization, is subsequent to androgen exposure in both male and female rats (MacLusky and Naftolin, 1981; McEwen, 1983; Toran-Allerand, 1984; Dohler, 1986). Alternatively, feminization represents the intrinsic pattern of neural structural and behavioral organization and results from the absence of perinatal androgen exposure.

The precise mechanism of brain sexual differentiation is currently unknown. Appropriate sexual differentiation occurs only after the differentiation of the gonads. Research in the last decade indicates that testicular androgens exert an organizational effect on the developing brain during a "critical" period that occurs in the late fetal or early postnatal period (McEwen, 1983; Dohler, 1986). The ambient androgenic hormonal milieu acts upon the neural tissue during this critical period to induce permanent and irreversible changes in the organization of the brain (MacLusky and Naftolin, 1981; Toran-Allerand, 1984). During this critical period of time, the plasma androgen levels are generally higher in males than in females (Warren et al., 1973, 1984; Habert and Picon, 1982), and the exposure of the nondifferentiated central nervous system to the disparate fetal androgens presumably induces the phenotypic differentiation of a broad spectrum of neuroendocrine and behavioral responses appropriate to the respective genotype (Stahl et al., 1978; Weisz and Ward, 1980; Toran-Allerand, 1984).

Sexually Dimorphic Structures of the Central Nervous System

In excess of 45 various sex differences in brains have been described, most of which are located within the hypothalamus-preoptic area (HPOA), hippocampus, and amygdala (McEwen, 1983). These sex differences occur from the interaction of steroid hormones on a number of cellular mechanisms, some of which include an increase in neuronal cell number and size (Gorski et al., 1978; Pfaff, 1966; Dorner and Staudt, 1968, 1969; Hellman et al., 1976), an increase in the length and branching of dendrites and dendritic fields (Greenough et al., 1977; Ayoub et al., 1982), alterations in distribution of synapses (Raisman and Field, 1973; Nichizuka and Arai, 1981), an increase in the regional density of axonal innervation (Loy and Milner, 1980; Milner and Loy, 1982), and alterations in somatic ultrastructure, including the number of intramembranous particles and endo- and pinocytotic pits (Naftolin et al., 1988). One morphological structure related to brain sexual differentiation is the sexually dimorphic nucleus of the HPOA (SDN-POA).

SDN-POA-androgen-dependency

The SDN-POA is morphologically larger in male rats than in female rats, and is located within a region of the brain associated with regulation of neuroendocrine function (Silverman et al., 1979; Arendash and Gorski, 1983) and masculine sexual behavior (de Jong et al., 1989). Extensive experimental evidence indicates that perinatal androgen exposure mediates the morphological differentiation of this nucleus. Development and differentiation of the nucleus begin late in the fetal period and continue throughout the first week of postnatal life, coincident with a critical period for sexual differentiation of the central nervous system (Jacobson et al., 1981; Jacobson and Gorski, 1981). Castration of neonatal male rats permanently reduces the volume of the SDN-POA (Gorski et al., 1978; Jacobson et al., 1981). Replacement of testosterone by exogenous administration 1 day after neonatal castration restores the volume of the nucleus to the appropriate masculine size. On the other hand, treatment of neonatal female rats with a single dose of testosterone propionate significantly increases the volume of the feminine nucleus, but the volume of the SDN-POA is not as large as the male nucleus. The neonatal female rats must be continuously exposed to testosterone propionate through the late prenatal and postnatal periods in order for the SDN-POA volume to approach the size of genotypic males (Dohler et al., 1982a, b, 1984).

However, the process of sexual differentiation of neural structures is more complex than what seemed initially apparent. Although mechanisms by which testicular androgens irreversibly mediate CNS sexual differentiation remain elusive, it is known that it is actually estrogens, rather than androgens, that mediate the alterations seen in the SDN-POA. This has been experimentally demonstrated by the prenatal or postnatal treatment of female rats with diethylstilbestrol, a synthetic estrogen. Female rats that received diethylstilbestrol resulted in the development of a SDN-POA which is similar in volume to that of control male rats (Dohler et al., 1982a, b, 1984). Male rats treated either pre- or postnatally with cyproterone acetate, an androgen receptor antagonist, develop a nucleus having a normal male volume (Dohler, 1986). Intrahypothalamic testosterone or estradiol implants into neonatal female rates are equally effective in inducing masculine brain sexual differentiation (Christensen and Gorski, 1978).

"Aromatization hypothesis" and the role of estrogens

Experimental results suggest that androgens appear to act as the precursor for estrogen formation, and that it is the locally formed estrogens that mediate the differentiation of the neural structures. Local conversion of androgens to estrogens is accomplished by the activity of a cytochrome P450 enzyme called aromatase. The aromatization hypothesis asserts that local conversion of circulating androgens to estrogens is essential for masculinization of the central nervous system in the male rat (Naftolin et al., 1975; McEwen et al., 1977; MacLusky and Naftolin, 1981; McEwen, 1983; Dohler, 1986). The catalytic activity of aromatase is first detectable in the brain of 16-day-old fetal rats and will reach maximum levels within a day or two prior to birth (Reddy et al., 1974; George and Ojeda, 1982; MacLusky et al., 1985). Aromatase activity within the HPOA is regulated by androgens in the adult rodent, presumably through an androgen receptor (Roselli et al., 1984, 1987; Roselli and Resko, 1984). The regulation of aromatase activity by testosterone administration in the neonatal rat has not been confirmed (Rudeen and Paredez, 1989).

Administration of aromatase inhibitors and anti-estrogens yield data that also support the aromatase hypothesis. Aromatase inhibitors that block the conversion of testosterone to estradiol attenuate the masculinizing effects of both exogenous and endogenous testosterone, whereas anti-estrogens have a similar effect on sexual differentiation of neural structures (Luttge and Whalen, 1970; McDonald and Doughty, 1974; Booth, 1977a, b; Morali et al., 1978; Vreeburg et al., 1977). The data support the aromatization hypothesis insomuch that neural mechanisms in the rodent brain undergo masculinization under the influence of testosterone. Testosterone is intraneuronally aromatized into estradiol, and it is the estradiol, in part, along with the androgens or its metabolites, that masculinize the rodent brain. The mechanisms by which these steriods induce the dimorphic changes in the neuronal structures are poorly understood. There is experimental evidence indicating that gonadal steroids affect neuronal cell number, cellular growth, and synapse formation (Naftolin et al., 1988). Additionally, the effects of the steroids on the neurons may be elicited through enzymes regulating synaptic transmission (Luine et al., 1977), modulation of neurotransmitter receptor levels (Arimatsu et al., 1981), or the alteration of steroid hormone receptors (Vito et al., 1979; Vito and Fox, 1982; Handa et al., 1987).

According to the same "aromatization hypothesis," the female brain is protected from masculinization by a sex steroid binding protein called alpha-fetoprotein (AFP). AFP is the major fetal plasma protein in most vertebrates and is synthesized at very high rates during the perinatal period in the rodent (Olsson et al., 1977). During this period, AFP binds estrogens with high affinity, but fails to effectively bind androgens. It was thought that androgens from the fetal testes are free to enter the neurons and act as substrate for estrogen formation but that circulating estrogens of both males and females were sequestered by the AFP and unable to enter the cell to induce masculinization (McEwen et al., 1975). However, it was later demonstrated that some neurons may contain AFP (Toran-Allerand, 1982). Intraneuronal AFP is likely imported by the cell since AFP mRNA has not been found in the HPOA neurons (Schachter and Toran-Allerand, 1982). AFP may act as a carrier for the transport of estrogens into neurons and serve to attenuate free estrogen levels in females so that low levels of estrogens are continuously provided to the developing female brain (Toran-Allerand, 1984). Under these conditions, the low levels of estrogens present during the developmental period are essential for the normal "feminization" of the brain so that the neural substrates and subsequent synaptogenesis will respond later during adulthood to female sex hormones. In contrast, the influence of high levels of estrogens made available through intra-neuronal aromatization of high levels of androgens from the perinatal testes allow for the defeminization and normal masculinization of the male brain. Local conversion of androgens to estrogens in genotypically male neuronal tissue allows for specific action of estrogens at high concentrations in selective brain regions.

FETAL ETHANOL EFFECTS ON SEXUAL DIFFERENTIATION OF THE CENTRAL NERVOUS SYSTEM

Fetal Ethanol Exposure on Sexual Development and Behavior

Numerous animal studies demonstrate that fetal ethanol exposure produces effects on the developing endocrine system and that the effects persist in the adult animal. Kakihana et al. (1980) and Rose et al. (1981) demonstrated that in utero ethanol exposure resulted in the reduction of gonadal hormones and corticosterone levels in the blood. Adult males exposed to ethanol in utero had significantly reduced testicular development and lower plasma testosterone levels at 55 and 110 days of age indicating that the effects of prenatal ethanol exposure on the endocrine system last into adulthood (Parker et al., 1984). Altered secondary sexual development such as alterations in anogenital distance in mice and rats also has been demonstrated in offspring exposed to ethanol during gestation (Boggan et al., 1979; Chen and Smith, 1979).

Endocrine imbalance from prenatal alcohol exposure can possibly have long-term consequences (Anderson, 1981). Adult nonsexual dimorphic behavior and sexual dimorphic behavior has been demonstrated to be affected by prenatal ethanol exposure. McGivern et al. (1984) reported that prenatal alcohol exposure altered preference for saccharin in adult male and female rats. Female rats have a greater preference for saccharin solutions compared with male rats. Male offspring exposed to ethanol in utero display altered masculine behavior, such that the male saccharin solution consumption appears more "female-like" by increasing their preference to a saccharin solution. It was speculated that the demasculinization of the male behavior is due to decreased testosterone levels during fetal life. Sexual behavior is also affected since in the report cited above (Parker et al., 1984), adult male rats exposed to ethanol in utero showed significantly lowered sexual motivation and performance when paired with receptive female rats.

Fetal Ethanol Effects on Androgen-Dependent Central Nervous System Morphology

The relatedness of the SDN-POA to reproductive function and its dependency on androgens for masculine development indicate this to be a nucleus suited for evaluation of the effects of in utero ethanol on its development and differentiation. It was determined that the volume of the SDN-POA of male rats was significantly reduced by fetal ethanol exposure, an effect of ethanol on development of the central nervous system during gestation which persisted into adulthood (Rudeen, 1986). Furthermore, a significant reduction of the volume of the SDN-POA can be induced by ethanol exposure when the ethanol is provided either prenatally or postnatally, when compared with male rats not exposed to ethanol during the same developmental periods (Rudeen et al., 1986). The exposure to ethanol during gestation or during the postnatal period was specific to the androgen-dependent nucleus since ethanol exposure did not significantly reduce the volume of another nucleus, the nucleus of the anterior commissure. This nucleus is located in the same region of the brain as the SDN-POA, but has not been demonstrated to be sexually dimorphic or androgen-dependent in its development. These findings were corroborated by Barron et a. (1988) who found that both the volume and average area of SDN-POA neurons were markedly smaller in fetal alcohol-exposed 70–80-day-old male rats than in males whose mothers were on control diets during the gestational period. In this study, however, prenatal alcohol exposure did not significantly alter the volume or cell size in adult female rats, or the volume of the nucleus of the anterior commissure, in either sex.

The precise mechanism by which in utero ethanol exposure resulted in the reduction of the volume of the SDN-POA in males is not known. As discussed above, it is known that the ultimate development and differentiation (masculinization) of the SDN-POA is critically influenced by the milieu of circulating androgens present during the "critical period" for brain sexual differentiation (Gorski et al., 1978; Dohler et al., 1982a, b; Jacobson et al., 1981). It is conceivable that the mechanism that fetal ethanol exposure may have on the development and differentiation of the androgen-dependent structures of the brain may be related to an alteration in the endogenous levels of the sex steroids during this critical period. This would have long-term effects on the androgen-dependent structures in the central nervous system. Additionally, fetal ethanol exposure may alter the ability of androgen-dependent neurons to metabolize testosterone into the active metabolite, estrogen, which is responsible for the masculinization process.

Neuronal testosterone metabolism

It is hypothesized that the masculinization process of the central nervous system in the rat is dependent on the direct action of high levels of estradiol as produced from high levels of testosterone and estradiol (McEwen et al., 1977; Naftolin et al., 1975). Fetal ethanol exposure may alter the ability of the neuron to metabolize testosterone, or alter the ability of the neuron to bind testosterone, and therefore, sequester the androgen for the masculinization process. Initial studies measuring aromatase activity in the HPOA in 1-day-old male rats using a stereospecific radioenzymatic assay showed an elevation of the catalytic enzyme activity in the HPOA of ethanol exposure rats compared with that in rats whose mothers were exposed to control diets (Rudeen eta al., 1988). McGivern et a., (1988) has also reported that HPOA aromatase activity was elevated in fetal ethanol exposed rats when examined from day 18 of gestation until the first day of life.

In the adult brain, aromatase activity is induced by the presence of testosterone as a substrate (Roselli et al., 1984). Castration of adult male rats results in the depression of HPOA aromatase activity and aromatase activity in the HPOA in castrated animals is restored by testosterone administration (Rudeen and Paredez, 1989). The castration-induced reduction of catalytic activity of aromatase in adult rats fetally exposed to ethanol is greater than that of adult male rats from mothers given control diets during gestation. These data indicate that the enzyme is more sensitive to changes in the androgen substrate levels in the fetal ethanol exposed rats. However, neonatal male rats subjected to testosterone either for 1 day following birth or for the first 6 days of life did not show an induction of aromatase activity in the HPOA. Thus it appears that aromatase activity is influenced by testosterone in the adult HPOA, but the enzyme activity is not influenced by testosterone during the perinatal period of development in the male rat.

It has been hypothesized that since aromatase activity is also induced by dihydrotestosterone (DHT) (Roselli and Resko, 1984), that perhaps the increase in aromatase activity during the perinatal period (Rudeen et al., 1988; McGivern et al., 1988b) was due to an increase in DHT levels. Therefore, in a more critical investigation, the simultaneous catalytic activities of both aromatase and 5α-reductase (the enzyme metabolizing testosterone to DHT) were measured in the HPOA of neonatal male rats by a radiometric quantitation of steroid metabolites using high performance liquid chromatography (HPLC) and an on-line radiochromatographic detector (Kelce et al., 1990b). From these studies it was determined that neither the aromatase activity nor the reductase activity in the HPOA of neonatal male rats was altered by fetal ethanol exposure. These results indicate that the metabolism of testosterone by either aromatase or reductase in the HPOA of neonatal rats is not significantly altered by fetal ethanol exposure and probably does not contribute to changes in the neuronal endocrine milieu.

Preliminary data indicate that the number of testosterone receptors in the HPOA of fetal ethanol exposed 1-day-old male rats is reduced by 50% from the number of receptors in the rats whose mothers were given the control diet during gestation. Although the number of receptors are affected by fetal ethanol exposure, the affinity of the receptors remained relatively unchanged by any of the treatments during gestation (Rudeen and Ganjam, unpublished data).

Taken together, these data indicate that the disposition of testosterone in the HPOA of fetal ethanol exposed male rats is inconclusive. It seems that the aromatase activity following fetal ethanol exposure in neonatal male rat HPOA is either unchanged (Kelce et al., 1990b) or enhanced (Rudeen et al., 1988; McGivern et al., 1988b). Whether this has any direct effect on the ultimate production of estradiol in this neural area has yet to be determined. It was hypothesized that the formation of estradiol may be limited by the availability of testosterone for aromatization rather than alteration in testosterone metabolism in the HPOA by changes in the catalytic activity of either aromatase or reductase (Kelce et al., 1990b). This is logical since the number of testosterone receptors in the HPOA of fetal ethanol exposed rats were dramatically reduced.

Fetal ethanol effects on androgen levels

It has been well documented that both acute and chronic alcohol exposure lower sex steroid levels in adult males (Gordon et al., 1978; Van Thiel and Lester, 1976; Lester and Van Thiel, 1977; Fisher and Levitt, 1980). The effects of ethanol on sex steroid levels in the perinate also have been examined. Brain DHT levels have been reported to be decreased in perinatal male rats exposed to ethanol compared with the DHT levels observed in rats not exposed to ethanol (Kakihana et al., 1980). DHT is a non-aromatizable reduced product of testosterone metabolism and has potent androgen effects; however, its importance in neuronal differentiation is questionable. Although Kakihana et al. (1980) showed that testosterone levels were unchanged by ethanol exposure, Parker et al. (1984) demonstrated that prenatal ethanol exposure resulted in a reduction of blood testosterone levels in 55 and 110 day old male rats.

Perinatal testicular testosterone levels dramatically increase during gestation (G) day 17 in the male fetus to reach peak levels from G18 to birth, then gradually decrease during the first postnatal week. This is associated with increased testicular contents of androstenedione and progesterone, indicative of active biosynthesis of testosterone in the perinate during this period (Warren et al., 1984). The increase in blood testosterone levels during development begins on about G13 in the rat fetus, and reaches maximal levels on G18 and G19 (Warren et al., 1973; Habert and Picon, 1982). The androgenic perinatal surge continues after parturition during which testosterone biosynthesis and blood levels gradually decline.

Several studies have demonstrated that fetal ethanol exposure significantly depressed the neonatal rise of testosterone levels in whole body tissue (McGivern, 1988a) and blood (Rudeen and Kappel, 1985; Rudeen, 1989; Kelce et al., 1989). In the former study, tissue testosterone levels were determined in male fetuses on G17, G18, G19, and G20. While a significant rise in testosterone was observed on G18 in the body tissue of male rats derived from dams exposed to control diets during gestation, there was no evidence of a surge of testosterone during this period in alcohol-exposed neonatal male rats. Additionally, the response of the fetal testes to stimulation by luteinizing hormone (LH) on G18 and G22 was dramatically lower in testes from fetuses exposed to ethanol in utero compared with testosterone levels stimulated in response to LH in animals derived from control dams. In the latter study, blood testosterone levels were elevated in 1-day-old neonate male rats, but the rise in blood androgen levels was absent in 1-day-old neonate male rats exposed to ethanol in utero. By postnatal day (P) 7, the blood testosterone levels in the male rats from control mothers had declined to the same levels observed in 7-day-old male rats exposed to ethanol during gestation (Rudeen and Kappel, 1985). It is not known whether testosterone levels increased in ethanol-exposed male rats between P1 and P7, or if there was a complete loss of the perinatal testosterone surge in the fetal ethanol-exposed rats. The inhibition of the perinatal surge of tissue and blood testosterone in fetal ethanol-exposed male rats suggests that ethanol acts as a gonadotoxin to inhibit testosterone biosynthesis in the perinatal testes. The reduction of testosterone during the critical period for sexual differentiation of the brain ostensibly would result in demasculinization of the brain as observed both structurally and behaviorally in fetal ethanol-exposed male rats.

Perinatal effects of ethanol on testicular steriodogenesis

It is the Leydig cells in the interstitial compartment of the neonatal rat testes that are responsible for the production of the perinatal testosterone surge. The biosynthesis of testosterone beginning from pregnenolone was assessed in testes of neonates from fetal ethanol-exposed animals and male rats whose mothers were exposed to control diets (Kelce et al., 1989). The catalytic activities of 3β-hydroxysteroid dehydrogenase/isomerase, which converts pregnenolone to progesterone (P_4); 17α-hydroxylase, which converts progesterone to 17α-hydroxyprogesterone; and $C_{17,20}$-lyase, which converts 17α-hydroxyprogesterone to androstenedione, were each measured by radiometric quantitation of the steroid metabolites by isocratic HPLC. Using this methodology, it was found that fetal ethanol exposure resulted in the significant reduction of the catalytic activity of only *one* of the enzymes in the biosynthesis of testosterone, that being 17α-hydroxylase activity. Associated with the reduction in enzyme activity was a reduction in the serum testosterone levels in the male. Interestingly, the effects of fetal ethanol exposure on 17α-hydroxylase activity were not permanent. By P20, the catalytic activity of the enzyme was not significantly lower in the fetal ethanol-exposed animals than in control animals. The differences in testicular 17α-hydroxylase activity among animals in the three groups was even less at P40 and P60.

The measurable effect of ethanol on the steroid biosynthesis in neonatal animals and not in older animals can be explained by the presence of two types of Leydig cells present in the testes at the different ages. The concept of two apparently distinct populations of Leydig cells is not novel. Fetal-type and adult-type Leydig cell populations are separate cell generations that are developmentally unrelated (Kerr and Knell, 1988), with the fetal-type Leydig cell population persisting, to some extent, in the adult testes (Zirkin and Ewing, 1987). During testicular differentiation, the Leydig cells appear to be of mesenchymal origin (Christensen, 1975) and attain characteristics typical of steroid producing cells during the prenatal period (Lording and deKrester, 1972). The cellular origin of the adult-type Leydig cells is believed to be derived from pre-existing mesenchyme-like cells of the extracordal compartment of the testes (Moon and Hardy, 1973). After P28, the Leydig cell population is due primarily to the division of morphologically recognizable Leydig cells (Hardy et al., 1989). The disappearance of the effect of ethanol on testicular steroidogenesis by P20 suggests that the effects of fetal ethanol exposure on testosterone biosynthesis are restricted to the fetal-type Leydig cell population, and on the synthesis and release of testosterone specifically in the male perinate during the critical period of testosterone production.

This specific effect of ethanol exposure on testosterone biosynthesis in the neonatal testes was further demonstrated by the acute administration of ethanol to neonatal male rats from mothers on control diets during gestation (Kelce et al., 1990a). In this study, the increase in the dose of alcohol administered to neonatal male rats on day 1 of life was increased from 0, 1, or 2 gm/kg body weight given intraperitoneally. Associated with the increased blood ethanol levels was a decrease in serum testosterone levels; this was most evident in 1-day-old rats and occurred to a lesser extent in P20 and P40 rats. As demonstrated in animals exposed to ethanol in utero, ethanol-naive neonatal male rats given a dose of 1 mg/kg body weight of ethanol exhibited 17α-hydroxylase activity that was significantly lower than the catalytic activity of the enzyme in animals that did not receive ethanol. Ethanol exposure reduced the catalytic activity of 17α-hydroxylase in the neonatal male rat in a dose-responsive manner since the 2 gm/kg ethanol dose further reduced the enzyme activity in the testes of these animals. The same doses of ethanol did not effectively reduce 17α-hydroxylase activity in 20- and 40-day-old male rats, corroborating the previous data indicating that the fetal-type Leydig cell was more sensitive to ethanol than the adult-type Leydig cell. Again, these data indicate that testosterone biosynthesis in the perinatal male animal is susceptible to ethanol exposure, even to a greater degree than the effects of ethanol on testosterone biosynthesis in older animals. Most importantly, these investigations demonstrate that ethanol induces a specific reduction in the catalytic activity of one enzyme in the biosynthesis of testosterone. The reduction of the catalytic activity of 17α-hydroxylase by ethanol exposure obviously results in the measurable decrement in serum testosterone levels during the critical period for brain sexual differentiation.

CONCLUSIONS

Collectively, the data indicate that fetal ethanol exposure results in structural and behavioral alterations of the central nervous system. These data also provide initial evidence for a hormonal mechanism by which fetal ethanol exposure induces alterations in the brain sexual differentiation that results in an apparent demasculinization effect. The process by which this occurs is depicted diagrammatically in Figure 1. Ethanol, when consumed by a pregnant female rat during the critical period for brain sexual differentiation (G18–P5), passes rapidly through the placental barrier (1) and enters the fetal circulation. Fetal ethanol levels equal or exceed that of the mother and partitions throughout all tissue compartments of the fetus, including the testes (2), since ethanol penetrates the interstitial tissue of the testes at a rate comparable to blood (Salonen and Eriksson, 1989). Within the interstitium of the testes, the ethanol gains access to the Leydig cells where testosterone biosynthesis occurs (3) at a high rate during the critical period for masculine brain sex differentiation. Inspection of the catalytic activity of the enzymes involved in the biosynthesis of testosterone from pregnenolone indicates that the activity of only one of the enzymes, 17α-hydroxylase, is affected by ethanol (4). The catalytic activity of this enzyme is significantly reduced, resulting in lowered production and secretion of blood testosterone (5). The decreased secretion of testosterone into the systemic circulation reduced levels of testosterone reaching the central nervous system, most importantly at the HPOA, an androgen-dependent area of the brain. An increase in the circulating levels of testosterone is apparently responsible, at least in part, for the masculinization process of the androgen-dependent areas of the brain (6). The reduction of the amount of testosterone available to the appropriate dimorphic neurons may be confounded by another effect of ethanol on the neuron that reduces the actual numbers of androgen receptors in the cell. Alternatively, the reduction in the number of androgen receptors may result from a lower level of circulating testosterone. Whatever the reason, the end result is an effect of fetal ethanol exposure to reduce the amount of testosterone available for aromatization. Intracellular testosterone metabolism in this brain area in the neonate is yet unclear (7). It appears that there is no loss of aromatase activity (biochemical plasticity in response to lowered substrate levels) and that the direction of testosterone metabolism through aromatization to estradiol, or reduction to DHT is not changed by ethanol exposure (8). The final result is presumably a reduction in intracellular estradiol levels essential for alteration of the cellular genomic expression necessary for the masculinization of the neuron. Without adequate stimulation by estradiol, the complete masculinization process during the critical period for sexual differentiation does not occur (9). The result is an expression of long-term structural changes in the brain concomitant with alterations in sexually dimorphic behaviors in young and adult animals.

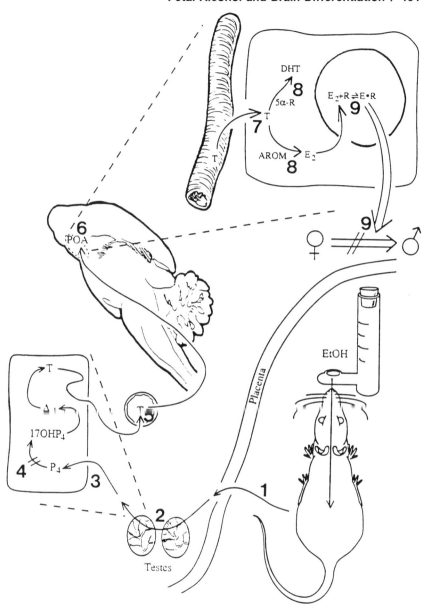

Fig. 1. Diagrammatic depiction of the hormonal mechanism for fetal ethanol-induced alterations in androgen-dependent neural tissue. EtOH, ethanol; P_4, progesterone; 170HP$_4$, 17α-hydroxyprogesterone; $_{\Delta_4}$, androstenedione; T, testosterone; POA, hypothalamic preoptic area containing the sexually dimorphic nucleus; DHT, dihydrotestosterone; AROM, aromatase; 5α-R, 5α-reductase; E_2, estradiol. See text for complete explanation.

This is only *one* hypothetical mechanism by which fetal ethanol exposure results in structural and functional alteration of the central nervous system. Since this is a hormonal mechanism and affects only the androgen-dependent structures of the brain, the ultimate effects of fetal ethanol exposure on sexual differentiation of the brain are limited to several factors. These factors include the period of time during which ethanol exposure occurs and the amount of ethanol present at the critical period for brain differentiation. In the former situation, androgen-dependent brain structures would not be affected if ethanol was not present during the period of fetal testosterone secretion important for the masculinization process. Furthermore, it appears that the synthesis and secretion of testosterone during the critical period is dose-dependent, being reduced to a greater level when the dose of ethanol is higher. Although this implies that the lower levels of ethanol may not significantly alter testosterone secretion, the amount of reduction of testosterone that is required to affect the masculinization process in the brain is not known.

Although many investigators have identified one loci of ethanol toxicity in other systems, there is little information on the precise molecular mechanism of ethanol on testosterone biosynthesis in the process of sexual brain differentiation. Important questions concerning the effects of ethanol on the genomic expression of the mRNA encoding the 17α-hydroxylase enzyme and the genomic alterations that occur during neuronal masculinization that are affected by changes in testosterone and/or estradiol content have yet to be addressed. Such experiments are important to determine the effects of fetal ethanol exposure on brain development and sexual differentiation.

ACKNOWLEDGMENTS

The author wishes to thank Drs. W. Kelce and V.K. Ganjam for their collaborative efforts in this project, and Ms. S. Paredez and C. Kappel for their technical contributions. This work was supported by NIAAA grants AA00107 and AA05893.

REFERENCES

Abel EL (1984): "Fetal Alcohol Syndrome/Fetal Alcohol Effects." New York: Plenum Press.

Abel EL, Jacobson S, Sherwin BT (1983): In utero alcohol exposure: Functional and structural brain damage. Neurobehav Toxicol Teratol 5:363–366.

Anderson RA (1981): Endocrine balance as a factor in the etiology of the fetal alcohol syndrome. Neurobehav Toxicol Teratol 3:89–104.

Arendash GW, Gorski RA (1983): Evidence for the existence of a sexually dimorphic nucleus in the preoptic area of the rat. Brain Res Bull 10:147–154.

Ayoub DM, Greenough WT, Juraska JM (1982): Sex differences in dendritic structure in the preoptic area of the juvenile macaque monkey brain. Science 219:-197–198.

Barnes DE, Walker DW (1981): Prenatal ethanol exposure permanently reduces the number of pyramidal neurons in rat hippocampus. Dev Brain Res 1:333–340.

Barron S, Tieman SB, Riley EP (1988): Effects of prenatal alcohol exposure on the sexually dimorphic nucleus of the preoptic area of the hypothalamus in male and female rats. Alcohol Clin Exp Res 12:59–64.

Boggan WO, Randall CL, Dodds HM (1979): Delayed sexual maturation in female C57/6J mice prenatally exposed to alcohol. Res Commun Chem Pathol Pharmacol 23:117–125.

Bonthius DJ, West JR (1990): Alcohol-induced neuronal loss in developing rats increased brain damage with binge exposure. Alcohol Clin Exp Res 14:107–118.

Booth JE (1977a): Sexual behavior of male rats injected with the anti-oestrogen MER-25 during infancy. Physiol Behav 19:35–39.

Booth JE (1977b): Sexual behavior of neonatally castrated rats injected during infancy with estrogen and dihydrotestosterone. J Endocr 72:135–141.

Caritis SN, Edelstone DI, Mueller-Heubach E (1979): Pharmacological inhibition of preterm labor. Am J Obstet Gynecol 133:557–578.

Chen JJ, Smith ER (1979): Effects of prenatal alcohol on sexual differentiation and open-field behavior in rats. Horm Behav 13:219–231.

Christensen AK (1975): Leydig Cells. In Greep RO, Astwood EB (eds): "Handbook of Physiology." Washington, D.C: American Physiology Society, pp 57–94.

Christensen LW, Gorski RA (1978): Independent masculinization of neuroendocrine systems by intracerebral implants of testosterone or estradiol in the neonatal female rat. Brain Res 146:325–340.

Clarren S, Ellsworth C, Sumi M, Streissguth A, Smith DW (1978): Brain malformations related to prenatal exposure to ethanol. J Pediatr 92:64–67.

Clarren SK (1981): Recognition of fetal alcohol syndrome. JAMA 245:1436–1439.

Clarren SK, Astley SJ, Bowden DM (1988): Physical anomalies and developmental delays in nonhuman primate infants exposed to weekly doses of ethanol during gestation. Teratology 37:561–569.

Crockett SA, Kiernan JA (1973): Acceleration of peripheral nervous regeneration in the rat by exogenous triiodothyronine. Exp Neurol 39:389–394.

Davis JN, Martin B (1982): Sympathetic ingrowth in the hippocampus: Evidence for regulation by mossy fibers in thyroxine-treated rats. Brain Res 247:145–148.

de Jong FH, Louwerse AL, Ooms MP, Evers P, Endert E, Van dePoll NE (1989): Lesions of the SDN-POA inhibit sexual behavior of male Wistar rats. Brain Res Bull 23:483–492.

Dilts PV (1970): Placenta transfer of ethanol. Am J Obstet Gynecol 107:1195–1198.

Dohler KD (1986): A special case of hormonal imprinting, the neonatal influence of sex. Experientia 42:759–769.

Dohler KD, Coquelin A, Davis F, Hines M, Shryne JE, Gorski RA (1982a): Differentiation of the sexually dimorphic nucleus in the preoptic area of the rat brain is determined by the perinatal hormonal environment. Neurosci Lett 33:295–298.

Dohler KD, Hines M, Coquelin A, Davis F, Shryne JE, Gorski RA (1982b): Pre- and postnatal influence of diethylstilbestrol on differentiation of the sexually dimorphic nucleus in the preoptic area of the female rat brain. Neuroendocr Lett 4:361–365.

Dohler KD, Srivastava SS, Shryne JE, Jarzab B, Sipos A, Gorski RA (1984): Differentiation of the sexually dimorphic nucleus in the preoptic area of the rat brain is inhibited by postnatal treatment with an estrogen antagonist. Neuroendocrinology 38:297–301.

Dorner G, Staudt J (1968): Structural changes in the preoptic anterior hypothalamic area of the male rat following neonatal castration and androgen substitution. Neuroendocrinology 3:136–140.

Dorner G, Staudt J (1969): Structural changes in the hypothalamic ventromedial nucleus of the male rat following neonatal castration and androgen treatment. Neuroendocrinology 4:278–281.

Ernhart CB, Sokal RJ, Martier S, Moron D, Nadler J, Ager W, Wolf A (1987): Alcohol teratogenicity in the human: A detailed assessment of specificity, critical period, and threshold. Am J Obstet Gynecol 156:33–39.

Ficher M, Levitt DR (1980): Testicular dysfunction and sexual impotence in the alcoholic rat. J Steroid Biochem 13:1089–1095.

Fuchs F, Fuchs AR, Poblete VF, Risk A (1967): Effect of alcohol on threatened premature labour. Am J Obstet Gynecol 99:627.

Gartner U, Ryden G (1972): The elimination of alcohol in the premature infant. Acta Pediatr Scand 61:720–721.

George FW, Ojeda SR (1982): Changes in aromatase activity in the rat brain during embryonic, neonatal and infantile development. Endocrinology 111:522–529.

Gordon GG, Southren AL, Lieber CS (1978): The effects of alcoholic liver disease and alcohol ingestion on sex hormone levels. Alcohol Clin Exp Res 2:250–264.

Gorski RA, Gordon J, Shryne JE, Southam AM (1978): Evidence for a morphological sex difference within the medial preoptic area of the rat brain. Brain Res 148:-333–346.

Gottesfeld Z, Garcia CJ, Chronister RB (1987): Perinatal, not adult, hypothyroidism suppresses dopaminergic axon sprouting in the deafferented olfactory tubercle of adult rat. J Neurosci Res 18:568–573.

Gottesfeld Z, Silverman PB (1990): Developmental delays associated with prenatal alcohol exposure are reversed by thyroid hormone treatment. Neurosci Lett 109:42–47.

Greenough WT, Carter CS, Steerman C, DeVoogd TJ (1977): Sex differences in dendritic patterns in hamster preoptic area. Brain Res 126:63–72.

Habert R, Picon R (1982): Control of testicular steroidogenesis in the fetal rat: Effect of decapitation on testosterone and plasma luteinizing hormone-like activity. Acta Endocrinol 99:466–473.

Handa RJ, Roselli CE, Horton L, Resko JA (1987): The quantitative distribution of cytosolic androgen receptors in microdissected areas of the male rate brain: Effects of estrogen treatment. Endocrinology 121:233–240.

Hannigan JH, Bellisario RL (1990): Lower serum thyroxine levels in rats following prenatal exposure to ethanol. Alcohol Clin Exp Res 14:456–460.

Hanson JW, Jones KL, Smith DW (1976): Fetal alcohol syndrome: Experience with 41 patients. JAMA 235:1458–1460.

Hardy MP, Zirkin BR, Ewing LL (1989): Kinetic studies on the development of the adult population of Leydig cells in testes of the puberal rat. Endocrinology 124:762–770.

Hellman RE, Ford DH, Rhines RK (1976): Growth in hypothalamic neurons as reflected by nuclear size and labeling with 3H-uridine. Psychoendocrinology 1:389–397.

Idanpaan-Heikkila JE, Fritchie GE, Ho BT, McIsaac WM (1971): Placental transfer of C^{14}-ethanol. Am J Obstet Gynecol 110:426–428.

Idanpaan-Heikkila JE, Jouppila P, Akerblom HK, Isoaho R, Kauppila E, Koivisto M (1972): Elimination and metabolic effects of ethanol in mother, fetus and newborn infant. Am J Obstet Gynecol 112:387–393.

Jacobson CD, Csernus VJ, Shryne JE, Gorski RA (1981): The influence of gonadectomy, androgen exposure, or a gonadal graft in the neonatal rat on the volume of the sexually dimorphic nucleus of the preoptic area. J Neurosci 1:1142–1147.

Jacobson CD, Gorski RA (1981): Neurogenesis of the sexually dimorphic nucleus of the preoptic area in the rat. J Comp Neurol 196:519–529.

Jones K, Smith DW (1973): Recognition of the fetal alcohol syndrome in early infancy. Lancet 2:999–1001.

Jones K, Smith DW, Ulleland CN, Streissguth AP (1973): Pattern of malformation in offspring of alcoholic mothers. Lancet 1:1267–1271.

Jung AL, Roan Y, Temple AR (1980): Neonatal death associated with acute transplacental ethanol intoxication. Am J Dis Child 134:419–420.

Kakihana R, Butte JC, Moore JA (1980): Endocrine effects of maternal alcoholization: Plasma and brain testosterone, dihydrotestosterone, estradiol, and corticosterone. Alcohol Clin Exp Res 4:57–61.

Kelce WR, Ganjam VK, Rudeen PK (1990a): Inhibition of testicular steroidogenesis in the neonatal rat following acute ethanol exposure. Alcohol 7:75–80.

Kelce WR, Ganjam VK, Rudeen PK (1990b): Effects of prenatal ethanol exposure on the enzymatic activity of 5α-reductase and aromatase in the neonatal rat hypothalamic preoptic area. J Steroid Biochem 35:103–106.

Kelce WR, Rudeen PK, Ganjam VK (1989): Prenatal ethanol exposure alters steroidogenic enzyme activity in newborn rat testes. Alcohol Clin Exp Res 13:617–621.

Kelley SJ, DJ Bonthius, JR West (1987): Developmental changes in alcohol pharmacokinetics in rats. Alcohol Clin Exp Res 11:281–286.

Kerr JB, Knell CM (1988): The fate of fetal Leydig cells during the development of the fetal and postnatal rat testes. Development 103:535–544.

Kesaniemi YA (1974): Metabolism of ethanol and acetaldehyde in intact rats during pregnancy. Biochem Pharmacol 23:1157–1162.

Kornguth S, Rutledge J, Sunderland E, Seigel F, Carlson I, Smollens J, Juhl U, Young B (1979): Impeded cerebellar development and reduced serum thyroxine levels, associated development, and reduced serum thyroxine levels associated with fetal alcohol intoxication. Brain Res 177:346–360.

Kotkoskie LA, Norton S (1989): Cerebral cortical morphology and behavior in rats following acute prenatal ethanol exposure. Alcohol Clin Exp Res 13:776–781.

Lester R, Van Thiel DH (1977): Gonadal function in chronic alcoholic men. Adv Exp Biol Med 85:399–414.

Lording DW, deKrester DM (1972): Comparative ultrastructural and histochemical studies of the interstitial cells of the rat testis during fetal and postnatal development. J Reprod Fertil 29:261–269.

Loy R, Milner TA (1980): Sexual dimorphism in extent of axonal sprouting in hippocampus. Science 208:1282–1284.

Luine V, McEwen B, Black J (1977): Effect of 17 β-estradiol on hypothalamic tyrosine hydroxylase activity. Brain Res 120:188–192.

Luttge WG, Whalen RE (1970): Dihydrotestosterone, Androstenedione, testosterone: Comparative effectiveness in masculinizing and defeminizing reproductive systems in male and female rats. Horm Behav 1:265–281.

MacLusky NJ, Naftolin F (1981): Sexual differentiation of the central nervous system. Science 211:1294–1303.

MacLusky NJ, Philip A, Hulburt C, Naftolin F (1985): Estrogen formation in the developing rat brain: Sex differences in aromatase activity during early postnatal life. Psychoneuroendocrinology 10:355–361.

Mann LI, Bhakthavathsalan A, Liu M, Makowski P (1975): Placental transport of alcohol and its effect on maternal and fetal acid-base balance. Am J Obstet Gynecol 122:837–844.

McDonald PG, Doughty C (1974): Effect of neonatal administration of different androgens in the female rat: Correlation between aromatization and the induction of sterilization. J Endocr 61:95–103.

McEwen B (1983): Gonadal steroid influences on brain development and sexual differentiation. In Greep RO (ed): "Reproductive Physiology IV." Baltimore, MD: University Park Press, pp 99–145.

McEwen BS, Lieberburg I, Chaptal C, Krey LC (1977): Aromatization: Important for sexual differentiation of the neonatal rat brain. Horm Behav 9:249–263.

McEwen BS, Plapinger L, Chaptal C, Gerlach J, Wallach G (1975): The role of fetoneonatal estrogen binding proteins in the association of estrogen with neonatal brain cell nuclear receptors. Brain Res 96:400–407.

McGivern RF, Clancy AN, Hill MA, Noble EP (1984): Prenatal alcohol exposure alters adult expression of sexually dimorphic behavior in the rat. Science 224:896–898.

McGivern RF, Raum WJ, Salido E, Redei E (1988a): Lack of prenatal testosterone surge in fetal rats exposed to alcohol: Alterations in testicular morphology and physiology. Alcohol Clin Exp Res 12:243–247.

McGivern RF, Roselli CE, Handa RJ (1988b): Perinatal aromatase activity in male and female rats: Effect of prenatal alcohol exposure. Alcohol Clin Exp Res 12:769–772.

Miller MW (1986): Effects of alcohol on the generation and migration of cerebral cortical neurons. Science 233:1308–1311.

Miller MW (1988): Effect of prenatal exposure to ethanol on the development of cerebral cortex. I. Neuronal generation. Alcohol Clin Exp Res 12:440–449.

Milner TA, Loy R (1982): Hormonal regulation of axonal sprouting in the hippocampus. Brain Res 243:180–185.

Moon Y-S, Hardy UH (1973): The early differentiation of the testes and interstitial cells in the fetal pig, and its duplication in organ culture. Am J Anat 138:253–268.

Morali G, Larsson K, Beyer C (1978): Inhibition of testosterone-induced sexual behavior in the castrated male rat by aromatase blockers. Horm Behav 9:203–211.

Naftolin F, MacLusky NJ, Leranth CZ, Sakamoto HS, Garcia-Segura LM (1988): The cellular effects of estrogens on neuroendocrine tissues. J Steroid Biochem 30:195–207.

Naftolin F, Ryan KJ, Davies IJ, Reddy VV, Flores F, Petro Z, Kuhn M (1975): The formation of estrogens by central neuroendocrine tissues. Rec Prog Horm Res 31:295–319.

Nichizuka M, Arai Y (1981): Sexual dimorphism in synaptic organization in the amygdala and its dependence on neonatal hormone environment. Brain Res 212:31–38.

Nunez EA, Benassayag C, Savu L, Vallete G, Jayle MF (1976): Serum binding of some steroid hormones during development in different animal species. Discussion of the biological significance of this binding. Ann Biol Anim Biochem Biophys 16:491–501.

Nyquist-Battie C, Gochee A (1985): Alterations in the development of the main olfactory bulb of the mouse after ethanol exposure. Int J Dev Neurosci 3:211–222.

Olsson M, Lindahl G, Ruoslahti E (1977): Genetic control of alpha-fetoprotein synthesis in the mouse. J Exp Med 145:819–827.

Palmer RH, Ovellette EM, Warner L, Leichtman SR (1974): Congenital malformations in offspring of a chronic alcoholic mother. Pediatrics 53:490–494.

Parker S, Mahendra U, Gavaler JS, Van Thiel DH (1984): Adverse effects of ethanol upon the adult sexual behavior of male rats exposed in utero. Neurobehav Toxicol Teratol 6:289–293.

Pfaff DW (1966): Morphological changes in the brains of adult male rats after neonatal castration. Endocrinology 36:415–416.

Raisman G, Field PM (1973): Sexual dimorphism in the neuropile of the preoptic area of the rat and its dependence on neonatal androgen. Brain Res 54:1–29.

Reddy VVK, Naftolin F, Ryan KJ (1974): Conversion of androstenedione to estrone by neural tissues from fetal and neonatal rats. Endocrinology 94:117–121.

Rose JC, Meis PJ, Castro MI (1981): Alcohol and fetal endocrine function. Neurobehav Toxicol Teratol 3:105–110.

Roselli CE, Ellinwood WE, Resko JA (1984): Regulation of brain aromatase activity in rats. Endocrinology 114:192–200.

Roselli CE, Horton LE, Resko JA (1987): Time-course and steroid specificity of aromatase induction in rat hypothalamus-preoptic area. Biol Reprod 37:628–633.

Roselli CE, Resko JA (1984): Androgens regulate brain aromatase activity in adult male rats through a receptor mechanism. Endocrinology 114:2183–2189.

Rudeen PK (1986): Reduction of the volume of the sexually dimorphic nucleus of the preoptic area by in utero ethanol exposure in male rats. Neurosci Lett 72:363–368.

Rudeen PK (1988): Fetal ethanol exposure in the rat: A mechanism for brain defects. In Kuriyama K, Takada A, Ishii H (eds): "Biomedical and Social Aspects of Alcohol and Alcoholism." New York: Elsevier, pp 859–862.

Rudeen PK, Creighton JA (1989): Mechanisms of central nervous system alcohol-related birth defects. In Sun GY, Rudeen PK, Wood WG, Wei TII, Sun A Y (eds): "Molecular Mechanisms of Alcohol." Clifton, NJ: Humana Press, pp 147–165.

Rudeen PK, Creighton JA, Kelce W, Ganjam VK (1988): Fetal ethanol effects on aromatase activity in the hypothalamic-preoptic area in the male neonatal brain. Soc Neurosci Abstr 14:284.

Rudeen PK, Kappel CA (1985): Blood and brain testosterone and estradiol levels in neonatal male rats exposed to alcohol in utero. Biol Reprod 32:75.

Rudeen PK, Kappel CA, Lear K (1986): Postnatal or in utero ethanol exposure reduction of the volume of the sexually dimorphic nucleus of the preoptic area in male rats. Drug Alcohol Depend 18:247–252.

Rudeen PK, Paredez S (1989): Aromatase activity (AA) in the hypothalamic/preoptic area of neonatal male and female rats: Testosterone (T) and ethanol (EtOH) exposure. Soc Neurosci Abstr 15:89.

Salonen I, Eriksson CJP (1989): Penetration of ethanol into the male reproductive tract. Alcohol Clin Exp Res 13:746–751.

Schachter BS, Toran-Allerand CD (1982): Intraneuronal alpha-fetoprotein and albumin are not synthesized locally in developing brain. Dev Brain Res 5:93–98.

Scheff SW, Hoff SF, Anderson KJ (1987): Altered regulation of lesion-induced synaptogenesis by adrenalectomy and corticosterone in young adult rats. Exp Neurol 93:456–470.

Serio M, Motta M, Zanisi M, Martini L (1984): Sexual differentiation: Basic and clinical aspects, Serono Symposia, Vol 11, Raven Press, pp 1–368.

Silverman AJ, Krey LW, Zimmerman EA (1979): A comparative study of the luteinizing hormone releasing hormone (LHRH) neuronal networks in mammals. Biol Reprod 20:98–100.

Sokol RJ (1981): Alcohol and abnormal outcomes of pregnancy. Can Med Assoc J 125:143–148.

Sokol RJ, Abel EL (1988): Alcohol-related birth defects: Outlining current research opportunities. Neurotoxicol Teratol 10:183–186.

Stahl F, Gotz F, Poppe I, Amendt P, Dorner G (1978): Pre- and early postnatal testosterone levels in rat and human. In Dorner G, Kawakami M (eds): "Hormones and Brain Development." Amsterdam: Elsevier/North Holland Biomedical Press, pp 99–110.

Sulik KK, Johnston MC, Webb MA (1981): Fetal alcohol syndrome: Embryogenesis in a mouse model. Science 214:936–938.

Toran-Allerand CD (1982): Regional differences in intraneuronal localization of alpha-fetoprotein in the developing mouse brain. Dev Brain Res 5:213–217.

Toran-Allerand CD (1984): On the genesis of sexual differentiation of the central nervous system: Morphogenetic consequences of steroidal exposure and possible role of alpha-fetoprotein. Prog Brain Res 61:63–98.

Tillner I, Majewski F (1978): Furrows and dermal ridges of the hand in patients with alcohol embryopathy. Hum Genet 42:307–314.

Van Thiel DH, Lester R (1976): Alcoholism: Its effect on hypothalamic pituitary gonadal function. Gastroenterology 71:318–327.

Vito CC, Fox TO (1982): Androgen and estrogen receptors in embryonic and neonatal rat brain. Dev Brain Res 2:97–110.

Vito CC, Wieland SJ, Fox TO (1979): Androgen receptors exist throughout the "critical period" of brain sexual differentiation. Nature 282:308–310.

Volk B, Maletz J, Tiedemann M, Mall G, Klein C, Berlet HH (1981): Impaired maturation of Purkinje cells in the fetal alcohol syndrome in the rat. Light and electron microscopic investigations. Acta Neuropathol 54:19–29.

Vreeburg JTM, Van derVaart PDM, Van derSchoot P (1977): Prevention of central defeminization, but not masculinization in male rats by inhibition neonatally of oestrogen biosynthesis. J Endocr 74:375–382.

Warren DW, Haltmeyer GC, Eik-Nes KB (1973): Testosterone in the fetal rat testes. Biol Reprod 8:560–565.

Warren DW, Huhtaniemi IT, Tapanainen J, Dufau ML, Catt KJ (1984): Ontogeny of gonadotropin receptors in the fetal and neonatal rat testes. Endocrinology 114:470–476.

Weisz J, Ward IL (1980): Plasma testosterone and progesterone titers of pregnant rats, their male and female fetuses and neonatal offspring. Endocrinology 106:306–316.

West JR, Hodges A, Black AC, Jr (1981): Prenatal exposure to ethanol alters the organization of hippocampal mossy fibers in rats. Science 211:957–959.

West Jr, Hodges CA (1983): Permanent hippocampal mossy fiber hyperdevelopment following prenatal ethanol exposure. Neurobehav Toxicol Teratol 5:139–150.

Zirkin BR, Ewing LL (1987): Leydig cell differentiation during maturation of the rat testis: A stereological study of cell number and ultrastructure. Anat Rec 219:157–163.

Development of the Central Nervous System:
Effects of Alcohol and Opiates, pages 189–207
© 1992 Wiley-Liss, Inc.

9

Ethanol-Induced Teratology and Second Messenger Signal Transduction

SAM N. PENNINGTON

Department of Biochemistry, East Carolina University, Greenville, North Carolina

INTRODUCTION

This chapter focuses on molecular changes occurring in the fetal central nervous system (CNS) as the result of prenatal exposure to ethanol. The discussion emphasizes the effects that such changes have on cell proliferation, migration, and differentiation, and on the ensuing fetal development. No attempt is made to distinguish between the effects of ethanol and those of acetaldehyde. In several cases, references are made to the effect of ethanol on adult CNS tissue because of the relative lack of systematic biochemical studies of ethanol's effect on the fetal CNS.

Background on FAS

The early, modern description of the fetal alcohol syndrome (FAS) was made in 1968 (Lemoine et al., 1968), and FAS was formally defined by Jones and Smith in 1973 (Jones et al., 1973; Jones and Smith, 1975). Subsequently, there has developed a extensive body of data describing the effects of in utero ethanol exposure on pre- and postnatal development. FAS and alcohol-related birth defects (ARBD) have been reviewed from both the clinical and experimental viewpoints. A 1982 paper (Colangelo and Jones, 1982) provided a wide-ranging review of the neurological ramifications of FAS. This paper gave a valuable overview of both the early clinical and experimental literature, including various inferences drawn from the CNS effects of ethanol in adult brain. Likewise, another view (Dow and Riopelle, 1987) provided an excellent outline of the development of the CNS and reviewed the effects of ethanol on the CNS. As pointed out in these reviews and others (Sandor, 1979; Streissguth et al., 1980; Sokol, 1982; Jones, 1986; Abel and Sokol, 1987), there exist significant clinical data and a wide variety of histological/histochemical data, but there remains a lack of fundamental molecular data. Thus, the molecular processes responsible for the retarded development of the central nervous system in fetal alcohol syndrome are essentially unknown.

Growth Retardation and Behavioral Teratology

The authors of most reviews of FAS share the conclusion that, in both humans and in animal models, ethanol exposure during pregnancy causes a variety of adverse outcomes with fetal growth suppression being the single most common ethanol-related deficit (Abel and Dintcheff, 1978). This growth retardation is especially pronounced in the CNS. Intrauterine growth retardation as a result of ethanol exposure is found in all animals models of ARBD, including animals exposed to ethanol on a single day of gestation (Goodlett et al., 1989; Poltorak et al., 1990). The growth inhibition also occurs in cross-fostered animals as well as in transplanted embryos (Checiu and Sandor, 1987). Multiple factors have been found to impact on and/or to modify ethanol-induced growth suppression. Thus, in both human and animal studies, such diverse parameters as maternal smoking (Harlap and Shiono, 1980), maternal nutrition (Detering et al., 1981), fetal hypothermia (Henderson et al., 1980), dehydration (Leichter and Lee, 1984), number of pregnancies (Dexter et al., 1983), peak blood alcohol levels (BAL), and binge drinking versus chronic consumption (Pierce and West, 1986a; Pierce and West, 1986b) have all been shown to influence the magnitude of the fetal growth response to ethanol. However, it remains to be determined how these factors are translated into the molecular events responsible for the CNS hypoplasia associated with fetal ethanol exposure.

Even in the absence of the full FAS (as defined by a set of craniofacial malformations, growth retardation, and mental retardation), the developing human CNS appears to be particularly sensitive to ethanol-induced growth suppression, and fetal ethanol exposure has been found to result in a high incidence of mental retardation (Abel and Sokol, 1987) and/or behavioral deficits that do not respond well to therapy (Darby et al., 1981; Streissguth et al., 1986). Thus, the correlation of mental retardation with small brain size is strongest at high levels of maternal alcohol consumption, but data suggest that CNS effects that are manifested later in life, such as learning disabilities or behavioral deficits, may occur at lower maternal doses (Streissguth et al., 1980).

Animal model studies provide compelling evidence that fetal exposure to ethanol causes growth suppression of the developing CNS and results in motor, sensory, and behavioral defects (Abel, 1979; Driscoll et al., 1980; Streissguth et al., 1986; Gilliam et al., 1987; Molina et al., 1987; Meyer et al., 1990). Specific ethanol-related anomalies in the structure of various brain areas and brain cell types have also been reported (Woodson and Ritchey, 1979; Detering et al., 1981; Hammer and Scheibel, 1981; West and Hodges-Savola, 1983; Rudeen et al., 1986; Pierce and West, 1987; Mohamed et al., 1987; Miller, 1986, 1987, 1988, 1989; Kotkoskie and Norton, 1989; Bonthius and West, 1990; Guerri et al., 1990; Miller and Potempa, 1990; also see Chapter 5), but these changes are not always correlated with unambiguous changes in cell function (Shoemaker et al., 1980). At the cellular level, ethanol-induced growth suppression is known to be associated with a prolonged G_1 phase of the cell cycle (Miller, 1989; Cook et al., 1990a, b; Guerri et al., 1990;), while the S (synthetic) and M (mitotic) phases are little affected. In some CNS proliferative zones, there are no changes in cell cycle but rather changes in the number of cycling cells (Miller and Nowakowski, 1991). In a series of papers (Miller, 1986, 1987, 1988, 1989; Miller et al., 1990), Miller has described the effects of in utero ethanol exposure on the histological development of fetal brains, including the generally inhibitory effects of ethanol on the generation, proliferation, migration, and distribution of neurons.

Several studies (Ramp et al., 1975; Shoemaker et al., 1980; Sandor, 1979; Vaema and Persaud, 1982; Pennington et al., 1983; Pennington et al., 1985; Pennington and Kalmus, 1987; Beeker et al., 1988; Pennington, 1988a; Pennington, 1988b) have used the chick embryo as a model for investigating the mechanism of ethanol-induced fetal growth inhibition. Because the chick embryo is a non-placental model, it is believed to negate alcohol-induced changes in maternal and placental physiology and to thus allow examination of the "direct" fetal effects of ethanol. In this model, a single dose of ethanol given at the start of incubation (day 0) results in a significant growth inhibition in the embryo on days 5–10 of development (hatching = day 21 to 22). Brain growth is inhibited by alcohol in this model, and the growth inhibition is highly correlated with blood ethanol levels (Pennington et al., 1985). Pharmacological treatments that either elevate or reduce the blood alcohol levels result in a corresponding increase or decrease, respectively, in the brain hypoplasia (Pennington, 1988a). Metabolic clearance of the ethanol dose as the fetal liver matures results in the return of the growth rate to normal or slightly higher levels (Pennington and Kalmus, 1987); at hatching, the ethanol-treated animals are not significantly smaller than vehicle-dosed controls (Pennington and Kalmus 1007). However, at hatching, the ethanol-treated chicks have statistically significant behavioral deficits including delayed hatching and piping relative to the vehicle-dosed controls (Means et al., 1986, 1988, 1989).

MOLECULAR CHANGES ASSOCIATED WITH FAS

Studies using several models have provided insight into the biochemical changes associated with ethanol-induced suppression of fetal brain growth. The wide variety of molecular mechanisms associated with various aspects of fetal alcohol syndrome have recently been reviewed (Schenker et al., 1990). As suggested by that review and others, there exist a multitude of possible molecular interactions between ethanol and developing tissue. At the molecular level, several laboratories have shown that ethanol causes a general depression in the rates of protein and DNA synthesis (Woodson and Ritchey, 1979; Dreosti et al., 1981; Pennington et al., 1985; Rawat, 1985; Pennington and Kalmus, 1987; Guerri et al., 1990). In addition, changes in fetal nutrient flow have been reported as a result of altered placental physiology. These changes include drug-induced placental hyperplasia (Gordon et al., 1985; Aufrere and Le Bourhis, 1987), altered amino acid uptake (Thadani et al., 1977; Fisher et al., 1981; Gordon et al., 1985; Snyder et al., 1989), altered carbohydrate absorption (Snyder et al., 1986), and changes in zinc transport (Kumar, 1982; Ghishan and Greene, 1983), but little is known of the mechanism by which these changes occur. The many "positive" results obtained from these studies suggest that the effect of ethanol in any given tissue may involve multiple mechanisms of pathology.

Because the exact sequence of molecular events responsible for the growth inhibitory effects of ethanol are unknown, it is not possible to predict which mothers or fetuses will respond adversely to ethanol exposure or if there are time periods or an ethanol dose that represent "no risk" during a given pregnancy. Thus, ethanol-elicited CNS growth suppression is a preventable cause of mental retardation, but at the present time, abstinence is the only preventive measure. For these reasons, it is important to identify the molecular events by which ethanol inhibits fetal growth.

Hormones, Fetal Growth, and Ethanol

A wide spectrum of maternal, placental, and fetal hormones is known to regulate fetal growth and development, and these hormone/signal systems may impact fetal growth in several ways. Among the hormones known to influence cellular mitotic activity and/or cell growth are platelet-derived growth factor (PDGF), nerve growth factor (NGF), epidermal growth factor (EGF), prostaglandins (PGs), insulin, insulin-like growth factors (IGFs), and the adrenergic hormones. As would be expected for such a diverse group of potent biological agents, these systems are intensely studied because of their ability to regulate a multitude of physiological functions. The biochemical process by which most of these nonsteroid hormones exert their effects can be arbitrarily divided into the steps of hormone release, hormone binding by a specific receptor, internalization of the hormone signal, generation of a hormone second messenger whose intensity (concentration) reflects the presence and/or relative concentration of the hormone, activation of a specific protein kinase by the second messenger, and covalent modification of various proteins by the kinase catalytic activity with resulting alterations in one or more physiological processes. An important finding has been the observation that there are distinct changes in the various molecular steps of this hormone signaling pathway as a result of fetal exposure to ethanol (Colangelo and Jones, 1982; Pennington et al., 1983; Randall and Anton, 1984; Pennington et al., 1985; Pennington and Kalmus, 1987; Randall et al., 1987; Beeker et al., 1988; Pennington, 1988b; Fielder et al., 1989; Okonmah et al., 1989; Anton et al., 1990; Dow and Riopelle, 1990; Hoek and Rubin, 1990; Balduini and Costa, 1990; Pennington, 1990; Poltorak et al., 1990; Wigal et al., 1990).

These changes include drug-induced anomalies in hormone levels. As an illustration, growth-inhibited brains of chick embryos dosed with ethanol have been shown to contain significantly higher levels of the E-type prostaglandins, with the increase apparently corresponding to lower prostaglandin dehydrogenase (PGDH) activity during the early stages of development (Pennington et al., 1985). Following clearance of the ethanol, the growth rate returned to normal, and the return to normal growth status was paralleled by a return of the prostaglandin E levels to normal. However, the decrease in tissue PGE levels was not the result of an increase in PGDH activity, because this enzyme activity remained depressed in the brains of alcohol-treated embryos throughout the time period studied (days 7 to 15). Simultaneous administration of a prostaglandin synthesis inhibitor (indomethacin) with the ethanol prevented the brain hypoplasia (Pennington et al., 1985), and others have reported that prostaglandin synthesis inhibitors, including aspirin and indomethacin, prevent alcohol-induced birth defects (Randall and Anton, 1984; Randall et al., 1987). However, in the chick embryo, this treatment also lowered blood alcohol levels (Pennington, 1988a). Thus, although the pharmacological treatment lowered PGE levels, the exact molecular mechanism by which indomethacin prevented the ethanol-induced growth inhibition is unclear. Furthermore, the administration of a long-lasting PGE_2 analog (dimethyl-PGE_2) failed to induce significant growth suppression in this model (Pennington, 1990), suggesting that the increased levels of the hormone-like PGE_2 alone was not sufficient to inhibit brain growth in the chick embryo. It should also be noted that other laboratories (Bonthius and West, 1989) have reported that, in the rat, aspirin given with the ethanol dose actually enhanced the growth inhibition induced by the alcohol, making it unclear whether or not PGs play the same role in regulating growth in all species.

Ethanol, Adenylate Cyclase, and Cyclic AMP

Certainly the most intensely studied second messenger system with respect to the effects of ethanol is the adenylate cyclase/cAMP system. Numerous laboratories have investigated the effects of ethanol on adenylate cyclase activity and the resulting effects on tissue cAMP status. The CNS, gut, kidney, and platelets have been the most widely studied tissues (Greene et al., 1971; Israel et al., 1972; Kuriyama and Israel, 1973; Volicer and Gold, 1973; Mashiter et al., 1974; Jauhonen et al., 1975; Volicer and Gold, 1975; Orenberg et al., 1976; Redos et al., 1976; Atkinson et al., 1977; Kuriyama, 1977; Shen et al., 1977; Breese et al., 1979; French et al., 1979; Harper and Brooker, 1980; Hynie et al., 1980; Hawley et al., 1981; Rabin and Molinof, 1981; Smith et al., 1981; Biddulph et al., 1982; Mena et al., 1982; Von-Hungen and Baxter, 1982; Lucchi et al., 1983; Rabin and Molinof, 1983; Seitz et al., 1983; Goldyne, 1984; Luthin and Tabakoff, 1984; Okuda et al., 1984; Rius et al., 1986; Hwang et al., 1987; O'Dell et al., 1983; Scawen et al., 1982; Myking et al., 1987; Rabin et al., 1987; Lykouras et al., 1988; Tabakoff et al., 1988; Valverius et al., 1988; Rabe et al., 1990; Rabin, 1990a, b; Rubin and Hoek, 1990). Far fewer labs have studied the effect of ethanol on the enzymatic degradation of cAMP by phosphodiesterase, but these studies have reported a nearly universal lack of effect of ethanol on phosphodiesterase (Kuriyama, 1977; Pennington, 1988b).

Using primarily an adult rodent model, Tabakoff and co-workers (Luthin and Tabakoff, 1984; Tabakoff et al., 1988; Valverius et al., 1988; Rabe et al., 1990) have studied the acute and chronic effects of ethanol on brain adenylate cyclase and cAMP levels. This group has shown that alcohol alters the function of the beta-adrenergic receptor as well as the coupling of this receptor to the cyclase enzyme. In the fetus, a similar interaction has been reported between ethanol and this receptor (Wigal et al., 1990). In this study, the interaction of ethanol with fetal membrane receptors was apparently specific to the beta-adrenergic receptor as little change was observed in the muscarinic receptor upon exposure to ethanol. However, in vitro exposure of neonatal rat brain tissue to high levels of ethanol (500 mM) resulted in inhibition of muscarinic receptor-mediated hydrolysis of phosphoinositide, but it had no effect on adult brain hydrolysis (Balduini and Costa, 1990). In fact, in adult brain, ethanol has been reported to activate the phophoinositide-specific phospholipase C (Hoek and Rubin, 1990). Kelly et al. (1989) have also reported that exposure of neonatal rats to ethanol during the brain growth spurt leads to alterations in hippocampal muscarinic receptor numbers in the animals as adults and that this change is associated with behavioral deficits in these animals.

The effect of alcohol on in vivo cAMP levels has likewise been widely studied (Kuriyama and Israel, 1973; Volicer and Gold, 1973; Orenberg et al., 1976; Breese et al., 1979; Weitbrecht and Cramer, 1980; Hawley et al., 1981; Rabe et al., 1990; Rabin, 1990a, b), but the results were much less clear cut. Multiple laboratories have reported increased (Volicer and Gold, 1975; Lucchi et al., 1983, 1984), decreased (Shen et al., 1983; Pennington, 1990a), or no change in tissue cAMP levels (Redos et al., 1976; Von-Hungen and Baxter, 1982) as the result of ethanol exposure, with the results dependent to some degree on the animal model and on the method or duration of ethanol dosing.

PC-12 cells have been used as a model of the effect of ethanol on neuronal cell adenylate cyclase activity and tissue cAMP content. PC-12 cells chronically exposed to ethanol showed lowered responsiveness to 2-chloroadenosine-induced stimulation of cAMP content (Rabin, 1990b). On the other hand, broken cell preparations showed no difference in adenylate cyclase activity, a finding similar to that reported for the effect of ethanol on embryonic chick brain adenylate cyclase activity exposed to ethanol in ovo (Pennington, 1988b). Rabin has also reported a similar finding in primary cultures of neonatal rat cerebella (Rabin, 1990a). However, it has been observed by others (Rabe et al., 1990) that sublines of PC-12 cells differ in their response to chronic ethanol exposure with respect to the effect on cAMP content. Thus, any extrapolation of the effect of ethanol in a given cell line or type to another tissue may be complicated by variable interactions.

Relatively few studies of the effects of ethanol on fetal CNS adenylate cyclase/cAMP have been reported (Mena et al., 1982; Pennington et al., 1983; Pennington et al., 1985; Pennington, 1988b; Pennington, 1990). Using a paradigm that did not include pair feeding, Mena and coworkers (Mena et al., 1982) found no difference in brain cAMP levels in day-21 fetuses or in day-1 and day-4 neonates. In chick embryos dosed with physiologically appropriate levels of ethanol (up to 1.5g/kg), it was observed that there was a down regulation of the responsiveness of brain adenylate cyclase to stimulation by exogenous PGs (Pennington, 1988b), but the levels of cAMP were repeatedly found to be elevated (Pennington et al., 1983, 1985; Pennington and Kalmus, 1987; Pennington, 1988b). Recently, the increase in cAMP has been shown to be the result of a rapid post mortem synthesis of cAMP in this model (Pennington, 1990), and the in vivo effect of chronic ethanol is now thought to involve a decrease in cAMP levels during early CNS development. Furthermore, these studies showed that unless the brain tissue was isolated in liquid nitrogen, there was a significantly greater postmortem accumulation of cAMP in the drug-treated brains than in the control brains, suggesting that there were drug-related changes in the membrane environment of the adenylate cyclase protein. Relevant to tissue preparation, it is important to note that treated embryos did have measurable blood ethanol levels at sacrifice but that the process of tissue preparation removed essentially all traces of ethanol such that the changes in biochemical function observed in this model were in the absence of ethanol per se. Likewise in this model, other drugs that inhibit fetal CNS growth, e.g. nicotine, showed a similar effect on cAMP, i.e., a lowering of in situ CNS cAMP content and a more rapid post mortem accumulation of cAMP (Pennington, unpublished observations).

Ethanol and Fetal Brain Protein Kinase

The adult CNS contains several types of protein kinases, including those regulated by known intermediaries and kinases for which the second messenger molecules are unrecognized. These protein kinases play vital roles in neuronal signal transduction in adult CNS (Wilson, 1980), and researchers have examined the effects of ethanol on several of these systems, including the cAMP-dependent protein kinase activity of adult brain (Kuriyama et al., 1976; Kuriyama, 1977; Gonzales et al., 1986; Rius et al., 1986; Rabin et al., 1987; Tabakoff et al., 1988; Valverius et al., 1988; Deitrich et al., 1989; Rabin, 1990a; Rubin and Hoek, 1990). It should be noted, however, that the effect of fetal ethanol exposure on cAMP-dependent protein kinase activity has not been systematically examined.

As in the mature CNS, the developing brain contains several types of protein kinases, with cAMP-dependent protein kinase again being the best studied. In both adult and fetal brains, the cAMP-dependent protein kinase enzyme complex occurs in two major molecular forms, protein kinase I (PK-AI) and protein kinase II (PK-AII). Both enzymes exist as inactive tetramers, i.e., holoenzymes, containing two regulatory (R) and two catalytic (C) subunits (R_2C_2). The catalytic subunits are released from the holoenzyme as a result of the binding of cAMP by the regulatory subunit (Fig. 1). PK-AI and PK-AII have similar C subunits but differ in the structure of the R subunits (RI and RII). A distinct RII has been reported in brain (Erlichman et al., 1980). In the adult brain, high levels of PK-AII activity are associated with neuronal cell function in all areas of the brain while lower levels of PK-AI activity are located primarily in glial cells. In the fetal brain, PK-AII appears to be the more prevalent form of the

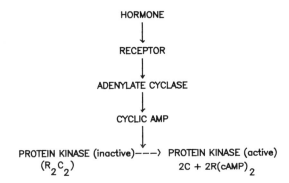

Fig. 1. Representation of the cAMP-dependent protein kinase cascade. Membrane components, including G-protein subunits, are not shown nor is the phosphorylation of regulatory subunit (R) by the catalytic subunit represented.

enzyme. Cyclic AMP-dependent kinases are also found predominantly in the cytoplasm of most cells, but in the adult and fetal brain, the activity appears to be equally distributed between the cytoplasmic and particulate (synaptic) fractions.

Cyclic AMP-dependent protein kinase

As described above, fetal ethanol exposure alters tissue cAMP levels, a result that appears to have significant impact on protein kinase activity. In addition, ethanol might also be anticipated to have a direct effect on the function of the kinase proteins. Based upon the data to be discussed below, it appears that ethanol has both direct and indirect (second messenger) effects on the activity of protein kinases. Although ethanol has been reported to have no effect on either basal or cAMP-stimulated kinase catalytic activity toward an exogenous substrate (histone II-B) in the developing brain (Pennington, 1988b), the phosphorylation of several endogenous brain proteins was altered by ethanol exposure (Beeker et al., 1988). For example, the basal and cAMP-stimulated autophosphorylation of cAMP-dependent protein kinase regulatory subunit (RII) was significantly lowered by ethanol (Beeker et al., 1988). Furthermore, the binding of cAMP by RII was also reduced by ethanol exposure (Pennington, 1988b), suggesting that ethanol had produced a down regulation in the regulatory activity of the cAMP-dependent kinase and a selective loss of catalytic (phosphorylating) activity. These studies suggested not only that the developing chick brain contained primarily protein kinase A-II (PK AII), but likewise suggested that ethanol exposure altered only the kinase activity associated with the cytoplasmic fraction. Therefore, the ethanol-induced loss of cAMP-stimulated kinase activity appeared to be a specific effect on the cytoplasmic fraction enzyme and not simply a redistribution of the activity between the cytoplasmic and particulate fractions. In a similar manner, nicotine, another growth inhibitory drug, also decreased brain protein kinase II regulatory activity (Fig. 2), suggesting that the loss of tissue cAMP and cAMP binding activity are common factors associated with drug-induced growth suppression in the CNS. These data not withstanding, a sustained-dose form of cAMP did not exhibit a growth stimulatory response in the chick embryo model (Fig. 3).

Tyrosine kinases

A variety of growth-related hormones are known to mediate their physiological action via the activation of tyrosine kinases, often with a resulting

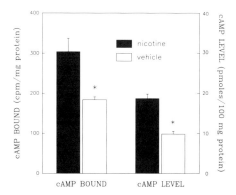

Fig. 2. The effect of a single dose of nicotine (2.0 mg/egg) on the cyclic AMP content and cyclic AMP binding activity of embryonic brain on day 7. The embryos were growth inhibited (data not shown) and the decrease in cyclic AMP content and binding activity are both significant ($P < 0.05$).

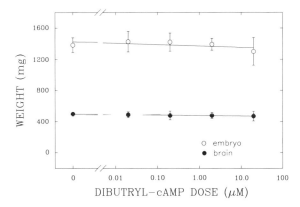

Fig. 3. The effect of a sustained dose form of cyclic AMP (dibutryl cAMP) on embryo weight. The dose was administered on day 0 and the embryos killed on day 7. There are no significant differences.

critical impact on fetal energy metabolism. For example, insulin, insulin-like growth factors, and epidermal growth factor all activate tyrosine kinases and mediate fetal growth, as well as directly or indirectly influencing fetal energy metabolism. Unfortunately, the biochemical mechanisms by which these hormonal signals are transduced into normal growth is poorly understood. Thus, it is difficult to study pathological changes in a system for which the normal physiology is not well defined. Furthermore, the effects of ethanol exposure on fetal hormones that activate tyrosine kinases have not been widely reported. Fielder and coworkers (Fielder et al., 1989) have examined the effects of prenatal ethanol treatment on maternal and fetal prolactin, growth hormone, and insulin, but found no profound changes as the result of ethanol consumption.

Fetal energy metabolism

Although the second messenger system is not well understood, one of the important pathophysiological results of fetal alcohol exposure is an alteration in fetal energy metabolism. Little is known of the molecular regulatory mechanisms by which the changes in fetal energy metabolism occur, but they might be presumed to involve tyrosine kinase-mediated events. The second messages that regulate fetal energy metabolism are unknown, but there are considerable data to suggest that ethanol-induced changes are important. For example, in regenerating tissue, various investigators (Gerhart et al., 1988; Henderson et al., 1989) have reported that ethanol blocks the ability of epidermal growth factor (EGF) to induce carbohydrate metabolism. Because the action of EGF is necessary for facial/cranial development, these workers suggested that such an effect in the fetus could result in the facial malformations associated with FAS. In regenerating tissue, the mechanism by which ethanol inhibits growth appears to involve specific molecular events rather than a general suppression of protein synthesis. Ethanol also inhibits growth in this model without altering the transcription of certain protooncogenes known to play a central role in cell proliferation (Diehl et al., 1990).

Whatever the mechanism, altered fetal energy metabolism has been shown to be an important molecular mechanism by which ethanol suppresses the growth of the CNS. For example, several studies (Snyder et al., 1986; Vingan et al., 1986; Miller and Dow-Edwards, 1988; Singh et al., 1988; Pullen et al., 1988) have shown that maternal ethanol intake results in abnormal placental glucose transport such that fetal:maternal glucose ratios were significantly lower in the ethanol-treated group. This decreased fetal:maternal glucose ratio was positively correlated with growth suppression. In one of the few published reports on the direct effects of ethanol on fetal cellular energy metabolism (Singh et al., 1990), alcohol appeared to inhibit glucose uptake in fetal rat brain cells grown in culture, but to have little effect on other insulin mediated events.

In brains of adult rats exposed to ethanol as fetuses, changes in glucose utilization (Vingan et al., 1986; Miller and Dow-Edwards, 1988) and an abnormal response to glucose loading (Lopez-Tejero et al., 1989) have been reported. Depending on the brain area and cell layer examined, increased or decreased glucose uptake/utilization was observed, with an overall decrease in glucose utilization being the predominant finding.

Ethanol exposure also has been shown to alter fetal brain glucose (glycogen) stores, with both increased and decreased tissue glycogen being found, depending on the dose received by the developing embryo (Delphia et al., 1978). Little change has been reported in fetal conversion of alanine to glucose as the result of fetal alcohol exposure (Sharma and Rawat, 1989), suggesting that ethanol does not alter fetal gluconeogenic activity.

It is important to note that for both the fetal and adult glucose uptake/utilization studies, the use of carbohydrate to isocalorically replace ethanol in the diet results in the the pair-fed controls receiving a diet extremely high in carbohydrates, and this fact has been suggested to influence the experimental outcome (Nguyen et al., 1990), at least for some paradigms.

Protein kinase C

An expanding body of data suggests that both acute and chronic exposure to ethanol may cause significant changes in the calcium and phospholipid-dependent protein kinase (PK-C). A variety of changes in adult brain and liver PK-C have been reported (Gonzales et al., 1986; Gonzales and Crews, 1988; Battaini et al., 1989; Hoek and Rubin, 1990) as the result of ethanol exposure, but limited data are available as to the effects of ethanol on fetal PK-C. As described above, ethanol alters the receptor-mediated generation of phosphoinositide second message, with both increase and decrease receptor responsiveness being reported (Kelly et al., 1989; Balduini and Costa, 1990; Hoek and Rubin, 1990).

Astroglial cells grown in culture have been shown (Skwidh and Shain, 1990) to respond to acute ethanol exposure by redistributing their PK-C activity from the cell cytosol to the membrane fraction with no change in total cellular activity. Such changes in PK-C may also result in changes in the PK-A responsiveness, as reports of both stimulatory (Magnaldo et al., 1988) and inhibitory interactions (Teitelbaum, 1990) between PK-C and PK-A have appeared.

SUMMARY

The interaction of ethanol and second messenger-mediated hormone systems appears to involve a number of distinct molecular changes. For example, studies have suggested that ethanol elevates PGE levels in embryonic brain and that indomethacin protects against this increase, but that indomethacin also enhances the clearance of the ethanol dose. Furthermore, a sustained-dose form of PGE_2 was not effective in inducing growth suppression. Together, these results suggest a pharmacokinetic mechanism of action for indomethacin in the chick model. It has also been observed that aspirin actually enhances the growth inhibition induced in rat pups exposed to ethanol during the early postnatal period. Changes are not observed in all fetal hormones as a result of ethanol exposure.

Ethanol exposure is known to alter a variety of membrane-associated signaling systems, including the adenylate cyclase pathway. Chronic ethanol exposure stimulates adenylate cyclase activity in a number of tissue preparations including adult brain. This increase in adult brain cyclase activity is not further elevated by beta adrenergic compounds. For the embryonic chick brain, it was observed that ethanol caused no changes in the in vitro activity of adenylate cyclase and phosphodiesterase. Adenylate cyclase activity from ethanol-treated brains, however, was significantly less responsive to stimulation by exogenous PGE_2, suggesting a down regulation. Studies on changes in brain levels of cAMP in response to chronic ethanol exposure are inconclusive. In adult tissue preparations, chronic ethanol dosing has been reported to elevate, to lower, and to have no effect on brain cAMP levels.

Significant data do suggest that ethanol may directly alter the activity of the cAMP-dependent protein kinase enzyme, and lower basal cAMP levels as well, at least in fetal tissue. Ethanol-induced decreases in cAMP levels were associated with decreases in basal protein kinase phosphorylating activity toward endogenous brain protein substrates. Furthermore, ethanol decreased the binding of added cAMP and suppressed the ability of exogenous cAMP to stimulate catalytic activity, suggesting a direct effect on the kinase.

Satisfactory resolution of the question as to the role of second messenger levels in ethanol-induced fetal brain hypoplasia must await further studies at the molecular level. Current data certainly imply that this area could be a fertile focus for research if appropriate models and ethanol dose levels are studied in a systematic manner.

ACKNOWLEDGMENTS

This work was supported in part by PHS grant AA-05813 (NIAAA).

REFERENCES

Abel EL (1979): Prenatal effects of alcohol on adult learning in rats. Pharmacol Biochem Behav 10:239–243.

Abel EL, Dintcheff BA (1978): Effects of prenatal alcohol exposure on growth and development in rats. J Pharmacol Exp Ther 207:916–921.

Abel EL, Sokol RJ (1987): Incidence of fetal alcohol syndrome and economic impact of fas-related anomalies. Drug Alcohol Depend 19:51–70.

Anton RF, Becker HC, Randall CL (1990): Ethanol increases PGE and thromboxane production in mouse pregnant uterine tissue. Life Sci 46:1145–1153.

Atkinson JP, Sullivan TJ, Kelly JP, Parker CW (1977): Stimulation by alcohols of cyclic AMP metabolism in human leukocytes. J Clin Invest 60:284–294.

Aufrere G, Le Bourhis B (1987): Effect of alcohol intoxication during pregnancy on foetal and placental weight: Experimental studies. Alcohol Alcohol 22:401–407.

Balduini W, Costa LG (1990): Developmental neurotoxicity of ethanol: In vitro inhibition of muscarinic receptors-stimulated phosphoinositide metabolism in brain from neonatal but not adult rats. Brain Res 512:248–252.

Battaini F, Del Vesco R, Gononi S, Trabucchi M (1989): Chronic alcohol intake modifies phorbol ester binding in selected rat brain areas. Alcohol 6:169–172.

Beeker K, Deans D, Elton C, Pennington SN (1988): Ethanol-induced growth inhibition in embryonic chick brain is associated with changes in cyclic AMP-dependent protein kinase regulatory subunit. Alcohol Alcohol 23:477–482.

Biddulph DM, Wrenn RW, Currie MG, Hubbard WR (1983): Enhancement by ethanol of parathyroid-hormone-stimulated cyclic AMP accumulation in isolated renal tubules. Mineral Electrolyte Metab 9:76–81.

Bonthius DJ, West JR (1989): Aspirin augments alcohol in restricting growth in the neonatal rats. Neurotoxicol Teratol 11:135–143.

Bonthius DJ, West JR (1990): Alcohol-induced neuronal loss in developing rats: Increased brain damage with binge exposure. Alcoholism (NY) 14:107–118.

Breese GR, Lundberg D, Mailman RB, Frye GD, Mueller RA (1979): Effect of ethanol on cyclic nucleotides in vivo: Consequences of controlling motor and respiratory changes. Drug Alcohol Depend 4:321–326.

Checiu M, Sandor S (1987): The effect of ethanol upon early development in mice and rats. Morphol Embryol 33:13–18.

Colangelo W, Jones DG (1982): The fetal alcohol syndrome: A review and assessment of the syndrome and its neurological sequelae. Prog Neurobiol 19:271–314.

Cook RT, Keiner J, Yen A, Fishbaugh J (1990a): Ethanol-induced growth inhibition and growth adapation in vitro. Cell cycle delays in late Gl. Alcohol Alcohol 25:33–43.

Cook RT, Keiner JA, Yen A (1990b): Ethanol causes accelerated Gl arrest in differentiating HL-60 cells. Alcohol Clin Exp Res 14:695–703.

Darby B, Streissguth AP, Smith DW (1981): A preliminary follow-up of 8 children diagnosed fetal alcohol syndrome in infancy. Neurobehav Toxicol Teratol 3:157–159.

Deitrich R, Bludeau PA, Baker RC (1989): Investigations of the role of protein kinsae C in the acute sedative effects of ethanol. Alcoholism (NY) 13:737–745.

Delphia JM, Negulesco JA, Finan E (1978): The effect of ethanol on cerebral glycogen levels in the chick embryo. Res Commun Chem Pathol Pharmacol 21:347–350.

Detering N, Collins R, Hawkins R, Ozand P, Karahasan A (1981): Comparative effects of ethanol and maturation on the development of catecholamine neurons: A long lasting effect in the hypothalamus. J Neurochem 36:2094–2096.

Dexter J, Tumbleson M, Decker J, Middleton C (1983): Comparison of the offspring of three serial pregnancies during voluntary alcohol consumption in Sinclair (S-1) minature swine. Neurobehav Toxicol 5:229–231.

Diehl AM, Thorgeirsson SS, Steer CJ (1990): Ethanol inhibits liver regeneration in rat without reducing transcripts of key protooncogenes. Gastroenterology 99:-1105–1112.

Dow KE, Riopelle RJ (1987): Neurotoxicity of ethanol during prenatal development. Clin Neuropharmacol 10:330–341.

Dow KE, Riopelle RJ (1990): Specific effects of ethanol on neurite-promoting proteoglycans of neuronal origin. Brain Res 508:40–45.

Dreosti IE, Ballard FJ, Belling GB, Record IR, Manuel SJ, Hetzel BS (1981): The effect of ethanol and acetaldehyde on DNA synthesis in growing cells and on fetal development in the rat. Alcohol Clin Exp Res 5:357–362.

Driscoll CD, Chen JS, Riley EP (1980): Operant DRL performance in rats following prenatal alcohol exposure. Neurobehav Toxicol 2:207–211.

Erlichman J, Sarkar D, Fleischer N, Rubin CS (1980): Identification of two subclasses of type II cAMP-dependent protein kinases. J Biol Chem 255:8179–8184.

Fielder PJ, Robleto DO, Ogren L, Talamantes F (1989): Ethanol consumption during pregnancy in mice: Effects on hormone concentrations. Am J Physiol 257:E561–E566.

Fisher SE, Barnicle MA, Steis B, Holzman I, Van Thiel DH (1981): Effects of acute ethanol exposure upon in vivo leucine uptake and protein synthesis in the fetal rat. Pediatr Res 15:355–339.

French SW, Ihrig TJ, Pettit NB (1979): Effect of alcohol on the plasma cAMP response to glucagon. Res Commun Chem Pathol Pharmacol 26:209–212.

Gerhart MJ, Reed BY, Veech RL (1988): Epidermal growth factor binding in the presence of ethanol. Adv Alcohol Subst Abuse 7:209–211.

Ghishan FK, Greene HL (1983): Fetal alcohol syndrome: Failure of zinc supplementation to reverse the effect of ethanol on placental transport of zinc. Pediatr Res 17:529–531.

Gilliam DM, Stilman A, Dudek BC, Riley EP (1987): Fetal alcohol effects in long- and short-sleep mice: Activity, passive advoidance, and in utero ethanol levels. Neurotoxicol Teratol 9:349–357.

Goldyne ME (1984): Leukotrienes: Clinical significance. J Am Acad Dermatol 10:659–668.

Gonzales RA, Crews FT (1988): Effects of ethanol in vivo and in vitro on stimulated phosphoinositide hydrolysis in rat cortex and cerebellum. Alcohol Clin Exp Res 12:94–98.

Gonzales RA, Theiss C, Crews FT (1986): Effect of ethanol on stimulated inositol phospholipid hydrolysis in rat brain. J Pharmacol Exp Ther 237:92–98.

Goodlett CR, Mahoney JC, West JR (1989): Brain growth delays following a single day of alcohol exposure in the neonatal rat. Alcohol 6:121–126.

Gordon BH, Streeter ML, Rosso P, Winik M (1985): Prenatal alcohol exposure: Abnormalities in placental growth and fetal amino acid uptake in the rat. Biol Neonate 47:113–119.

Greene HL, Herman RH, Kraemer S (1971): Stimulation of jejunal adenyl cyclase by ethanol. J Lab Clin Med 78:336–342.

Guerri C, Saez R, Sancho-tello m, de Aquilera M, Renau-Piquera J (1990): Ethanol alters astrocyte development: A study of critical periods using primary cultures. Neurochem Res 15:559–565.

Hammer RP, Scheibel AB (1981): Morphologic evidence for a delay of neuronal maturation in fetal alcohol exposure. Exp Neurol 74:587–596.

Harlap S, Shiono PH (1980): Alcohol, smoking, and incidence of spontaneous abortions in the first and second trimester. Lancet 1:173–176.

Harper JF, Brooker G (1980): Alcohol potentiation of isoproterenol-stimulated cyclic AMP accumulation in rat parotid. J Cyclic Nucleotide Res 6:51–62.

Hawley RJ, Major LF, Schulman ES, Trocha PJ, Takenga JK, Catravas GN (1981): Cerebrospinal fluid cyclic nucleotides and GABA do not change in alcohol withdrawal. Life Sci 28:295–299.

Henderson GI, Baskin GS, Horbach J, Porter P, Schenker S (1989): Arrest of epidermal growth factor-dependent growth in fetal hepatocytes after ethanol exposure. J Clin Invest 84:1287–1294.

Henderson GI, Hoyumpa A, Rothschild M, Schenker S (1980): Effect of ethanol and ethanol-induced hypothermia on protein synthesis in pregnant and fetal rats. Alcohol Clin Exp Res 4:165–177.

Hoek JB, Rubin E (1990): Alcohol and membrane-associated signal transduction. Alcohol Alcohol 25:143–156.

Hwang DH, Chanmugam P, Hymel G, Boudreau M (1987): Effects of chronic ethanol ingestion on arachidonic acid metabloism in rat tissues and in vitro effects of ethanol on cAMP in platelets. Prostaglandins Med 26:299–305.

Hynie S., Lanefelt F, Fredholm B (1980): Effect of ethanol on human lymphocyte levels of cyclic AMP in vitro: Potentiation of the response to isoproterenol, PGE2, or adenosine stimulation. Acta Pharmacol Toxicol 47:58–65.

Israel MA, Kimura H, Kuriyama K (1972): Changes in activity and hormonal sensitivity of brain adenyl cyclase following chronic ethanol administration. Experientia 28:1322–1323.

Jauhonen VP, Savolainen MJ, Hassinen IE (1975): Cyclic AMP-linked mechanisms in ethanol induced derangements of metabolism in rat liver and adipose tissue. Biochem Pharmacol 24:1879–1883.

Jones K.L. (1986): Fetal Alcohol Syndrome. Pediatr Rev 8:122–126.

Jones KL, Smith DW (1975): The fetal alcohol syndrome. Teratol 12:1–10.

Jones KL, Smith DW, Ulleland CN, Streissguth AP (1973): Patterns of malformation in offspring of chronic alcoholic mothers. Lancet 1:1267–1271.

Kelly SJ, Black AC, West JR (1989): Changes in muscarinic cholinergic receptors in the hippocampus of rats exposed to ethyl alcohol during the brain growth spurt. J Pharmacol Exp Ther 249:798–804.

Kotkoskie LA, Norton S (1989): Morphometric analysis of developing rat cerebral cortex following acute prenatal ethanol exposure. Exp Neurol 106:283–288.

Kumar SP (1982): Fetal alcohol syndrome. Ann Clin Lab Sci 12:254–257.

Kuriyama K (1977): Ethanol-induced changes in activities of adenylate cyclase, guanylate cyclase and cyclic adenosine 3'5'-monophosphate dependent protein kinase in the brain and liver. Drug Alcohol Depend 2:335–348.

Kuriyama K, Israel MA (1973): Effect of ethanol administration on cyclic 3', 5'-adenosine monophosphate metabolism in brain. Biochem Pharmacol 22:2919–2922.

Kuriyama K, Nakagawa K, Muramatsu M, Kakita K (1976): Alterations of cerebral protein kinase activity following ethanol administration. Biochem Pharmacol 25:2541–2542.

Leichter J., Lee M (1984): Does dehydration contribute to retarded fetal growth in rats exposed to alcohol during gestation?. Life Sci 35:2105–2111.

Lemoine P, Harousseau M, Borteyru JP, Menuet JC (1968): Les enfants de parents alcooliques. Anomolies observees. A propos de 127 cas. Quest Med 21:476–482.

Lopez-Tejero D, Llobera M, Herrera E (1989): Permanent abnormal response to glucose load after prenatal ethanol exposure in rats. Alcohol 6:469–473.

Lucchi L., Covelli V, Anthopoulou H, Spano PF, Trabucchi M (1983): Effect of chronic ethanol treatment on adenylate cyclase activity in rat striatum. Neurosci Lett 40:187–192.

Lucchi L, Govoni S, Trabucchi M (1984): Age related differences in dopamine-stimulated adenylate cyclase sensitivity to in vivo chronic ethanol treatment. Alcohol 1:263–267.

Luthin GR, Tabakoff B (1984): Activation of adenylate cyclase by alcohols requires the nucleotide-binding protein. J Pharmacol Exp Ther 228:579–587.

Lykouras L, Markianos M, Moussas G (1988): Plasma cyclic AMP in non-abstinent, chronic alcoholics. Relation to clinical parameters. Drug Alcohol Depend 21:7–9.

Magnaldo I, Pouyssegur J, Paris S (1988): Thrombin exerts a dual effect on stimulated adenylate cyclase in hamster fibroblast, an inhibition via a GTP-binding protein and a potentiation via activation of protein kinase C. Biochem J 253:711–719.

Mashiter K, Mashiter G, Field JB (1974): Effect of PGE1, ethanol and TSH on the adenylate cyclase activity of beef thyroid plasma membranes and cyclic AMP content of dog thyroid slices. Endocrinol 94:370–376.

Means LW, Burnette M, Pennington SN (1988): The effect of embryonic ethanol exposure on detour learning in the chick. Alcohol 5:305–308.

Means LW, Henson JL, Pennington SN (1986): The effects of ethanol on embryonic and hatching behaviors in the chick. IRCS Med Science 14:142–143.

Means LW, McDaniel K, Pennington SN (1989): Embryonic ethanol exposure impairs detour learning in the chick. Alcohol 6:327–330.

Mena MA, Salinas M, Del Rio RM, Herrera E (1982): Effects of maternal ethanol ingestion on cerebral neurotransmitters and cyclic AMP in the rat offspring. Gen Pharmacol 13:241–248.

Meyer LS, Kotch LE, Riley EP (1990): Alterations in gait following ethanol exposure during the brain growth spurt in rats. Alcoholism (NY) 14:23–27.

Miller MW (1986): Effects of alcohol on the generation and migration of cerebral cortical neurons. Science 233:1308–1311.

Miller MW (1987): Effect of prenatal exposure to alcohol on the distribution and time of origin of corticospinal neurons in the rat. J Comp Neurol 257:372–382.

Miller MW (1988): Effect of prenatal exposure to ethanol on the development of cerebral cortex: I. Neuronal generation. Alcohol Clin Exp Res 12:440–449.

Miller MW (1989): Effects of prenatal exposure to ethanol on neocortical development: II. Cell proliferation in the ventricular and subventricular zones of the rat. J Comp Neurol 287:326–338.

Miller MW, Chiaia NL, Rhoades RW (1990): Intracellular recording and injection study of corticospinal neurons in the rat somatosensory cortex: Effect of prenatal exposure to ethanol. J Comp Neurol 297:91–105.

Miller MW, Dow-Edwards DL (1988): Structural and metabolic alterations in rat cerebral cortex induced by prenatal exposure to ethanol. Brain Res 474:316–326.

Miller MW, Nowakowski RS (1991): Effect of prenatal exposure to ethanol on the cell cycle kinetics and growth fraction in the proliferative zones of the fetal rat cerebral cortex. Alcohol Clin Exp Res (in Press).

Miller MW, Potempa G (1990): Numbers of neurons and glia in mature rat somatosensory cortex: Effects of prenatal exposure to ethanol. J Comp Neurol 293:92–102.

Mohamed S, Nathaniel D, Nanthaniel E, Snell L (1987): Altered Purkinje cell maturation in rats exposed prenatally to ethanol. Exp Nerurol 97:35–52.

Molina L, Hoffman H, Spear L, Spear N (1987): Senorimotor maturation and alcohol responsiveness in rats prenatally exposed to alcohol during gestation day 8. Neurotoxicol Teratol 9:121–128.

Myking O, Aakvaag A, Digranes O (1987): Androgen-estrogen imbalance in men with chronic alcoholism and fatty liver. Alcohol Alcohol 22:7–15.

Nguyen T, Chi CW, Larkin EC, Rao GA (1990): Low liver glycogen content in alcoholic rats due to depressed carbohydrate ingestion. Biochem Arch 6:217–221.

O'Dell BL, Browning JD, Reeves PG (1983): Plasma levels of prostaglandin metabolites in zinc-deficient female rats near term. J Nutr 113:760–765.

Okonmah AD, Brown JW, Fishman LM, Carballeira A, Soliman KFA (1989): Influence of ethanol on fetal brain cholinergic enzyme activities. Pharmacology 39:367–372.

Okuda C, Miyazaki M, Kuriyama K (1984): Alterations in cerebral beta-adrenergic receptor-adenylate cyclase system induced by halothane, ketamine and ethanol. Neurochem Int 6:237–244.

Orenberg EK, Zarcone VP, Renson JF, Barchas JD (1976): The effect of ethanol ingestion on cyclic AMP, homovanillic acid, and 5-hydroxylindoacetic acid in human cerebrospinal fluid. Life Sci 19:1669–1676.

Pennington SN (1988a): Alcohol metabolism and fetal brain hypoplasia. Alcohol 5:91–94.

Pennington SN (1988b): Ethanol-induced growth inhibition: The role of cyclic AMP dependent protein kinase. Alcohol Clin Exp Res 12:125–130.

Pennington SN (1990): Molecular changes associated with ethanol-induced growth suppression in the chick embryo. Alcohol Clin Exp Res 14:832–837.

Pennington SN, Allen Z, Runion J, Farmer P, Rowland L, Kalmus G (1985): Prostaglandin synthesis inhibitors block alcohol-induced fetal hypoplasia. Alcohol Clin Exp Res 9:433–437.

Pennington SN, Boyd JW, Kalmus G, Wilson R (1983): The molecular mechanism of fetal alcohol syndrome (FAS) I. Ethanol-induced growth suppression. Neurobehav Toxicol 5:259–262.

Pennington SN, Kalmus G (1987): Brain growth during ethanol-induced hypoplasia. Drug Alcohol Depend 20:279–286.

Pierce D, West JR (1986a): Alcohol-induced microencephaly during the third trimester equivalent: Relationship to dose and blood alcohol concentration. Alcohol 3:185–191.

Pierce D, West JR (1986b): Blood alcohol concentration: Critical factor in producing fetal alcohol effects. Alcohol 3:269–272.

Pierce D, West JR (1987): Differential deficits in regional brain growth induced by postnatal alcohol. Neurotoxicol Teratol 9:129–141.

Poltorak M, Freed WJ, Casanova MF (1990): Prenatal exposure to ethanol causes a delay in the developmental expression of neurofilament epitopes in cerebellum. Pharmacol Biochem Behav 35:693–698.

Pullen GL, Singh SP, Snyder AK (1988): Growth patterns of the offspring of alcohol fed rats. Growth Dev Aging 52:85–89.

Rabe CS, Giri PR, Hoffman PL, Tabakoff B (1990) Effect of ethanol on cyclic AMP levels in intact PC-12 cells. Biochem Pharmacol 40:565–571.

Rabin RA (1990a): Direct effects of chronic ethanol exposure on beta-adrenergic and adenosine-sensitive adenylate cyclase activities and cyclic AMP content in primary cerebellar cultures. J Neurochem 55:122–128.

Rabin RA (1990b): Chronic ethanol exposure of PC-12 cells alters adenylate cyclase activity and intracellular cyclic AMP content. J Pharmacol Exp Ther 252:1021–1027.

Rabin RA, Baker R, Deitrich R (1987): Effects of chronic ethanol exposure on adenylate cyclase activities in the rat. Pharmacol Biochem Behav 26:693–697.

Rabin RA, Molinof PB (1981): Activation of adenylate cyclase by ethanol in mouse striatal tissue. J Pharmacol Exp Ther 216:129–134.

Rabin RA, Molinof PB (1983): Multiple sites of action of ethanol on adenylate cyclase. J Pharmacol Exp Ther 227:551–556.

Ramp WK, Murdock WC, Gonnerman WA, Peng TC (1975): Effects of ethanol on chicks in vivo and on chick embryo tibiae in organ culture. Calcif Tissue Res 17:195–203.

Randall CL, Anton RF (1984): Aspirin reduces alcohol-induced prenatal mortality an malformations in mice. Alcohol Clin Exp Res 8:513–515.

Randall CL, Anton RF, Becker HC (1987): Effect of indomethacin on alcohol-induced morphological anomalies in mice. Life Sci 41:361–369.

Rawat AK (1985): Nucleic acid and protein synthesis inhibition in developing brain by ethanol in the absence of hypothermia. Neurobehav Toxicol Teratol 7:161–166.

Redos JD, Hunt WA, Catravas GN (1976): Lack of alteration in regional brain adenosine-3′,5′-cyclic monophosphate levels after acute and chronic treatment with ethanol. Life Sci 18:989–992.

Rius R, Govoni F, Trabucchi M (1986): Cyclic AMP-dependent protein phosphorylation is reduced in rat striatum after chronic ethanol treatment. Brain Res 365:355–359.

Rubin R, Hoek JB (1990): Inhibition of ethanol-induced platelet activation by agents that elevate cyclic AMP. Thromb Res 58:625–632.

Rudeen PK, Kappel C, Lear K (1986): Postnatal or in utero ethanol exposure reduction of the volume of the sexually dimorphic nucleus of the preoptic area in male rats. Drug Alcohol Depend 18:247–252.

Sandor S (1979): The prenatal noxious effect of ethanol. Rev Roum Morphol Embryol Physiol 225:211–223.

Scawen SD, Darbyshire J, Harvey MJ, Atkinson T (1982): The rapid purification of 3-hydroxybutyrate dehydrogenase and malate dehydrogenase on triazine dye affinity matrices. Biochem J 203:699–705.

Schenker S, Becker HC, Randall CL, Philips DK, Baskin GS, Henderson G.I. (1990): Fetal alcohol syndrome: Current·status of pathogenesis. Alcohol Clin Exp Res 14:635–647.

Seitz HK, Simon B, Czygan P, Veith S, Kommerell B (1983): Effect of chronic ethanol ingestion on the cyclic AMP system of the upper gastrointestinal tract in the rat. Alcohol Clin Exp Res 7:369–371.

Sharma A, Rawat AK (1989): Toxicological consequences of chloroquine and ethanol on the developing fetus. Pharmacol Biochem Behav 34:77–82.

Shen A, Jacobyansky A, Pathman D, Thurman RG (1983): Changes in brain cyclic AMP levels during chronic ethanol treatment and withdrawal in the rat. Eur J Pharmacol 89:103–110.

Shen A, Jacobyansky A, Smith T, Pathman D, Thurman RG (1977): Cyclic adenosine 3′, 5′-monophosphate, adenylate cyclase and physical dependence on ethanol: Studies with tranylcypromine. Drug Alcohol Depend 2:431–440.

Shoemaker WJ, Koda LY, Shoemaker CA, Bloom FE (1980): Ethanol effects in chick embryos: Cerebellar purkinje neurons. Neurobehav Toxicol 2:239–242.

Singh SP, Pullen GL, Snyder AK (1988): Effect of ethanol on fetal fuels and brain growth. J Lab Clin Med 112:704–710.

Singh SP, Snyder AK, Eman S (1990): Effects of ethanol on hexose uptake by cultured rat brain cells. Alcohol Clin Exp Res 5:741–745.

Skwidh S, Shain W (1990): Ethanol and diolein stimulate PK-C translocation in astroglial cells. Life Sci 47:1037–1042.

Smith TL, Jacobyansky A, Shen A, Pathman D, Thurman RG (1981): Adaptation of cyclic AMP generating system in rat cerebral cortical slices during chronic ethanol treatment and withdrawal. Neuropharmacol 20:67–72.

Snyder AK, Singh SP, Pullen GL (1986): Ethanol-induced intrauterine growth retardation: Correlation with placental glucose transfer. Alcohol Clin Exp Res 10:167–170.

Snyder AK, Singh SP, Pullen GL, Eman S (1989): Effects of maternal ethanol ingestion on the uptake of alpha-aminoisobutryic acid by fetal rat liver, lung and brain. Biol Neonate 56:277–282.

Sokol RJ (1982): Alcohol and pregnancy: A clinical prespective for laboratory research. Subst Alcohol Actions/Misuse 3:183–186.

Streissguth AP, Barr H, Sampson P, Parrish-Johnson J, Kirchner G, Martin D (1986): Attention, distraction and reaction time at age 7 years and prenatal alcohol exposure. Neurobehav Toxicol Teratol 8:717–725.

Streissguth AP, Landesman-Dwyer S, Martin JC, Smith DW (1980): Teratogenic effects of alcohol in humans and laboratory animals. Science 209:353–361.

Tabakoff B, Hoffman P, McLaughlin A (1988): Is ethanol a discriminating substance?. Semin Liver Dis 8:26–35.

Teitelbaum I (1990): Cyclic AMP monophosphate and diacylglycerol. J Clin Invest 86:46–51.

Thadani PV, Lau C, Slotkin TA, Schanberg SM (1977): Effects of maternal ethanol ingestion on amine uptake into synaptosomes of fetal and neonatal rat brain. J Pharmacol Exp Ther 200:292–297.

Vaema PK, Persaud TVN (1982): Protection against ethanol-induced embryonic damage by administering gamma-linolenic and linoleic acids. Prostaglandins Med 8:641–645.

Valverius P, Hoffman P, Tabakoff B (1988): Effects of chronic ethanol ingestion on mouse brain beta-adrenergic receptors (BAR) and adenylate cyclase. Adv Alcohol Subst Abuse 7:99–101.

Vingan RD, Dow-Edwards DL, Riley EP (1986): Cerebral metabolic alterations in rats following prenatal alcohol exposure: A deoxyglucose study. Alcohol Clin Exp Res 10:22–26.

Volicer L, Gold BI (1973): Effect of ethanol on cyclic AMP levels in the rat brain. Life Sci 13:269–280.

Volicer L, Gold BI (1975): Interactions of ethanol with cyclic AMP. Adv Exp Biol Med 56.211–23T.

Von-Hungen K, Baxter CF (1982): Sensitivity of rat brain adenylate cyclase to activation by calcium and ethanol after chronic exposure to ethanol. Biochem Biophys Res Comm 106:1078–1082.

Weitbrecht W, Cramer H (1980): Depression of cyclic AMP and cyclic GMP in cerebrospinal fluid of rats after acute administration of ethanol. Brain Res 200:-478–480.

West JR, Hodges-Savola CA (1983): Permanent hippocampal mossy fiber hyperdevelopment following prenatal ethanol exposure. Neurobehav Toxicol 5:139–150.

Wigal SBE, Amsel A, Wilcox RE (1990): Fetal ethanol exposure diminishes hippocampal beta-adrenergic receptor density while sparing muscarinic receptors during development. Dev Brain Res 55:161–169.

Wilson J (1980): Protein phosphorylation: Involvement in brain function. In Kumar S (ed): "Brain Biochemistry." New York: Pergamon Press, pp 523–544.

Woodson PM, Ritchey SJ (1979): Effects of maternal alcohol consumption on fetal brain cell number and cell size. Nutr Rep International 20:225–228.

Development of the Central Nervous System:
Effects of Alcohol and Opiates, pages 209–219
© 1992 Wiley-Liss, Inc.

10

Structure and Function of the Endogenous Opiate Systems: An Overview

HENRY KHACHATURIAN AND MICHAEL E. LEWIS
Neuroimaging and Applied Neuroscience Research Branch, National Institute of Mental Health, Rockville, Maryland (H.K.); Cephalon, Inc., West Chester, Pennsylvania (M.E.L.)

INTRODUCTION

The endogenous opiate systems are composed of three distinct neuronal groups widely distributed throughout the neuraxis. Each opiate neuron contains one or more distinct precursor molecules, namely, proopiomelanocortin (POMC), proenkephalin, and prodynorphin (Fig. 1). Each of these precursors is enzymatically cleaved into several bioactive end-products which are released at the synaptic terminals of opiatergic neurons. The opiate peptides act upon several subclasses of opiate receptors, μ, δ, and κ, to exert their physiological effects. Opiates affect numerous brain functions, e.g., nociception, cardiovascular regulation, respiration, neuroendocrine and neuroimmune activity, thermoregulation, and consummatory, sexual, aggressive, locomotor, and hedonic behavior, as well as learning and memory (Adler et al., 1988; Herz and Millan, 1988; Khachaturian et al., 1988; Martinez et al., 1988; Pasternak, 1988; Stefano, 1989).

The anatomical distribution and functional significance of opiate neuronal systems are described in this chapter. The distribution of the brain opiate systems, opiate receptors, and their functional implications have been the subject of intense investigation in the last two decades. Here, we attempt to provide the reader with a broad overview of some of the most significant findings to date. In addition to the specific reviews appearing in this volume, the following reviews also contain specific details about topics covered in this chapter: Khachaturian et al., 1985a; Petrusz et al., 1985; Fallon and Leslie, 1986; Mansour et al., 1988; Weihe et al., 1988; Illes, 1989; Stengaard-Pedersen, 1989; and Loh and Smith, 1990.

STRUCTURE OF THE ENDOGENOUS OPIATE SYSTEMS
Proopiomelanocortin

The bioactive peptides of the proopiomelanocortin (POMC) precursor include β-endorphin, adrenocorticotrophic hormone (ACTH) and α-melanocyte stimulating hormone (α-MSH). POMC is synthesized in the

PRO-OPIOMELANOCORTIN

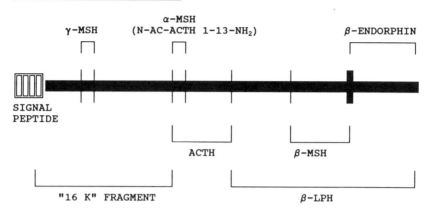

PRO-ENKEPHALIN

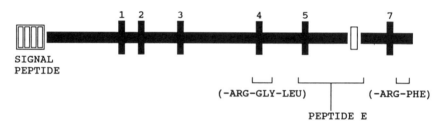

PRO-DYNORPHIN

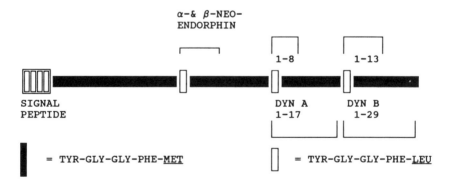

Fig. 1. The structure of the three opioid precursor molecules is presented in this schematic drawing. The opiate-active core sequence tyr-gly-gly-phe-met is represented in both POMC and proenkephalin, while the opiate-active core sequence tyr-gly-gly-phe-leu is found in both pro-enkephalin and prodynorphin. See text for abbreviations.

pituitary and the brain of several species, including rat, monkey, and human (Khachaturian et al., 1985a; Ibuki et al., 1989). By far, the major biosynthetic site is the pituitary gland. Immunocytochemical studies have long revealed the co-existence of β-endorphin and ACTH in anterior lobe corticotrophs and β-endorphin and α-MSH in intermediate lobe melanotrophs (Bloom et al., 1977). Biochemical studies have elucidated the protein structure of the POMC precursor and its products (Mains et al., 1977; Roberts and Herbert, 1977). Lastly, the complete structure of POMC has been deduced by molecular biological techniques (Nakanishi et al., 1979).

In the brain, POMC is synthesized in the arcuate nucleus of hypothalamus and the nucleus tractus solitarius in the medulla (Khachaturian et al., 1985b). Immunocytochemical studies have demonstrated the co-existence of β-endorphin, ACTH, and α-MSH in the arcuate neurons (Bloom et al., 1978; Watson et al., 1978a,b), thus demonstrating the similarity between the brain and the intermediate pituitary in the processing of this precursor (Watson and Akil, 1980). POMC is also found in neurons of the nucleus tractus solitarius (Schwartzburg and Nakane, 1983). The latter POMC neurons form local, rostral, and caudal projections, e.g., to the parabrachial nuclei, and to the spinal cord (Tsou et al., 1986).

The arcuate POMC neurons have extensive projections (Khachaturian et al., 1985b). Rostral projections course through and/or innervate periventricular diencephalic and telencephalic structures, including several hypothalamic nuclei, preoptic area, septum, and bed nucleus of stria terminalis. Lateral projections traverse through the medial and basal hypothalamus, coursing into and innervating the medial amygdala. Projections to the thalamus course through the periventricular regions. Caudal projections of POMC neurons course through the mesencephalon and innervate the periaqueductal gray and other brainstem regions. Tract-tracing techniques have shown that the source of periaqueductal gray POMC fibers are neurons situated in the rostral 3/5 of the arcuate nucleus (Yoshida and Taniguchi, 1988). In the brainstem, the parabrachial nuclei, nuclei reticularis gigantocellularis and raphe magnus, nucleus tractus solitarius, dorsal motor nucleus of the vagus nerve, and other nuclei are also innervated by POMC fibers.

Proenkephalin

This precursor is the source of several opiate peptides, including leucine-enkephalin (L-enkephalin), and methionine-enkephalin (M-enkephalin). L-enkephalin and M-enkephalin were first isolated from the brain (Hughes et al., 1975), and their molecular structure was deduced through cloning and sequencing of cDNA from proenkephalin mRNA (Comb et al., 1982; Gubler et al., 1982; Noda et al., 1982). Immunocytochemical studies to date have shown these two peptides to be distributed similarly in every region of the brain (Elde et al., 1976; Bloom et al., 1978; Watson et al., 1978a).

Proenkephalin neurons are found throughout the brain in several species (Haber and Elde, 1982; Khachaturian et al., 1983a,b; McGinty et al., 1984; Haber and Watson, 1985; Fallon and Leslie, 1986; Simerly et al., 1988; Cassell and Gray, 1989; Chung et al., 1989; Ibuki et al., 1989; Walker et al., 1989). Some enkephalin neurons form local circuits; others have wide projections (Nahin, 1988). Enkephalin perikarya can be seen in the cerebral cortex, hippocampus, amygdala, septum, hypothalamus, pons, medulla, and spinal cord. In most instances, enkephalins coexist or have synaptic interactions with other transmitters (acetylcholine, epinephrine, norepinephrine, serotonin, γ-aminobutyric acid, and substance P), and probably have a cotransmitter or neuromodulator role (Hokfelt et al., 1986; Ibuki et al., 1988; Senba et al., 1988; Shinoda et al., 1988; Weihe et al., 1988; Milner et al., 1989; Murakami et al., 1989; Pickel et al., 1989).

Prodynorphin

This precursor, like proenkephalin, gives rise to several opiate active peptides. These include dynorphin A, dynorphin B, and α-neo-endorphin. Prodynorphin neurons are found throughout the brain and spinal cord. In addition, prodynorphin can be seen colocalized with leutinizing hormone and follicle stimulating hormone in the pituitary anterior lobe (Seizinger et al., 1983; Khachaturian et al., 1986). Prodynorphin peptides were first extracted and sequenced from the pituitary and hypothalamus (Goldstein et al., 1979; Kangawa et al., 1981; Fischli et al., 1982; Kilpatrick et al., 1982), and confirmed using prodynorphin cDNA (Kakidani et al., 1982). Numerous immunocytochemical studies confirmed the coexistence of prodynorphin peptides in the same neurons (Watson et al., 1983; Weber and Barchas, 1983).

Immunocytochemical studies have revealed dynorphin neuronal system to be distributed widely throughout the neuraxis in a number of species (Khachaturian et al., 1982, 1985a; Vincent et al., 1982; Weber and Barchas, 1983; McGinty et al., 1984; Haber and Watson, 1985; Fallon and Leslie, 1986; Abe et al., 1988; Cho and Basbaum, 1988; Ibuki et al., 1989; Miller and Seybold, 1989). In the magnocellular neurons of the hypothalamus, dynorphin A is colocalized with arginine-vasopressin (Watson et al., 1981, 1982a, b). Prodynorphin neurons are seen in the cerebral cortex, striatum, amygdala, hippocampus, hypothalamus, mesencephalon, pons, medulla, and spinal cord. Prodynorphin fibers are seen in the globus pallidus, substantia nigra, raphe, and other nuclei. Dynorphin neurons form both local circuits and long-tract projections (Nahin, 1988; Zardetto-Smith et al., 1988). Like proenkephalin, prodynorphin peptides are also frequently found to be colocalized with other transmitters (substance P, enkephalin), and thus might have a cotransmitter or neuromodulator role in several central nervous system (CNS) functions (Sasek and Elde, 1986; Tuchscherer and Seybold, 1989).

FUNCTION OF THE ENDOGENOUS OPIATE SYSTEMS

There are numerous studies on the physiological and behavioral effects of opiate peptides, or nonpeptide opiate agonists or antagonists (Mansour et al., 1988; Olson et al., 1989). Still, it has been difficult to draw any firm conclusions regarding the function of opiate receptor subtypes in the brain. The same can be said for the functional roles of opiates during development; however, these studies have proven more successful in providing information on possible functional roles of these systems (McDowell and Kitchen, 1987). In this chapter, an attempt has been made to highlight some of the better known functional roles of the multiple opiate peptide/receptor systems in the CNS, i.e., the endogenous pain control system and extrapyramidal motor system.

Endogenous Pain Control System

The endogenous pain control system was first characterized by studies showing that electrical stimulation of the brain can reduce pain responsiveness in humans and other species (Mayer et al., 1971; Hosobuchi et al., 1977; Richardson and Akil, 1977a,b). This so-called stimulation-produced analgesia (SPA) can be reversed by naloxone and shows cross-tolerance with morphine (Akil et al., 1972, 1978; Mayer and Hayes, 1975). The brain stimulation sites for analgesia include the periaqueductal gray and other sites where there are abundant β-endorphin immunoreactive fibers (Basbaum and Fields, 1984). Furthermore, SPA increases β-endorphin levels in the cerebrospinal fluid (Akil et al., 1978; Hosobuchi et al., 1979). However, β-endorphin is only one of many opiate and non-opiate systems so far implicated in the regulation of nociception (for reviews, see Akil et al., 1984; Basbaum and Fields, 1984).

These early investigations of the endogenous pain control system had primarily emphasized the role of μ receptors since the most common opiate analgesics have the greatest affinity for this class of receptors. However, μ receptor agonists exhibit many undesirable side effects, including dependence, tolerance, respiratory depression, and nausea. In order to overcome these difficulties, there has recently been an increased effort to understand the role of κ opiate receptors in endogenous pain control mechanisms (Millan, 1990). Selective κ agonists like the arylacetamides U50488H and PD117302 are antinociptive in both the brain and spinal cord (Millan, 1990). Unfortunately, κ agonists also induce dysphoric and psychotomimetic effects and therefore are less likely to prove clinically significant. Nevertheless, κ agonists stimulate spinal and supraspinal κ receptor-mediated antinociception, and selective κ antagonists such as nor-binaltorphine should allow studies of the role of κ receptors in the mediation of physiological (e.g. stress-induced) analgesia.

Extrapyramidal Motor System

Even before the discovery of endogenous opiate systems, it was well known that opiate administration could alter motor function. The administration of morphine or β-endorphin into the mesencephalic A10 dopamine neuron region can produce locomotor activation (Joyce and Iversen, 1979). Microinjection of morphine into the nucleus accumbens, which is innervated by A10 dopamine neurons, results in a dose-dependent locomotor response, with catalepsy followed by locomotor activation (Costall et al., 1978). Yet, the effects of opiates on locomotor activity depend critically on the stage of development (McDowell and Kitchen, 1987). Opiate receptor subtypes in different brain regions show different maturation patterns, and the physical state of μ receptors appears to also change during maturation, which may have functional consequences (McDowell and Kitchen, 1987; McLean et al., 1989).

More recently, molecular biological approaches have proven useful in the analysis of opiate interactions with the extrapyramidal dopamine system. These studies have focused on the effects of dopamine agonists or antagonists on opiate neuronal activity as measured by changes in levels of opiate peptides or their precursor mRNAs. Chronic administration of the dopamine receptor antagonist haloperidol results in an increase in both the level of M-enkephalin peptide as well as proenkephalin mRNA in the striatum (Sabol et al., 1983; Hong et al., 1985; Angulo et al., 1986; Sivam et al., 1986; Romano et al., 1987). Conversely, administration of the dopamine agonists apomorphine, amphetamine, or cocaine, results in an increase in prodynorphin peptide levels in the striatum and substantia nigra (Li et al., 1986; Hanson et al., 1990; Trujillo and Akil, 1990). Taken together, these results indicate that striatal proenkephalin and prodynorphin systems are oppositely regulated by dopamine systems. It is also interesting to speculate that increases in dopamine activity are followed by increased κ and μ receptor activation, and that decreases in dopamine activity are followed by increased δ receptor activation.

In summary, it appears that the multiple opiate systems in the striatum can be differentially influenced by dopamine activity, and that, in turn, the nigrostriatal dopamine system can be differentially influenced by the activation of different opiate receptor types. The striatonigral dynorphin pathway is a particularly attractive target for functional studies (Thompson et al., 1990). Such an approach, particularly with combined studies at the systems and molecular levels, will undoubtedly prove more useful in allowing investigators to unravel the complex relationships between opiate and dopamine systems, receptor activation, and gene expression.

ACKNOWLEDGMENTS

The authors wish to acknowledge the valuable and continued inspiration of C. Howard, to whose memory this chapter is respectfully dedicated. They also thank Mrs. Mary Lou Prince for preparing Figure 1.

REFERENCES

Abe J, Okamura H, Kitamura T, Ibata Y, Minamino N, Matsuo H, Paull WK (1988): Immunocytochemical demonstration of dynorphin (PH-8P)-like immunoreactive elements in the human hypothalamus. J Comp Neurol 276:508–513.

Adler MW, Geller EB, Rosow CE, Cochin J (1988): The opioid system and temperature regulation. Ann Rev Pharmacol Toxicol 28:429–49.

Akil H, Mayer DJ, Liebeskind JC (1972): Comparison chez le rat entre l'analgesie induite par stimulation de la substance grise periaqueducale et al analgesie morphinique. CR Acad Sci (Paris) 274:3603–3605.

Akil H, Richardson DE, Barchas JD, Li CH (1978): Appearance of β-endorphin-like immunoreactivity in human ventricular cerebrospinal fluid upon analgesic electrical stimulation. Proc Natl Acad Sci USA 75:5170–5172.

Akil H, Watson SJ, Young E, Lewis ME, Khachaturian H, Walker JM (1984): Endogenous opioids: Biology and function. Ann Rev Neurosci 7:223–255.

Angulo JA, Davis LG, Burkhart BA, Christoph GR (1986): Reduction of striatal dopaminergic neurotransmission elevates striatal proenkephalin mRNA. Eur J Pharmacol 130:341–343.

Basbaum AI, Fields HL (1984): Endogenous pain control systems: Brainstem spinal pathways and endorphin circuitry. Ann Rev Neurosci 7:309–234.

Bloom FE, Battenberg E, Rossier J, Ling N, Guillemin R (1978): Neurons containing β-endorphin exist separately from those containing enkephalin: Immunocytochemical studies. Proc Natl Acad Sci USA 75:1591–1595.

Bloom FE, Battenberg E, Rossier J, Ling N, Leppaluoto J, Vargo TM, Guillemin R (1977): Endorphins are located in the intermediate and anterior lobes of the pituitary gland, not in the neurohypophysis. Life Sci 20:43–48.

Cassell MD, Gray TS (1989): Morphology of peptide-immunoreactive neurons in the rat central nucleus of the amygdala. J Comp Neurol 281:320–333.

Cho HJ, Basbaum AI (1988): Increased staining of immunoreactive dynorphin cell bodies in the deafferented spinal cord of the rat. Neurosci Lett 84:125–130.

Chung K, Briner RP, Carlton SM, Westlund KN (1989): Immunohistochemical localization of seven different peptides in the human spinal cord. J Comp Neurol 280:158–170.

Comb M, Seeburg PH, Adelman J, Eiden L, Herbert E (1982): Primary structure of human Met- and Leu-enkephalin precursor and its mRNA. Nature 295:663–666.

Costall B, Fortune DH, Naylor RJ (1978): The induction of catalepsy and hyperactivity by morphine administered directly into the nucleus accumbens of rats. Eur J Pharmacol 49:49–64.

Elde R, Hokfelt T, Johansson O, Terenius L (1976): Immunohistochemical studies using antibodies to leucine enkephalin: Initial observations on the nervous system of the rat. Neuroscience 1:349–351.

Fallon JH, Leslie FM (1986): Distribution of dynorphin and enkephalin peptides in the rat brain. J Comp Neurol 249:293–336.

Fischli W, Goldstein A, Hunkapiller M, Hood L (1982): Two "big" dynorphins from porcine pituitary. Life Sci 31:1769–1772.

Goldstein A, Tachibana S, Lowney LI, Hunkapiller M, Hood L (1979): Dynorphin-(1–13), an extraordinarily potent opiod peptide. Proc Natl Acad Sci USA 76:6666–6670.

Gubler U, Seeburg P, Hoffman BJ, Gage LP, Udenfriend S (1982): Molecular cloning establishes proenkephalin as precursor of enkephalin-containing peptides. Nature 295:206–208.

Haber SN, Elde R (1982): The distribution of enkephalin immunoreactive fibers and terminals in the monkey central nervous system. Neuroscience 7:1049–1095.

Haber SN, Watson SJ (1985): The comparative distribution of enkephalin, dynorphin and substance P in the human globus pallidus and basal forebrain. Neuroscience 14:1011–1024.

Hanson GR, Midgley LP, Bush LG, Johnson M, Gibb JW (1990): Comparison of responses by neuropeptide systems in rat to the psychotropic drugs, methamphetamine, cocaine and PCP. NIDA Res Monogr 95:348.

Herz A, Millan MJ (1988): Endogenous opioid peptides in the descending control of nociceptive responses of spinal dorsal horn neurons. Prog Brain Res 77:263–273.

Hokfelt T, Holets VR, Staines W, Meister B, Melander T, Schalling M, Schultzburg M, Freedman J, Bjorklund H, Olson L, Lindh B, Elfvin L-G, Lundberg JM, Lindgren JA, Samuelsson B, Pernow B, Terenius L, Post C, Everitt B, Goldstein

M (1986): Coexistence of neuronal messengers—an overview. Prog Brain Res 68:33–70.

Hong JS, Yoshikawa K, Kanamatsu T, Sabol SL (1985): Modulation of striatal enkephalinergic neurons by antipsychotic drugs. Fed Proc 44:1535–2539.

Hosobuchi Y, Adams JE, Linchitz R (1977): Pain relief by electrical stimulation of the central grey matter in humans and its reversal by naloxone. Science 197:-183–186.

Hosobuchi Y, Rossier J, Bloom FE, Guillemin R (1979): Stimulation of human periaqueductal grey for pain relief increases immunoreactive β-endorphin in ventricular fluid. Science 203:279–281.

Hughes J, Smith TW, Kosterlitz HW, Fothergill LA, Morgan BA, Morris HR (1975): Identification of two related pentapeptides form the brain with potent opiate agonist activity. Nature 258:577–579.

Ibuki T, Okamura H, Miyazaki M, Kimura H, Yanaihara N, Ibata Y (1988): Colocalization of GABA and [met]enkephalin-arg^6-gly^7-leu^8 in the rat cerebellum. Neurosci Lett 91:131–135.

Ibuki T, Okamura H, Miyazaki M, Yanaihara N, Zimmerman EA, Ibata Y (1989): Comparative distribution of three opioid systems in the lower brainstem of the monkey *(Macaca fasciculata)*. J Comp Neurol 279:445–456.

Illes P (1989): Modulation of transmitter and hormone release by multiple neuronal opioid receptors. Rev Physiol Biochem Pharmacol 112:139–233.

Joyce EM, Iversen SD (1979): The effect of morphine applied locally to mesencephalic dopamine cell bodies on spontaneous motor activity in the rat. Neurosci Lett 14:207–212.

Kakidani H, Furutani Y, Takahashi H, Noda M, Morimoto Y, Hirose T, Asai M, Inayama S, Nakanishi S, Numa S (1982): Cloning and sequence analysis of cDNA for porcine β-neo-endorphin/dynorphin precursor. Nature 298:245–249.

Kangawa K, Minamino N, Chino N, Sakakibara S, Matsuo H (1981): The complete amino acid sequence of α-neo-endorphin. Biochem Biophys Res Commun 99:871–878.

Khachaturian H, Day R, Watson SJ, Akil H (1988): Opioid peptides in the hypothalamus-pituitary-adrenal axis: Neuroendocrine anatomy. In Barchas JD, Bunney WE (eds): "Perspectives in Psychopharmacology: A Collection of Papers in Honor of Earl Usdin." New York: Alan R. Liss, pp 233–247.

Khachaturian H, Lewis ME, Hollt V, Watson SJ (1983a): Telencephalic enkephalinergic systems in the rat brain. J Neurosci 3:844–855.

Khachaturian H, Lewis ME, Schafer M-KH, Watson SJ (1985a): Anatomy of CNS opioid systems. Trends Neurosci 8:111–119.

Khachaturian H, Lewis ME, Tsou K, Watson SJ (1985b): β-endorphin α-MSH, ACTH, and related peptides. In Bjorklund A, Hokfelt T (eds): "Handbook of Chemical Neuroanatomy, Vol. 4: GABA and Neuropeptides in CNS, Part I." Amsterdam: Elsevier, pp 216–272.

Khachaturian H, Lewis ME, Watson SJ (1983b): Enkephalin systems in diencephalon and brainstem of the rat. J Comp Neurol 220:310–320.

Khachaturian H, Sherman TG, Lloyd RV, Civelli O, Douglas J, Herbert E, Akil H, Watson SJ (1986): Prodynorphin is endogenous to the anterior pituitary and is co-localized with LH and FSH in the gonadotrophs. Endocrinology 119:1409–1411.

Khachaturian H, Watson SJ, Lewis ME, Coy DH, Goldstein A, Akil H (1982): Dynorphin peptide immunocytochemistry in the rat central nervous system. Peptides 3:941–954.

Kilpatrick DL, Wahlstrom A, Lahm HW, Blacher R, Udenfriend S (1982): Rimorphin, a unique, naturally occurring [leu]enkephalin-containing peptide found in association with dynorphin and α-neo-endorphin. Proc Natl Acad Sci USA 79:-6480–6483.

Li S, Sivam SP, Hong JS (1986): Regulation of the concentration of dynorphin A(1-8) in the striatonigral pathway by the dopaminergic system. Brain Res 398:390–392.

Loh HH, Smith AP (1990): Molecular characterization of opioid receptors. Ann Rev Pharmacol Toxicol 30:123–47.

Mains RE, Eipper EA, Ling N (1977): Common precursor to corticotropins and endorphins. Proc Natl Acad Sci USA 74:3014–3018.

Mansour A, Khachaturian H, Lewis ME, Akil H, Watson SJ (1988): Anatomy of CNS opioid receptors. Trends Neurosci 11:308–314.

Martinez JL Jr, Weinberger SB, Schulteis G (1988): Enkephalins and learning and memory: A review of evidence for a site of action outside the blood-brain barrier. Behav Neural Biol 49:192–221.

Mayer DJ, Hayes RL (1975): Stimulation-produced analgesia: Development of tolerance and cross-tolerance to morphine. Science 188:941–943.

Mayer DJ, Wolfle TL, Akil H, Carder B, Liebeskind JC (1971): Analgesia from electrical stimulation in the brainstem of the rat. Science 174:1351–1354.

McDowell J, Kitchen I (1987): Development of opioid systems: Peptides, receptors and pharmacology. Brain Res Rev 12:397–421.

McGinty JF, van der Kooy D, Bloom FE (1984): The distribution and morphology of opioid peptide immunoreactive neurons in the cerebral cortex of rats. J Neurosci 4:1104–1117.

McLean S, Rothman RB, Chuang DM, Rice KC, Spain JW, Coscia CJ, Roth BL (1989): Cross-linking of [125I]β-endorphin to μ-opioid receptors during development. Dev Brain Res 45:283–289.

Millan JM (1990): Kappa-opioid receptors and analgesia. Trends Pharmacol Sci 11:7076.

Miller KE, Seybold VM (1989): Comparison of met-enkephalin, dynorphin A, and neurotensin immunoreactive neurons in the cat and rat spinal cords: II. Segmental differences in the marginal zone. J Comp Neurol 279:619–628.

Milner TA, Pickel VM, Reis DJ (1989): Ultrastructural basis for interactions between central opioids and catecholamines. I. Rostral ventrolateral medulla. J Neurosci 9:2114–2130.

Murakami, S, Okamura H, Pelletier G, Ibata Y (1989): Differential colocalization of neuropeptide Y- and methionine-enkephalin-arg[6]-gly[7]-leu[8]-like immunoreactivity in catecholaminergic neurons in the rat brain stem. J Comp Neurol 281:-532–544.

Nahin RL (1988): Immunocytochemical identification of long ascending, peptidergic lumbar spinal neurons terminating in either the medial or lateral thalamus in the rat. Brain Res 443:345–349.

Nakanishi S, Inoue A, Kita T, Nakamura M, Chang ACY, Cohen S, Numa S (1979): Nucleotide sequence of cloned cDNA for bovine corticotropin-β-lipotropin precursor. Nature 278:423–427.

Noda M, Furutani Y, Takahashi H, Toyosato M, Hirose T, Inayama S, Numa S (1982): Cloning and sequence analysis of cDNA for bovine adrenal preproenkephalin. Nature 295:202–206.

Olson GA, Olson RD, Kastin AJ (1989): Endogenous opiates: 1988. Peptides 10:1253–1280.

Pasternak GW (1988): Multiple morphine and enkephalin receptors and the relief of pain. JAMA 259:1362–1367.

Petrusz P, Merchenthaler I, Maderdrut JL (1985): Distribution of enkephalin-containing neurons in the central nervous system. In Bjorklund A, Hokfelt T (eds): "Handbook of Chemical Neuroanatomy, Vol. 4: GABA and Neuropeptides in CNS, Part I." Amsterdam: Elsevier, pp 273–334.

Pickel VM, Chan J, Milner TA (1989): Ultrastructural basis for interactions between central opioids and catecholamines. II. Nuclei of the solitary tract. J Neurosci 9:2519–2535.

Richardson DE, Akil H (1977a): Pain reduction by electrical brain stimulation in man. (part one): Acute administration in periaqueductal and periventricular sites. J Neurosurg 47:184–194.

Richardson DE, Akil H (1977b): Pain reduction by electrical brain stimulation in man. (part two): Chronic self-administration in the periventricular grey matter. J Neurosurg 47:184–194.

Roberts JL, Herbert E (1977): Characterization of a common precursor to corticotropin and β-lipotropin: Identification of β-lipotropin peptides and their arrangement relative to corticotropin in the precursor synthesized in a cell-free system. Proc Natl Acad Sci USA 74:5300–5304.

Romano GJ, Shivers BD, Harlan RE, Howells RD, Pfaff DW (1987): Haloperidol increases proenkephalin mRNA levels in the caudate-putamen of the rat: A quantitative study at the cellular level using in situ hybridization. Mol Brain Res 2:33–41.

Sabol SL, Yoshikawa K, Hong JS (1983): Regulation of methionine-enkephalin precursor messenger RNA in rat striatum by haloperidol and lithium. Biochem Biophys Res Commun 113:391–399.

Sasek CA, Elde RP (1986): Coexistence of enkephalin and dynorphin immunoreactivities in neurons in the dorsal gray commissure of the sixth lumbar and first sacral spinal cord segments in rat. Brain Res 381:8–14.

Schwartzberg DG, Nakane PK (1983): ACTH-related peptide containing neurons within the medulla oblongata of the rat. Brain Res 276:351–356.

Seizinger BR, Grimm C, Hollt V, Herz A (1983): Evidence for a selective processing of proenkephalin B into different opioid peptide forms in particular regions of rat brain and pituitary. J Neurochem 42:447–457.

Senba E, Yanaihara C, Yanaihara N, Tohyama M (1988): Co-localization of substance P and met-enkephalin-arg[6]-gly[7]-leu[8] in the intraspinal neurons of the rat, with special reference to the neurons in the substantia gelatinosa. Brain Res 453:110–116.

Shinoda K, Michigami T, Awanr K, Shiotani Y (1988): Analysis of the rat interpeduncular subnuclei by immunocytochemical double-staining for enkephalin and substance P, with reference to the coexistence of both peptides. J Comp Neurol 271:243–256.

Simerly RB, McCall LD, Watson SJ (1988): Distribution of opioid peptides in the preoptic region: Immunohistochemical evidence for a steroid-sensitive enkephalin sexual dimorphism. J Comp Neurol 276:442–459.

Sivam SP, Strunk C, Smith DR, Hong JS (1986): Proenkephalin-A gene regulation in the rat striatum: Influence of lithium and haloperidol. Mol Pharmacol 30:186–191.

Stefano GB (1989): Role of opioid neuropeptides in immunoregulation. Prog Neurobiol 33:149–59.

Stengaard-Pedersen K (1989): Opioid peptides and receptors. Localization, interactions and relationships to other molecules in the rodent brain, especially the hippocampal formation. Prog Histochem Cytochem 20:1–119.

Thompson LA, Matsumoto RR, Hohmann AG, Walker JM (1990): Striatonigral prodynorphin: A model system for understanding opioid peptide function. Ann NY Acad Sci 579:192–203.

Trujillo KA, Akil H (1990): Changes in prodynorphin peptide content following treatment with morphine or amphetamine: Possible role in mechanisms of action of drug of abuse. NIDA Res Monogr 95:550–551.

Tsou K, Khachaturian H, Akil H, Watson SJ (1986): Immunocytochemical localization of pro-opiomelanocortin-derived peptides in the adult rat spinal cord. Brain Res 378:28–35.

Tuchscherer MM, Seybold VM (1989): A quantitative study of the coexistence of peptides in varicosities within the superficial laminae of the dorsal horn of the rat spinal cord. J Neurosci 9:195–205.

Vincent SR, Hokfelt T, Christensson I, Terenius L (1982): Dynorphin immunoreactive neurons in the central nervous system of the rat. Neurosci Lett 33:185–190.

Walker LC, Koliatsos VE, Kitt CA, Richardson RT, Rokaeus A, Price DL (1989): Peptidergic neurons in the basal forebrain magnocellular complex of the rhesus monkey. J Comp Neurol 280:272–282.

Watson SJ, Akil H (1980): Alpha-MSH in rat brain: Occurrence within and outside brain β-endorphin neurons. Brain Res 182:217–223.

Watson SJ, Akil H, Fischli W, Goldstein A, Zimmerman E, Nilaver G, van Wimersma Greidanus TB (1982a): Dynorphin and vasopressin: Common localization in magnocellular neurons. Science 216:85–87.

Watson SJ, Akil H, Ghazarossian VE, Goldstein A (1981): Dynorphin immunocytochemical localization in brain and peripheral nervous system. Proc Natl Acad Sci USA 78:1260–1263.

Watson SJ, Akil H, Richard CW, Barchas JD (1978a): Evidence for two separate opiate peptide neuronal systems. Nature 275:226–228.

Watson SJ, Khachaturian H, Akil H, Coy DH, Goldstein A (1982b): Comparison of the distribution of dynorphin systems and enkephalin systems in brain. Science 218:1134–1136.

Watson SJ, Khachaturian H, Taylor L, Fischli W, Goldstein A, Akil H (1983): Prodynorphin peptides are found in the same neurons throughout rat brain: Immunocytochemical study. Proc Natl Acad Sci USA 80:891–894.

Watson SJ, Richard CW, Barchas JD (1978b): Adrenocorticotropin in rat brain: Immunocytochemical localization in cells and axons. Science 200:1180–1182.

Weber E, Barchas JD (1983): Immunocytochemical distribution of dynorphin B in rat brain: Relation to dynorphin A and α-neo-endorphin. Proc Natl Acad Sci USA 80:1125–1129.

Weihe E, Nohr D, Hartschuh W (1988): Immunohistochemical evidence for a cotransmitter role of opioid peptides in primary sensory neurons. Prog Brain Res 74:189–199.

Yoshida M, Taniguchi Y (1988): Projection of pro-opiomelanocortin neurons from the rat arcuate nucleus to the midbrain central gray as demonstrated by double label staining with retrograde labeling and immunohistochemistry. Arch Histol Cytol 51:175–183.

Zardetto-Smith AM, Moga MM, Magnuson DJ, Gray TS (1988): Lateral hypothalamic dynorphinergic efferents to the amygdala and brainstem in rat. Peptides 9:1121–1127.

Development of the Central Nervous System:
Effects of Alcohol and Opiates, pages 221–254
© 1992 Wiley-Liss, Inc.

11

Behavioral Effects of Opiates During Development

GORDON A. BARR

*Department of Psychology, Biopsychology Doctoral Program, Hunter
College, City University of New York, and Department of Developmental
Psychobiology, New York State Psychiatric Institute, Columbia
University College of Physicians and Surgeons, New York, New York*

INTRODUCTION

This chapter reviews the behavioral effects of opiate drugs during development. Although many behavioral effects of opiates have been studied, there is a body of literature only for three: pain perception, feeding, and separation-induced (distress) vocalizations. This review will focus on those behaviors. Of these, the work on the ontogeny of opiate-induced analgesia is far better developed than the work on either feeding or separation-induced vocalizations. More attention is paid to that behavior in this chapter, and, hopefully, the analgesia studies can be used as a guide for further research into feeding and vocalization. More work has been conducted with the rat than with other species, hence, for the purposes of this review, the rat will be the "default" species. When data are from other species, that species will be identified. The emphasis is placed on more recent studies that have begun to examine the mechanisms by which these drugs act rather than on the more descriptive studies that simply describe the drug effects. The goal of this chapter is to emphasize the progress made in understanding how opiate drugs act on the developing organism and to point to areas where further study is needed.

WHY STUDY DEVELOPMENT?

The study of drug effects in immature animals is relatively new, especially those studies that examine the mechanisms by which drugs work to alter behavior. There are many reasons to address these problems. One strategy used to understand the neural bases of any behavior is to study its developmental history. Determining the changes in physiological and behavioral processes during ontogeny can provide clues about the neural organization of those functions. The appearance of neural circuits may correspond to the onset of specific behavioral functions, or neurobehavioral processes that are intertwined in adults may have separate developmental histories.

A second and equally important reason to study the neural bases of behavior in development is to understand behaviors and processes that are unique to young animals. The developing animal has a specific ecological and physiological niche and provides important examples of the adaptive strategies that the young use to thrive in this unique setting. Studying developmental strategies of the young allows us to understand how learning and the environment modify these early behaviors. Perhaps the best studied is sucking for milk which apparently is under different physiological control than is adult or infant feeding (Ellis et al., 1983; Hall, 1985; Blake and Henning, 1986; Rodriquez-Aendejas et al., 1986; Capuano, 1987).

Third, there is a large body of literature that suggests that the central nervous system of the developing animal responds differently to damage than does the adult animal (e.g., Hebb, 1949; D'Amato and Hicks, 1968; Goldman, 1974; Weber and Stelzner, 1977; Bregman and Goldberger, 1982, 1983; Barr et al., 1987a). In some instances, the immature nervous system can be more vulnerable to damage than is the adult animal (Bleier, 1969; Risling et al., 1983). This has been attributed to a variety of developmental differences, including lack of sustaining collaterals, less available trophic factors, and lower metabolic capabilities (see Jacobson, 1978). On the other hand, the central nervous system of the young animal can demonstrate greater neuroplasticity in response to injury. The young animal demonstrates an increased ability to recover functionally from physiological insult. This has been defined as the "infant lesion effect" and is seen in the young of a variety of species (Schneider, 1970; Goldman, 1974; Stelzner et al., 1975; Weber and Stelzner, 1977; Bregman and Goldberger, 1983) including humans (Witelson, 1987). The possible reasons for this include the ability to project axons around the damage to innervate the appropriate target or to project to normally inappropriate targets, to decreased retraction of excessive (exuberant) projections, or to less glial scarring (for reviews see Goldberger and Murray, 1985; Bregman, 1986; Goldberger, 1986; Stelzner et al., 1986). Many neurotransmitter systems demonstrate this plasticity, but the opioid system of the preweanling rat is an example of a neural system that is uniquely responsive to insult at early ages. Treatment with opiates during development results in permanent changes in morphological, behavioral, and biochemical measures (reviewed in McDowell and Kitchen, 1987; see also Chapter 14). Because plasticity is different in the infant than in the mature animal, it is important to understand how the regulatory rules and processes differ between the mature and immature nervous systems that permit the increased plasticity in infancy.

A fourth reason for the study of developing animals is that the immature organism provides a model system to analyze the relationships between neural systems and behavior. The use of maturing animals can provide information that cannot be easily obtained in adult animals. The developing animal is not simple; likely, it is not even simpler than the adult. But as behaviors, or the response to drugs, mature, those developmental changes can be related to neural development. Different tracts may develop with different time courses (e.g., nigrostriatal vs. mesocortical dopamine systems; Coyle and Campochiaro, 1976; Lorén et al., 1976; Schmidt et al., 1982); different targets may be innervated at different times (e.g., 5-HT projections to the dorsal cervical vs. lumbar spinal cord; Bregman 1987); and different subunits of a single system may mature at different ages (e.g. κ, μ, and δ opioid receptors, or pre- vs. postsynaptic processes; Pasternak et al., 1980; Zhang and Pasternak, 1981; Loughlin et al., 1985; Spain et al., 1985; Tavani et al., 1985; Barr et al., 1986; McDowell and Kitchen, 1987; Volterra et al., 1986; Petrillo et al., 1987).

Neural systems function differently in young and mature animals and studies of the neural regulation of behavior in infants can demonstrate phenomena that are not apparent in adults. This may be attributable to the differential maturity of some neural systems compared to others, and can provide opportunities to study the organization of neural circuits in a manner not possible in the adult. For instance, recent work on the changing role of the periaqueductal gray (PAG, see below) in the development of opiate-induced analgesia may provide insights on the function of the nucleus in this behavior because it appears to work quite differently in infants than in older animals.

The study of neuroanatomical and neuropharmacological mechanisms of behavior have benefited from advances in both concept and methodology. In the past 30 or so years, largely because of the advances in neuroanatomical methods used to map neurotransmitter systems, it has become apparent that neural tracts that contain the same neurotransmitter may subserve very different functions. This is perhaps best worked out for the monoamine neurotransmitter, dopamine. Anatomically, dopamine pathways can be divided into five separate systems (Cooper et al., 1986) and each has a distinct function. For example, the ascending nigrostriatal pathway is involved in motor control (Ungerstedt, 1974), the arcuate-hypophyseal system in regulation of anterior pituitary control (Lindvall and Björklund, 1974), and the mesencephalic limbic dopamine system in locomotor and motivational processes (Moore and Kelly, 1978). Conversely, single tracts and even single neurons contain multiple transmitters (Hökfelt et al., 1984, 1986). To understand accurately the behavioral function of distinct neurochemical systems, methods are required that assess the functional specificity of neuroanatomically and neurochemically diverse systems.

ISSUES IN THE STUDY OF BRAIN AND BEHAVIOR DURING DEVELOPMENT

The study of neural bases of behavior requires attention to a number methodological issues. These issues are important in studies of adult animals and in similar studies of infant animals. Studies of brain behavior relationships in developmental studies are often not performed because of the methodological difficulties in studying young animals and because of the conceptual biases of the investigators who are studying these problems (Barr, 1991). Because the structure of the brain is changing dynamically during development (Miller, 1988), studies of mechanism are more difficult in the infant animal than in the adult. The development of neural pathways involves more than the simple appearance of or an increase in the density of projections. It is clear that the maturity of a developing circuit often reflects not merely the presence or absence of a pathway, but rather a refinement of a series of events that might include exuberant projections, loss of connections and retraction of projections, cell death and so forth (O'Leary et al., 1981; Cunningham, 1982; Finlay et al., 1987). When done well, however, developmental studies can provide more information than comparable studies in the adult because one can relate changes in neural systems to changes in function.

One of the issues in the study of the function of opiate drugs during development is understanding the development of receptor types and endogenous opioid peptides in different anatomical regions of the brain and spinal cord. This topic is covered in Chapters 12 and 13; to give a single example, it was reported that various components of the opioid system developed differently in the forebrain v. the hindbrain (Tsang et al., 1982). Below I discuss some of the issues that are necessary to consider in understanding how neural systems regulate behavior in developing animals.

Systems Analysis

Behavior is the result of the integrated function of a number of neural circuits. These include input (sensory function), central processing, and output (motor function). The functional integrity of any neural system is dependent on the maturation of each component of that system (see for example, Hyson and Rubel, 1991). If the system under examination is not functional or functions differently when tested, it is not known whether that specific system is immature or whether some outflow component, several neurons away, has yet to develop. By analysis at several levels, some headway can be made towards solving this problem. A further complication is that these systems interact. In the extreme, the function of a neural circuit is dependent on the development of all neurons in the circuit. At an earlier developmental stage, the function of the system may differ from mature function depending on the completeness of the maturation of the system. The system functions, but less well, or at least differently, than the fully mature pathways. Furthermore, subcomponents of a particular system mature at different rates. The development of functional postsynaptic receptors may precede presynaptic release of the ligand. Receptor agonists may be effective, but drugs that act at the presynaptic terminal may not be, so that the neural system is not physiologically functional although some components are and some drugs are active. The study of the neural mechanisms of behavior, therefore, requires attention to all components of a system. Although important in studies in adult animals, it is of particular importance in infant animals. A full understanding of the mechanisms of any mammalian behavior, although not yet possible, requires analysis at all levels of a system, from the sensory input to motor output.

Differences in Drug Actions in Adult and Infant Animals

Both the pharmacodynamics and pharmacokinetics of drug action differ in young and mature animals. Studies, therefore, must take both factors into account to understand differences in drug effects between mature and immature animals.

Pharmacodynamic issues

Whereas drugs may target specific receptor types or binding sites in adults, are they as specific in infant animals? The data on which specificity has been determined for drugs are from adult animals. There are no guarantees that they are equally specific in immature animals. It is possible that the conformation of the receptor is different, such that the drug-receptor interaction is more or less specific. Studies on the development of opioid receptors, however, have repeatedly found that for a large number of ligands, the affinity of the ligand for its receptor remains constant as the density of binding sites changes (Pasternak et al., 1980; Zhang and Pasternak, 1981; Spain et al., 1985; Barr et al., 1986; Petrillo et al., 1987). Unfortunately, the number of drugs for which this has been demonstrated is limited, and the demonstration of that specificity and selectivity of the drug in immature animals is conspicuously absent from almost all the developmental pharmacological literature.

There are differences in drug action due to the immaturity of the neonate. Because drugs typically act at multiple receptor sites, if different receptor populations develop at different rates, the drugs may act at different sites in infant animals than in adult animals. Ideally, one should know the specificity of the ligand, the population of binding sites in the locus of stimulation, and the developmental time course of the receptor population at these loci. In practice, these data are rarely available. In the adult, morphine is a ligand for μ, δ, and κ receptors; in the immature organism, these receptor populations are incomplete. Therefore, the receptor mechanisms through which morphine acts cannot be known without further studies to assess biochemically and anatomically the maturation of these three receptor types and without the use of more specific ligands to assess the role of each opioid receptor.

Pharmacokinetic issues

The physiological absorption, disposition, and elimination of drugs in the infant differs from that of the adult. Therefore, the pharmacokinetics of drugs administered centrally or peripherally will differ. Care must be taken not to accept dose and time-course effects from adults uncritically. A particularly important factor is the immaturity of the blood-brain barrier. Drugs that do not cross from the periphery into the brain (or vice versa) in adults may readily do so in young animals (Saunders and Møllogård, 1984). Those studies that have measured brain concentrations of opiates (e.g., morphine) have reported decreasing concentrations from birth to adulthood (see below). This is likely due to the development of the blood-brain barrier, the maturation of enzymes, and somatic changes that alter distribution in various body tissues. A particular problem arises when a drug that has only a peripheral action and does not cross the blood-brain barrier in adults is administered to neonates. Clearly, these drugs could be acting centrally in the absence of a formed barrier. A more subtle problem is the assessment of dose-dependent effects during development following peripheral drug administration. Because of the immaturity of the blood-brain barrier, gastric function, liver enzymes and so forth, drugs will reach the central nervous system of the young animals in different concentrations than the adult. Therefore, any conclusion about pharmacodynamic changes requires a full consideration of pharmacokinetic actions.

The experiments described below are aimed at understanding the function of specific populations of neurons in behavior. They have for the most part studied the effects of opiates and to a great extent morphine and naloxone or naltrexone, but have not examined the maturation of the entire system. Yet to be described are the afferents, synaptology, and efferents for any brain site for any behavior. In part the work is too new; in part the brain is too complex. But the questions that the experiments and methods have raised are always the same: how are the neural systems at each level of the neurolaxis organized to function at different ages? With this question in mind, I will describe the data available to date on the role that opiates and opioid systems play in behavior during development.

ANALGESIA

The issue of how pain is processed and modulated at various levels of the neuroaxis has been the subject of intense study for decades, and significant progress has been made in the understanding of how painful sensations are perceived, processed, and dampened. The manner in which neural systems change during maturation to alter the processing of pain, and how pain processing differs between immature and adult organisms are important unresolved questions. Not long ago the prevailing medical opinion was that human infants do not perceive pain due to the immature state of their nervous system and, in particular, the lack of myelination of afferent nerve fibers. This assumption led directly to inappropriate withholding of analgesics for painful surgical treatments (Yaster, 1987). Although it is clear today that the neonate can feel pain, the use of postoperative analgesia remains less common for the infant-patient than for the adult. Little is known of the way the newborn processes pain, or whether and how endogenous pain modulatory systems work, and how the actions of analgesic drugs change during maturation (for recent reviews see Fitzgerald, 1987; Fitzgerald and McIntosh, 1989).

Methodological Issues for the Study of Analgesia
Characteristics of the noxious stimulus

Type of noxious stimulus. In studies conducted in adult animals, it has become increasingly clear that a full understanding of how opiates act to alter pain processing must take into account the type and intensity of the stimulus and how and where it is applied. There are differences in opiate effects among tests of analgesia that use mechanical (pressure) or thermal stimuli or inflammatory or interoceptive irritants such as hypertonic saline, acetic acid, or acetylcholine. Indeed, there is the question of whether or not young rats respond to these latter types of stimuli at all (Bronstein et al., 1986). As with adults, few groups use tests for nociception other than the tail flick (removal of the tail following application of the thermal stimulus to the tail) or hot plate (licking or removal of a paw after being placed on a hot surface) tests. Many groups have used noxious thermal stimuli (see below). Three groups have used noxious mechanical (pressure) stimuli (Kitchen and McDowell, 1985; Giordano and Barr, 1987; Allerton et al., 1989; Barr et al., 1989). Only Abbott and Guy (1990) have used other stimuli (i.e., the formalin test). In these developmental studies, there are differences in drug effects and in the anatomical loci involved in antinociception to mechanical and thermal stimuli, as has been reported in the adult (Abbott and Melzack, 1982; Kuraishi et al., 1983, 1985). Thus, any consideration of the effects of opiate drugs in infants requires attention to the type of noxious stimulus.

Intensity of noxious stimulus. In animal studies it is not possible to ascertain the subjective intensity of the stimulus. Response latency following application of the noxious stimulus, however, may provide a crude indication of pain perception, with more rapid withdrawal occurring in response to more intense stimulation. The response latency to withdraw a limb or tail from noxious heat or mechanical stimuli did not change from 3–14 days of age over a wide range of stimuli (Hughes, 1988; Hughes and Barr, 1988). At least one developmental study has examined different intensity stimuli (Zadina and Kastin, 1986). Over a range of stimuli, the effects of the manipulation (chronic treatment with β-endorphin) were *not* evident at low or high intensity stimuli but only at moderate intensities; likewise, the age of onset of analgesia to morphine is dependent in part on the intensity of the stimulus. The more intense the stimulus, the later the onset of analgesia, even though baseline latencies did not change with maturation (Giordano and Barr, 1987). Testing over a range of stimuli should be the minimum requisite to be able to draw conclusions about the effects of opiate drugs on pain processing.

Somatotopic changes during development

The site of application of the noxious stimulus is important. In infant rats, as in adults, the tail flick response is a reflex mediated within the local segments, but the hindlimb withdrawal response requires supraspinal processing (Yaksh, 1986; Paredes et al., 1990). The different effects of opiates depend on where the stimulus is applied, with the forepaw being more sensitive that the hindpaw or tail when opiates are administered peripherally, intraventricularly, or directly to brain tissue (Barr et al., 1987b; Tive and Barr, 1988). This likely reflects maturation of different levels of the neural axis and could, for example, mirror the ontogeny of descending bulbospinal inhibitory pathways (Fitzgerald and Koltzenberg, 1986; Bregman, 1987). Most of the data on processing of noxious sensory input have concentrated on lumbar spinal cord. For example, Fitzgerald and Koltzenberg (1986), in an elegant set of experiments, reported the late maturation of descending inhibition of dorsal horn neurons responding to noxious stimulation of the skin of the hindpaw. Because the maturation of putative descending inhibitory pathways develops in a caudad direction (Bregman, 1987), the question arises as to the development of descending inhibition at other levels of the spinal cord. In studies described below, it is apparent that analgesia occurs differentially, depending on the appendage that is tested and, by implication, the segmental levels at which processing is occurring.

Interaction of stimulus intensity and localization

A model of the theoretical effects of different anatomical pathways that mediate the processing of noxious stimuli of varying intensity is shown in Figure 1. Failure to appreciate the fact that the intensity of the stimulus can affect the analgesic effects of drug treatment has led to some confusion in the literature about "when" opiate-induced analgesias are first seen. (The question of "when" during development is likely not as important as the question of "how," and for this chapter "how" neural mechanisms and behavior change with maturation to result in changes in response to opiates.) Using withdrawal latency as a crude measure of intensity, it is apparent that equivalent doses of an opiate in both infant and adult animals will produce different levels of analgesia (Dykstra, 1985; Zadina and Kastin, 1986; Giordano and Barr, 1987). These relationships are depicted

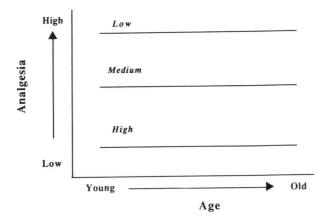

Fig. 1. Schematic diagram demonstrating that, in general, opiate drugs are more effective against lower intensity stimuli than higher intensity stimuli. As the intensity of the stimulus increases, as depicted by the three parallel lines, the amount of analgesia, shown on the abscissa, decreases. Although never directly tested, this appears to be consistent over a wide range of ages.

in Figure 1. In developmental studies, the intensity function can drastically alter the development of analgesia. For example, in Figure 2 it is demonstrated that as a rule, the forepaw is more sensitive to opiate-induced antinociceptive effects than are the hindpaws or tail (Barr et al., 1987b; Giordano and Barr, 1987). Moreover, there is an interaction between the intensity of the stimulus and the location at which it is applied (Fig. 3). If more intense stimuli are used, the developmental pattern of analgesia is rostral to caudal. When less intense stimuli are used, that developmental pattern is masked because of the effectiveness of the opiates. The forepaw is typically more sensitive than the tail, and because the withdrawal response to less intense stimuli is attenuated by opiates more easily than is the response to more intense stimuli, the results of an experiment are a function of both factors. The data generated and, therefore, the conclusion drawn are fully dependent on the parameters chosen in any experiment.

Site of action of the opiates

Because there are multiple sites that can act to modify pain processes, the site of action of the opiates is an important variable. Most studies have used peripheral injections. This insures that the drug will act on all levels of the neuroaxis, including opioid receptors in the spinal cord, at supraspinal sites to modulate the ascending pain signal, or at brain sites that

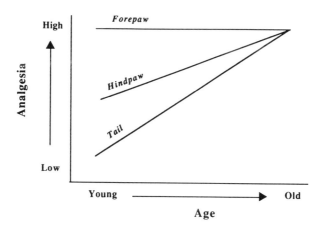

Fig. 2. This figure schematizes a result that we have repeatedly found—that at young ages, the forepaw is more sensitive to the effects of morphine than is either the hindpaw or tail. The latter two appendages vary somewhat in their sensitivity depending on age, drug, type, and intensity of stimulus, but in general the hindpaw is more sensitive to the antinociceptive effects of morphine than the tail. We believe this is the functional result of the postnatal development of descending inhibitory systems activated by supraspinal acting opiates. This differential sensitivity disappears as the animal matures.

project directly or indirectly to the dorsal horn of the spinal cord to produce analgesia. Less commonly, opiates have been administered directly to the brain either by intracerebroventricular (ICV) administration (Pasternak et al., 1980; Zhang and Pasternak, 1981; Kehoe and Blass, 1986a; Barr et al., 1987b;) or to specific brain nuclei using standard chemical stimulation procedures (Tive and Barr, 1988; Barr, 1991). Some studies have examined the site of action in the spinal cord by direct intrathecal administration (Allerton et al., 1989; Paredes et al., 1990) or by severing the spinal cord (Pasternak et al., 1980).

Experimental Data

Peripheral administration of opiates

I will summarize first the more descriptive data and then review the more mechanistic studies. Although the analgesic effects of opiates were among the first properties studied developmentally, until recently the studies have been descriptive, with less emphasis on understanding the changes in neural mechanisms during maturation. The neural locus at which the opiates act in infant animals is not known. In adult animals, opiate drugs can produce analgesia by acting in at least three different neural sites. First, they can act directly in the brain to inhibit ascending pain sensations. Second, they can act directly in the dorsal horn of the spinal cord. Third, opiates acting at brain sites can activate bulbospinal inhibitory projections that dampen nociceptive input at the level of the spinal cord. In this review we will concentrate on the latter two alterna-

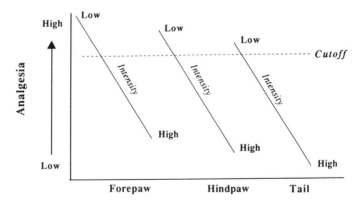

Fig. 3. This figure demonstrates the hypothetical interaction of the stimulus intensity and the appendage to which it is applied in young animals. Because low intensity stimuli are quite responsive to opiates, if those intensities are used, the rostral to caudal development of analgesia may be masked due to ceiling effects. Thus, the tail which is less sensitive to opiates in very young animals would be seen as no different from the forepaw if low intensity stimuli are used. The value of the cutoff depicted here is arbitrary and would depend on the age of the animal, the opiate, and the type of stimulus used.

tives, which have also been studied the most in the literature on adult animals (Basbaum and Fields, 1984).

Since the first reports demonstrating that opiates induced analgesia in infant animals (e.g., Kupferberg and Way, 1963), many studies have demonstrated an antinociceptive effect in immature animals (for a review see McDowell and Kitchen, 1987), including human infants (see Yaster, 1987). Studies that have examined analgesia at early ages have found that rat and κ mouse pups become more responsive to opioid-induced analgesia as they develop during the preweaning period (Johannesson and Becker, 1973; Auguy-Valette et al., 1978; Pasternak et al., 1980; Zhang and Pasternak, 1981; Spear et al., 1985; Barr et al., 1986; Alleva and Laviola, 1987; Giordano and Barr, 1987). The onset of analgesia can be quite abrupt, occurring within a single day (Spear et al., 1985; Barr et al., 1986). The exact pattern of analgesia depends on which region of the body is stimulated, the type and intensity of stimulus used, and the opiate that is given. Stimuli that are less intense or that are applied to rostral body parts are more sensitive to opiate-induced analgesia at earlier ages (Giordano and Barr, 1987; Barr et al., 1989; unpublished observations in my lab). From the end of the preweaning period to adulthood, the effect of peripherally administered opiates decreases, with the most potent effects being elicited in 20–21 day old rats and the effects declining with age (Johannesson and Becker, 1973; Nicák and Kohút, 1978). This may be due to different pharmacokinetics of morphine in the younger animal since brain levels of morphine in the weanling animal, is higher than levels in the adult.

The developmental course of analgesia differs for opiate ligands that prefer different receptor types (Pasternak et al., 1980; Zhang and Pasternak, 1981; Barr et al., 1986; Giordano and Barr, 1987; Helmstetter et al., 1988), in part because of the differential maturation of opioid receptor types (Bardo et al., 1986; Petrillo et al., 1987) and in part because different receptor types at different neuroanatomical sites mature at different ages (Kornblum et al., 1987; see also Chapter 12). In early work, Pasternak and co-workers reported that drugs that targeted high affinity opioid receptors produced analgesia that developed between 7 and 11 days of age. Morphine, for example, showed a 10–15-fold increase in potency from 2–3 days of age to 11 days of age and a 40-fold shift from 2–14 days of age. Other effective drugs that demonstrated the same pattern were β-endorphin and d-ala^2-met^5-enkephalinamide (Pasternak et al., 1980; Zhang and Pasternak, 1981). These data suggest that opioid receptors at both the spinal and/or supraspinal levels change postnatally. The analgesic effect of the opiates correlated with the gradual and relatively late appearance of a high affinity opioid binding site that Pasternak's group defined as the μ_1 opioid receptor. A lower affinity (defined as μ_2) opioid receptor was present in neonates and did not change in density during the first two postnatal weeks. This correlated with profound respiratory depression produced by morphine in 2 day olds, in the absence of analgesia.

Using similar logic, I and my colleagues described the development of μ and κ opioid receptors that correlated with the appearance of analgesia induced by morphine and ketocyclazocine (Barr et al., 1986). We found that, consistent with other data, a high affinity μ opioid receptor was present in low numbers at birth and developed linearly over the first 2 weeks of life. The κ opioid receptor was present in higher numbers at birth and did not increase substantially until the end of the second week. This differential development corresponded to changing patterns of analgesia induced by morphine and ketocyclazocine. Morphine's analgesic action first appeared between 10 and 14 days of age whereas ketocyclazocine and bremazocine were effective at 3 days of age and above (Kitchen and McDowell, 1985; Barr et al., 1986; Helmstetter et al., 1988). The relatively late onset of morphine-induced analgesia is due in part to the relative intense thermal stimulus used in that study (see Giordano and Barr, 1987 for a comparison of the effects of opiates on different intensity stimuli). Although these two drugs are not fully selective for μ and κ opioid receptors, the different patterns of analgesia, the lack of cross-tolerance, the inability of a δ opioid receptor antagonist to block their effects, and the different potencies of naloxone to antagonize each effect suggest that the different developmental patterns of analgesia were due to the differential development of μ and κ opioid receptor types (Barr et al., 1986; Giordano and Barr, 1987). Like Pasternak, we noted an early onset of respiratory depression induced by morphine following peripheral or ICV administration (but not intraspinal), suggesting that the analgesic effect and the decrease in respiratory rate induced by morphine are developmentally dissimilar and may be due to different interactions with these two receptor types. An alternate possibility, however, is that the two effects are mediated by the same receptor but that the receptor type develops in brain nuclei that control respiration prior to those that inhibit processing of noxious stimuli.

Intracerebroventricular administration

At least three groups have demonstrated analgesia after ICV injection of opiates in infant rats. Morphine (Kehoe and Blass, 1986a; Barr et al., 1987b), β-endorphin, and d-ala^2-met^5-enkephalinamide (Pasternak et al., 1980) injected directly to the lateral ventricle or cerebral cistern produced analgesia using tests of thermal or mechanical pain. Following lateral ventricle injection, the exact ontogenetic pattern of analgesia depended on the type and intensity of the stimulus and the region of the body tested (Barr et al., 1987b) (Fig. 4). As with peripheral administration, there is a rostral to caudal development of analgesia that may reflect the postnatal development of descending inhibitory bulbospinal projections to the dorsal horn of the spinal cord. Several doses of morphine or ketocyclazocine were injected into the lateral ventricle of 3-, 10-, and 14-day-old rat pups. When the mechanical test was used, mild analgesia appeared in the forepaw at 3 and 10 days of age. Analgesia to this mechanical stimulus first appeared in the hindpaw and tail at 10 days of age, a stage of development in which no analgesia was seen in these caudal body parts when the thermal stimulus was used. In the 3-day-old pups, morphine produced analgesia to the thermal stimulus only in the forepaw. Analgesia in the thermal test appeared in the hindpaw and tail only when the animals were 14 days of age.

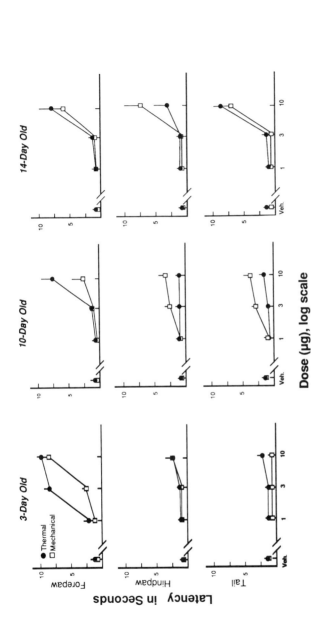

Dose (μg), log scale

Fig. 4. This figure shows the effects of morphine administered directly to the lateral ventricle of rat pups aged 3–14 days of age and tested with either a mechanical or thermal noxious stimulus. Description of the test protocol can be found in Hughes and Barr (1988). Cutoff was 10 seconds. In the forepaw, morphine was quite effective against both the mechanical and the thermal stimuli at all ages. It was ineffective in the hindpaw or tail in the 3-day-old pups. At 10 days of age, morphine increased the response latency to the noxious mechanical stimulus only and was equally potent in all three appendages. In contrast, morphine was still ineffective in the hindlimb and tail of the 10-day-old pups. At 14 days of age morphine produced antinociception in all cases. We believe that the pattern of analgesia seen reflects the recruitment of different descending pathways mediating antinociception to the two types of stimuli with an earlier maturation of the pathway subserving analgesia when the mechanical stimulus was used.

By 14 days of age analgesia was seen in all body parts to both stimuli. Ketocyclazocine had no effect when given ICV.

Intraspinal administration

Opiates produce analgesia in adult animals, including humans, when administered directly to the spinal cord (for review see Yaksh, 1986). Both μ and κ opioid receptors exist in the spinal cord of the early postnatal rat pup (Allerton et al., 1989; Attali et al., 1990), and thus it might be expected that μ and κ opiates would produce analgesia when administered directly to the spinal cord. When morphine is administered intraspinally to pre-weanlings, the pattern of analgesia observed again depends on the type of stimulus and its somatotopic presentation and on the age of the animal (Barr et al., 1989). In the 4-day-old pups, intrathecal injection of morphine produced analgesia when the thermal noxious stimulus was presented to the forepaw. Morphine had no effect in tests in which the hindpaw or tail was immersed in hot water (immersion tests). Intrathecal morphine produced analgesia against the mechanical stimulus in all three body parts at this age. In the 10-day-old rat, morphine was effective against the thermal stimulus in all three body parts; the effects of morphine were not assessed in the mechanical test (Figs. 5, 6). Although morphine binds preferentially to the μ opioid receptor, it interacts with all three types of opioid receptors. Two studies have examined the role of κ opioid receptors. Both ketocyclazocine, a κ opioid receptor preferring opiate, and the more specific U69593 produced dose-dependent antinociception to mechanical pressure (Allerton et al., 1989; Barr et al., 1989). The effects of U69593 were naloxone-reversible. EKC was less effective when tested with a noxious thermal stimulus. In adult animals, the arylacetamide ligands such as U69593 do not produce analgesia due to the apparent absence of those binding sites (termed κ_1) in spinal cord. In contrast, the spinal cord of the neonate has a significant concentration of κ_1 opioid receptors which can be demonstrated both in vivo and in vitro (Allerton et al., 1989). The behavioral results suggest that functional opioid receptors exist in the spinal cord as early as 4 days of age, but demonstrate subtle differences from analgesia induced by direct spinal injections in adult animals.

In vitro spinal cord preparations

Preparations that isolate the spinal cord of the infant rat with peripheral nerves or tail intact have demonstrated that μ and κ opioid receptors are capable of inhibiting nociceptive responses. In a recording of ventral root potentials evoked by stimulation of the dorsal root, skin, or tail (with pressure, capsaicin, or heat), a number of opiates depress the response to noxious stimulation (Yanagisawa et al., 1984; Briggs and Barnes, 1987; James et al., 1990). In the neonate, μ opioid receptor agonists such as [D-ALA^2,NMe-Phe^4, Gly-ol]-enkephalin (DAMGO) are most effective and more potent than κ opioid receptor preferring compounds such as U69569, PD117302, or U50488 (Briggs and Barnes, 1987; James et al., 1990). Morphine itself is effective, but not as potent as DAMGO or the κ agonists in these preparations (James et al., 1990). Morphine likely acts presynapti-

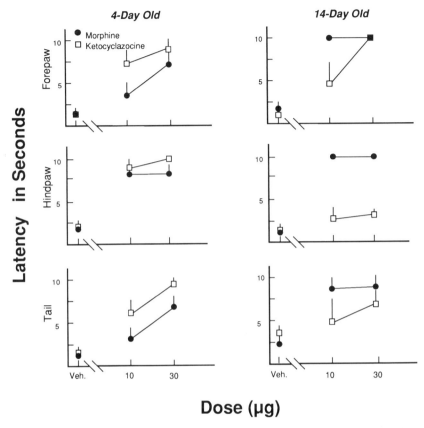

Fig. 5. These data show the result of the intrathecal administration of morphine or ketocyclazocine when a mechanical noxious stimulus was applied. Both drugs were effective although morphine was significantly more potent in the 14-day-old pups than was ketocyclazocine.

cally in the young animal as it is thought to do in the adult (Bell and Jaffe, 1986). Consistent with in vivo studies (Fitzgerald and Koltzenberg, 1986), there is evidence for a lack of descending inhibition in the flexor nerve reflex of young pups (Hori and Watanabe, 1987). δ-Agonists are ineffective and δ-blockers do not antagonize the effects of agonists including the enkephalins. This is consistent with the paucity of demonstrable δ opioid receptors in the spinal cord of the infant rat (Attali et al., 1990).

Periaqueductal gray

One important neural component of analgesic endogenous modulatory systems in the adult is the PAG of the midbrain. That the PAG produces profound analgesia when stimulated has been known for over 20 years

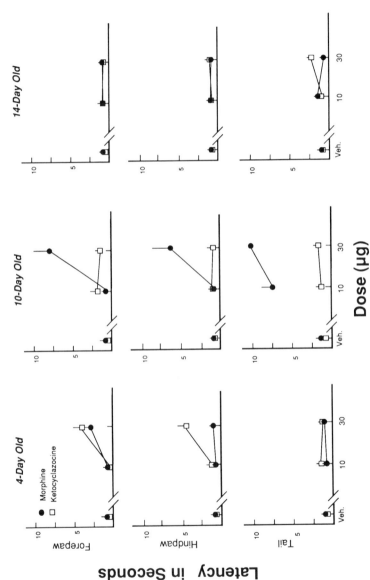

Fig. 6. These data demonstrate the result of intrathecal administration of morphine or ketocyclazocine when a thermal noxious stimulus was used. Both drugs were most effective in the forepaw in the 4-day-old pups and ketocyclazocine was not analgesic in the 10-day-old pups.

(Reynolds, 1969). Even the general manner by which this occurs—activation of medullary nuclei that project caudally and inhibit neurons responsive to nociceptive input in the dorsal horn of the spinal cord—is also known (Basbaum and Fields, 1984). What is not known are the details of its function and how the PAG interfaces with other pain modulatory systems, and virtually nothing is known of the neural pathways that mediate analgesia in the immature animal.

In these studies, rat pups aged 2, 9, or 13 days of age were implanted with chronic indwelling cannulas aimed at either the dorsal or ventral subareas of the PAG. On the next day they were injected with one of two doses of morphine or vehicle (200 η1 in all cases). Pups were tested with noxious mechanical or thermal stimuli applied to the forepaw, hindpaw, or tail (Hughes and Barr, 1988). The resultant analgesia was dependent upon the site of injection, age, location of the noxious stimulus, and the stimulus type. In follow-up experiments, PAG stimulation was combined with systemic naloxone treatment or intrathecal injection of the serotonergic or noradrenergic antagonist methysergide or phentolamine in initial steps to determine the mechanisms of the PAG induced analgesia.

Ventral sites. In 3-day-old rat pups, morphine induced significant levels of analgesia when administered to the ventral PAG. This analgesia appeared in a rostral to caudal direction as the animal matured, appearing first when tested with the thermal stimulus. At 3 days of age, analgesia was most potent against the thermal stimulus and was seen only in the forepaw. In 10-day-old pups, morphine was still effective against only the thermal stimulus, but the analgesic effect was evident in the thermal test in caudal body parts as well. No analgesia to the mechanical stimulus was seen in 3- or 10-day-old pups. In 14-day-old pups, morphine induced analgesia to the thermal and mechanical stimuli in all body parts.

Dorsal sites. Morphine administered to the dorsal PAG failed to induce analgesia against neither the mechanical nor the thermal stimulus until the animal was 14 days of age. At 2 weeks of age, analgesia was induced in all body parts by either stimulus. In all cases, morphine was less effective when administered to the dorsal PAG as compared to the ventral PAG (see Fig. 7).

One issue raised by studies of analgesia produced by stimulation of the PAG is whether the antinociceptive effects can be separated from a cluster of "aversive" behaviors that occur with stimulation (e.g., Jacquet and Lajtha, 1974, Oliveras et al., 1987). Oliveras et al. (1987) proposed that the ventral PAS was the only aspect of that nucleus that supported true analgesia. Stimulation of the dorsal region of the PAG produced avoidance responding, vocalization, and aversive-like behaviors. They postulated that the analgesic effect of dorsal PAG stimulation was secondary to these other behaviors. Several recent studies as well as results from my lab cast doubt on that interpretation (Morgan et al., 1987; Leão Borges et al., 1988; Tive and Barr, 1988). Benzodiazepines administered systematically (Morgan et al., 1987) or directly to the PAG (Leão Borges et al., 1988) attenuated the aversive effects of dorsal PAG stimulation without affecting the analgesia

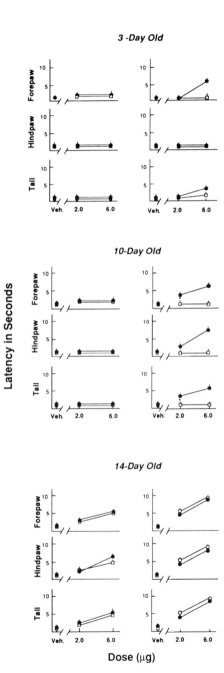

3 -Day Old

10-Day Old

14-Day Old

Latency in Seconds

Dose (μg)

produced by that stimulation. In developmental studies, aversive reactions did not accompany analgesia in pups 14 days of age or younger. In 21-day-old pups, however, stimulation of the PAG induced hyperreactivity, jumping, and vocalization in conjunction with analgesia (Tive and Barr, 1988). Consequently, both the benzodiazepine data and these developmental studies argue that dorsal PAG stimulation can produce analgesia that is independent from the aversiveness of the stimulation.

The production of analgesia can occur at multiple levels of the central nervous system that can be compartmentalized experimentally by restricting manipulation to a single level of the neuroaxis. This approach has been useful in the analysis of feeding behaviors (Ziegler, 1976) and has been extended to the study of feeding in the infant rat (Hall, 1985). In the studies presented above, the attempt is to isolate separate components of the central nervous system to observe the effects on analgesia during development. The difference between the feeding model and the model presented here is that because the final common path that activated is likely the spinal cord, manipulations "upstream" in the brain are dependent on maturation at the spinal cord level. By testing several different elements of the circuit (e.g., receptor, presynaptic process), crude models can be developed as to how the various levels of the central nervous system mature to inhibit painful sensations.

Summary of the data

Table I summarizes data that can be used to model the development of analgesia in the developing rat pup (Fig. 8). In the 3-day-old pup, analgesia was noted when morphine was injected into the ventral portion of the PAG or when glutamate was injected into the dorsal PAG (Tive and Barr, 1988). This implies the presence of the opioid receptor and descending pathway from the PAG to the rostral ventral medullary area (RVM; the specific nuclei that are involved are unknown) and to the rostral aspect of the spinal cord. Antinociception was not induced in more caudal sites and there is evidence of a lack of descending inhibition in young pups (Fitzgerald and Koltzenburg, 1986). The relevant receptors in the dorsal horn,

---

Fig. 7. These data, taken from Tive (1990), demonstrate the results of stimulation of either the dorsal PAG (left panel at each age) or the ventral PAG (right panel). The results when the thermal stimulus was applied are shown by the solid circles and the data when the mechanical stimulus was used are shown by the open squares. When administered to the dorsal PAG, morphine had no antinociceptive action until 14 days of age and was equally potent for both stimuli. When morphine was injected into the ventral PAG, a different pattern resulted. Morphine was effective in the forepaw only in the 3-day-old pups but only to the thermal noxious stimulus. There was no analgesia for the mechanical stimulus until 14 days of age. We conclude from these data that the PAG consists of two distinct areas that mediate analgesia differently and that the mechanisms by which the analgesia is produced differ for the two types of stimuli.

however, are not likely to be serotonergic or noradrenergic because direct administration of serotonin (5-HT) or norepinephrine (NE) to the cord at this age has no effect on the forepaw. NE and 5-HT are both analgesic in the hindpaw and tail, although their preferred stimuli are different. These receptors have not been linked to descending paths since the presynaptic components of that system have not been tested. Morphine given intrathecally at this age blocks the response to mechanical stimuli in all appendages but thermal stimuli only in the forepaw. Therefore, functional opioid receptors are present at the appropriate level of the spinal cord. In the 10-day-old pups, the relevant neural systems have matured and analgesia is seen in all body parts following ventral morphine or dorsal glutamate injections. Therefore, the receptors and pathways from the PAG to the RVM and then to the spinal cord can be considered functional. From postnatal day 10, serotonin and NE given intrathecally produce analgesia at all regions of the body that have been tested and to both stimuli except that intrathecal 5-HT and the mechanical stimulus applied to the forepaw are ineffective. Morphine was effective against the thermal stimulus at this age also; tests were not conducted with the mechanical stimulus at this age, but the κ agonist U69593 produced analgesia at the level of the spinal cord as early as 9 days of age (Allerton et al., 1989). In the 14-day-old pups, the major changes are the effectiveness of glutamate applied to the ventral PAG, the effectiveness of morphine into the dorsal PAG, and the puzzling lack of effect of intrathecal morphine when tested with the thermal stimulus. Because neither intrathecal 5-HT nor NE has been tested at this age, those receptors are present based on the studies that blocked these receptors in conjunction with PAG stimulation.

Description of the working model

In the schematic diagram presented in Figure 8, based on experimental data described above and summarized in Table 1, I have attempted to construct models that describe the changing pattern or analgesia during development. The panels present highly simplified and schematized diagrams of changes in neural circuits from the PAG to the RVM and subsequently to the spinal cord receptors during development. For illustration purposes, the spinal cord is divided into "mechanical" and "thermal" components, but with no implication that these are morphological distinctions. There are several assumptions that are made in this model. First, ascending systems have been ignored for simplicity. Second, other descending systems, many of which impact on the circuit presented here, are also ignored. For example, there is extensive anatomical and pharmacological evidence that other nuclei project to the PAG, RVM, and spinal cord and produce analgesia when stimulated. Finally, because all levels of the neuroaxis described in the model have not been examined, important data are missing. When PAG stimulation does not elicit analgesia, it is not known whether that is due to the immature state of the opioid receptor in the dorsal PAG or to some yet undeveloped link between that receptor and the spinal cord. In these cases, the entire circuit has been left out.

TABLE I. Summary of Experiments[a]

		Thermal			Mechanical		
	Age	FP	HP	T	FP	HP	T
IntraPAG							
Morphine							
Dorsal	3	0	0	0	0	0	0
	10	0	0	0	0	0	0
	14	+	+	+	+	+	+
Ventral	3	++	0	0	0	0	0
	10	++	++	++	0	0	0
	14	++	++	++	++	++	++
Glutamate							
Dorsal	3	0	0	0	+	0	0
	10	0	0	0	+	+	+
	14	++	++	++	++	++	++
Ventral	3	0	0	0	0	0	0
	10	0	0	0	0	0	0
	14	++	++	++	++	++	++
Intrathecal							
Morphine	4	+	0	0	++	++	++
	10	++	++	++	—	—	—
	14	0	0	0	++	++	++
Ketocyclazocine	4	+	+	0	++	++	++
	14	0	0	0	++	++	++
Norepinephrine	4	0	0	0	0	++	++
	10	+	++	++	++	++	++
Serotonin	4	0	++	++	0	0	0
	10	++	++	++	0	0	0
Intraventricular							
Morphine	4	++	0	0	++	0	0
	10	++	0	0	+	+	+
	14	++	++	++	++	++	++

[a]Summary of the data on the development of analgesia from experiments described in the text. The data are organized by the site of administration. "0" means that the drug was ineffective; "+" means statistically effective but not maximally so; "++" means that the drug was fully effective in producing analgesia, when "—" appears, there are no data available. The intraPAG data are from Tive and Barr (1988). The intrathecal data for the opiates, norepinephrine and serotonin are from Barr et al. (1987b), Hughes and Barr (1988), and Schwarz and Barr (1990), respectively. The intraventricular data are adapted from Pasternak et al. (1980) and Barr et al. (1987b).

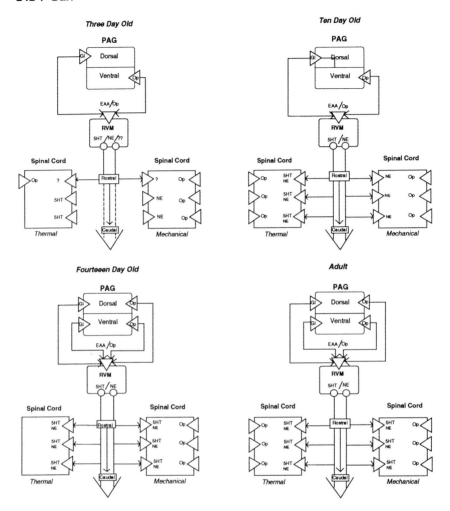

Fig. 8. This is a mythological portrait of a portion of the neural circuitry that mediates analgesia in rat pups of different ages. The scheme is based on models of others and is described in detail in the text of this chapter. EAA, excitatory amino acids; G1, glutamate; Op, opioid; triangles represent postsynaptic receptors; arrows represent axonal projections.

Before the third week of life, some aspect of the pathway from the PAG to the RVM and the descending spinal inhibitory systems is immature, since lesions of the dorsal lateral funiculus and intraventricular or intraPAG injections produce minimum analgesia (Fitzgerald and Koltzenberg, 1986; Tive and Barr, 1988; Barr et al., 1989), at least at lumbar and sacral levels of the spinal cord. Stimulation of the ventral PAG with morphine does produce analgesia in the forepaw. Hence, there is evidence for at least partial innervation by these descending pathways. It is not known, however, if the lack of effect is due to immaturity of the projections to the RVM or from the RVM to the spinal cord. Monoaminergic and opioid receptors are present, in the presumed absence of innervation, because intrathecal injections of agonists produce analgesia. By 10 days of age, there is some evidence for greater development of the descending pathways since PAG stimulation and intraventricular administration of morphine produce some analgesia. This pathway, however, may not be fully functional since the pattern of analgesia is not yet adult-like (Fitzgerald and Koltzenberg, 1986). Spinal cord receptors that have been studied are functional. By 14 days of age, the patterns of analgesia detected are similar to those described in the adult and thus within the limits of the procedures appear mature.

FEEDING

In adults, opioids are involved in the regulation of food intake. Agonists of μ and κ opioid receptors enhance ingestion and opioid antagonists suppress it (for review see Morley et al., 1983). Mammals suckle and this form of ingestion has a separate set of regulatory controls than does adult feeding (see Hall, 1985). Ingestion independent of the dam can occur in very young animals but the full complement of physiological mechanisms regulation ingestion in the immature animal is incomplete and different from those that regulate suckling. The role of opioid systems in the regulation of ingestion either on or off the nipple has only recently been studied. In the review below, intake from suckling the dam and from independent feeding paradigms are treated separately.

Suckling

The literature on the effects of opiates and opiate antagonists on suckling is neither plentiful nor consistent. With the exception of one group, the data are consistent in that opiate antagonists do not inhibit milk intake or suckling when the young pup is attached to the dam. Several studies, using a variety of doses of antagonists, experimental protocols, and dependent measures, have failed to find any effect of naloxone or naltrexone. This lack of effect occurs whether intake is measured by weight gain (Aroyewun and Barr, 1982, 1983; Capuano et al., 1990) or by any of several measures of attachment to the teat (Spear and Ristine, 1982; Blass et al., 1990). The exceptions, two studies by Sewell and colleagues, report that a number of antagonists, though not including naloxone or naltrexone which were not tested, inhibited intake as early as 1 day of age (Jackson and Sewell, 1984; Lal and Sewell, 1989). The reasons for this discrepancy are not clear, but they are not likely due to the level of deprivation, time of measurement, ambient temperature, or any other obvious methodological difference. It is possible that the reason is the use of different antagonists, but that possibility is mitigated by the report that naloxone inhibited intake is an earlier study (cited in Jackson and Sewell, 1984). If opiate antagonists do inhibit intake, there is some evidence that μ and κ opioid receptors, but not δ opioid receptors, are involved in the inhibitory effect in young pups (Jackson and Sewell, 1984). Such a finding might be expected given the late development of the δ opioid receptor (see Chapter 12). Although the effects of antagonists are unclear, the agonist met-enkephalin (but not leu-enkephalin) enhanced intake in mildly deprived 5-day-old rat pups (Lal and Sewell, 1989). I am unaware of any other studies on the effects of agonists on suckling.

Independent Ingestion

Naloxone failed to inhibit feeding off the nipple until 14 days of age in rats (Aroyewun and Barr, 1982, 1983; Spear and Ristine, 1982; Capuano et al., 1990). This led to the incorrect conclusion that the opioid receptors did not function in the regulation of independent ingestion until that age (Aroyewun and Barr, 1982, 1983). Morphine enhanced independent feeding as early as 3 days of age (Capuano et al., 1990). Hence, the relevant opioid receptors are functional early. The failure of naloxone to inhibit intake in the young pup is likely not due to the late development of receptors, but may result from the slow maturation of the presynaptic release of the opioid ligand. Without that release, naloxone is ineffective because there is no activity at the receptor to antagonize. Further complicating the interpretation of these data is a recent divergent report of inhibition of feeding by naloxone as early as 6 days of age (Blass et al., 1990). Those authors did not explore the discrepancies, and the reasons for the differences are not known.

Clearly, the literature on opioid control of intake is sparse. More studies are required, especially those that use agonists as well as antagonists. To date, there have been no attempts to localize the site of action of the opiates within the central nervous system, no work linking opiates to any specific physiological satiety mechanism (i.e., gastric fill) despite an increasing understanding of those mechanisms (for review see Phifer, 1991), and little attention has been paid to the role of specific opioid receptor types.

SEPARATION INDUCED VOCALIZATION

In a number of species, when the infants are separated from their mother and siblings, they emit a separation call that has been described as a signal of distress (Panksepp et al., 1980; Hofer and Shair, 1987). For some species (e.g., human, dog, chicken) the vocalization is within the receptive range of humans, whereas for other species (rat, mouse) it is ultrasonic. The separation call has been described as the earliest and most basic of all mammalian vocalizations (MacLean, 1985). At least for the rat, the ultrasonic vocalizations (USV) are differentially regulated, depending on the age of the pup. For the newborn, the cries are thermally regulated and are elicited by exposure to temperatures lower than that of the nest. As the pup matures, the levels of vocalization become less dependent on ambient temperature and more responsive to the presence or absence of conspecifics such as the dam or littermates.

Opiate drugs and endogenous opioids play an important regulatory role in the production of ultrasonic distress vocalizations in all species tested, but there is no consensus on the manner by which opioid systems regulate these vocalizations. Opiate agonists clearly reduce crying in a behaviorally specific and dose-dependent fashion, but opioid antagonists do not consistently alter baseline vocalizations except in the presence of a conspecific "companion."

Two different models have been postulated to explain how opioid systems are involved in distress vocalizations. In the first, originally delineated by Panksepp (for review, see Panksepp et al., 1980), opioid systems are viewed as the neural mediators by which the presence of the dam, littermates, and other cues in the nest normally quiet the young animal. Consequently, in the natural setting, opioid systems appear active. When the infant is socially isolated, opioids are no longer functioning and the infant responds to "withdrawal" with crying. The implications of this model are that opioid agonists should quiet the isolated infant, opioid antagonists should induce crying in the presence of cues that normally quiet the infant, and antagonists should not increase crying in the isolated animal because the endogenous system is not functioning.

The second model views the opioid system as normally quiescent. On isolation, the infant is stressed, and vocalizes. The stress of separation mobilizes the opioid systems and their activation leads to a quieting of the infant over time. The implication of this latter model is that opioid agonists quiet a distressed animal as predicted by the first model. But unlike the Panksepp model, opioid antagonists should increase vocalizations in the isolated animal but not in animals while they are in the nest. The data are not fully consistent with either scheme.

The administration of morphine and related opioid alkaloids and opiate peptides decreases crying in the separated infant dog (Panksepp et al., 1983), chick (Panksepp et al., 1978a,b), guinea pig (Herman and Panksepp, 1978), rat (Kehoe and Blass, 1986a; Cuomo et al., 1988; Carden and Hofer, 1990a,b), mouse (Albonetti et al., 1985), and monkey (Kalin et al., 1989). The range of opioids that is effective is impressive, and includes opiate alkaloids such as morphine, β-endorphin, several enkephalin peptides, and putative enkephalinase inhibitors. This opiate-induced suppression of vocalization is naloxone-reversible. Casomorphans, opiates found in milk, inhibit vocalization in chicks, but not rats (Panksepp et al., 1984; Cuomo et al., 1988). The effect in the chick is only partially naloxone-reversible. Why a constituent in milk would inhibit ultrasounds in a nonmammalian species but not a mammalian species (that feeds milk to its young) is puzzling.

There is evidence that both δ and μ opioid receptors are involved in the quieting effect, at least for pups 10 days of age and older. Intracisternal administration of DAMGO or DPDPE, which target μ and δ opioid receptors, respectively, decreased USV in 10- and 14-day-old pups (Carden et al., 1990). DAMGO is extraordinarily potent, having effects in the picomolar range. DPDPE had an effect on 10-day-old rat pups and its potency increased at 14 days. The increased potency of the δ opioid agonist is consistent with the proliferation of δ opioid binding sites during the second postnatal week (Spain et al., 1985; Petrillo et al., 1987). The increase in δ opioid receptors correlates with the change in the regulation of the calling from control by ambient temperature to control by the presence or absence of social companions. It is tempting to speculate that these receptors mediate the onset of the social control of separation distress. Kappa opioid agonists, in contrast, increase USV dramatically when given centrally (Carden et al., 1990) or peripherally (Kehoe et al., 1990).

The reliability of the effectiveness of opiate agonists is in stark contrast to the unreliability of the effect of the opioid antagonists naloxone and naltrexone. There are reports that opioid antagonists increase USV in isolated rat and mice pups (Robinson et al., 1985; Kehoe and Blass, 1986b), but others have reported a failure of the antagonists to increase calling (Gardner, 1985; Cramer et al., 1990; Winslow and Insel, 1991), and still others have reported inconsistent effects (Panksepp et al., 1978a). In the most extensive study, Carden tested pups aged 7, 10, 12, 14, and 16 days of age with a wide range of naloxone (0.5–5.0 mg/kg) and found no effect of any dose of naloxone at any age. This is, however, in contrast to her earlier finding that naloxone increased USV in 10-day-old pups (Carden and Hofer, 1990a). Others have reported anecdotally that the antagonist effect is ephemeral and waxes and wanes for unknown reasons. At times it is robust; at other times it is absent.

The reason for the variability of the effect of the opioid antagonist may be some environmental factor that has been overlooked, but it is also possible, in view of the differential effects of μ, δ, and κ opioid receptor agonists (Carden et al., 1990), that the opioid systems can both increase and decrease USV and that antagonists may vary in their effects depending on which receptor is preferentially antagonized. This is a function of the type of antagonist, the dose, and the activity of the endogenous system. A more clear answer to the inconsistent antagonist data may come from the use of antagonists that are more specific to each opioid receptor type.

What is more clear about the effect of naloxone and naltrexone is that they block the quieting effect of a conspecific. Carden (1990a) has reported that a littermate "comforts" the isolated pup and reduces USV. This is blocked by opioid antagonists. Likewise, Panksepp et al. (1985) have reported in chicks that naloxone was most effective in situations in which the chick was isolated and either tested with companions or exposed to mirrors. In this nonmammalian version of the companion effect, comfort provided by the mirror or conspecific was antagonized by the opioid blocker. Opioid antagonists can also antagonize "comfort" provided by other stimuli. Infusions of milk, sucrose, fat, and polysaccharides also quiet the distress vocalizations of isolated pups and the quieting effects are naloxone-reversible (Blass et al., 1987; Blass and Fitzgerald, 1988; Shide and Blass, 1989).

At this time, it is not possible to determine which of the two models, if either, is correct. It is clear that isolation is not a simple experience that elicits the release of opioids, although isolation does increase analgesia that can be reversed by naloxone (Spear et al., 1985; Kehoe and Blass,

1986b). The conditions under which separation from the cues that comfort the infant elicit or do not elicit opioid release remain to be specified.

One of the most interesting aspects of USV in the rat is that it is a uniquely developmental phenomenon. It disappears during the third week of life. Yet, paradoxically, few studies have used a developmental approach in the study of the effects of opiates on this behavior. For example, there is virtually no information about the effect of opiates on pups younger than 10 days of age even though there are dramatic changes occurring in both opioid systems and the physiological control of separation vocalizations. Moreover, there is virtually no information on the role of opiates in the termination of these vocalizations [although naloxone will not reinstate calling in an 18-day-old that has stopped ultrasounding (Carden and Hofer, unpublished data)]. Because this behavior is uniquely developmental and because it occurs during a period of rapid growth and change of the opioids, more developmental studies are necessary. Moreover, unlike the more recent work with analgesia, few studies have paid attention to the differential role of different opioid receptors and to the anatomical bases of the behavior. To my knowledge, only two studies (Carden et al., 1990; Kehoe et al., 1990) have used selective agonists. Which structures in the central nervous system are involved in the regulation of vocalizations in the young animal are not known (see Panksepp et al., 1980 for a discussion of brain sites involved in vocalization in the adult). The question arises as to how specific opioid systems at specific anatomical loci modulate distress vocalizations and how those anatomically and neurochemically unique systems change during the natural ontogenetic course of this behavior.

SUMMARY

Opiates act differently in the immature animal than in the adult. The study of those differences and what they tell us about the maturation and function of opioid neural systems is just beginning. Analgesia has been studied the most and that "story" is the most consistent and well developed. Other behaviors such as feeding and isolation vocalizations have been studied more recently and less intensively. The data are less consistent and the models less well developed. The difficulty in obtaining consistent effects on either USV, on suckling, or on independent feeding with either naloxone and naltrexone, even within the same lab, makes it imperative that these studies include the use of agonists as well. Because of the range of behaviors that opiates affect, there is much more to do.

ACKNOWLEDGMENTS

I thank my students who have worked on various aspects of the work described here, including Ola Aroyewun, Chris Capuano, Jim Giordano, Harry Hughes, Dorene Miya, and Leslie Tive. Special thanks are due to Bill Paredes, who, directly or indirectly, had a hand in most of this research. They did the bulk of the work that I described here. I particularly thank Susan Carden, Myron Hofer, Harry Shair, and Shaoning Wang for critical comments on drafts of this chapter. The work by the author and his students was supported in part by NIDA grant DA-15213, PSC-CUNY grants, and funds from the Biopsychology Doctoral program, City University of New York and from Hunter College. During the preparation of the manuscript the author was supported in part by NIDA grant DA-06600.

REFERENCES

Abbott FV, Guy E (1990): Development of formalin pain and morphine and amphetamine analgesia in infant rats. Abst Soc Neurosci 16:412.

Abbott FV, Melzack R (1982): Brainstem lesions dissociate neural mechanisms of morphine analgesia in different kinds of pain. Brain Res 251:149–155.

Albonetti ME, D'Udine B, Oliverio A (1985): D-amino acids influence ultrasonic calling in mice pups: Effects of D-phenylalanine and D-leucine. Neurosci Lett 57:233–236.

Allerton CA, Smith JAM, Hunter JC, Hill RG, Hughes, J (1989): Correlation of ontogeny with function of [3H]U69593 labelled κ opioid binding sites in the rat spinal cord. Brain Res 502:149–157.

Alleva E, Laviola, G (1987): Short-term and delayed behavioral effects of pre- and post-weaning morphine in mice. Pharmacol Biochem Behav 26:539–542.

Aroyewun O, Barr GA (1982): The effects of opiate antagonists on milk intake of preweanling rats. Neuropharmacology 21:757–762.

Aroyewun O, Barr GA (1983): Effects of chronic antenatal and postnatal narcotics on naloxone-induced anorexia in preweanling rats. Neuropharmacology 22:-329–336.

Attali B, Saya D, Vogel Z (1990): Pre- and postnatal development of opiate receptor subtypes in rat spinal cord. Dev Brain Res 53:97–102.

Auguy-Valette A, Cros J, Gouarderes C, Gout R, Pontonnier G (1978): Morphine analgesia and cerebral opiate receptors: A developmental study. BJ Pharmacol 63:303–308.

Bardo MT, Neiswander JL, Miller JS (1986): Repeated testing attenuates conditioned place preference with cocaine. Psychopharmacology 89:239–243.

Barr GA (1991): Neuropharmaco-ontogeny: Concepts and methods of study. In Shair H, Barr GA, Hofer MA (eds): "Methods and Concepts in Developmental Psychobiology." New York: Oxford University Press, pp 321–341.

Barr GA, Eckenrode TC, Murray M (1987a): Normal development and effects of early deafferentation on choline acetyltransferase, substance P, and serotonin-like immunoreactivity in the interpeduncular nucleus. Brain Res 418:301–313.

Barr GA, Miya D, Paredes W (1987b): Changing patterns of analgesia induced by lateral ventricle or spinal injections of morphine or ketocyclazocine in developing rats. Abst Soc Neurosci 13:1001.

Barr GA, Miya D, Paredes W (1989): Differences in analgesia induced by intrathecal and intracerebral morphine and ketocyclazocine in 3- and 14-day old rat pups. Paper presented to the International Narcotic Research Conference.

Barr GA, Paredes W, Erickson KL, Zukin RS (1986): K-opioid receptor-mediated analgesia in the developing rat. Dev Brain Res 29:145–152.

Basbaum AI, Fields HL (1984): Endogenous pain control systems: Brainstem spinal pathways and endorphin circuitry. Ann Rev Neurosci 7:309–338.

Bell JA, Jaffe JH (1986): Electrophysiological evidence for a presynaptic mechanisms of morphine withdrawal in the neonatal rat spinal cord. Brain Res 382:299–304.

Blake HH, Henning SJ (1986): Control of protein intake in the young rat. Physiol Behav 38:607–611.

Blass EM, Fillion TJ, Weller A, Brunson LN (1990): Separation of opioid from nonopioid mediation of affect in neonatal rats: Nonopioid mechanisms mediate maternal contact influences. Behav Neurosci 104:625–636.

Blass EM, Fitzgerald E (1988): Milk-induced analgesia and comforting in 10-day-old rats: Opioid mediation. Pharmcol Biochem Behav 29:9–13.

Blass EM, Fitzgerald E, Kehoe P (1987): Interactions between sucrose, pain and isolation distress. Pharmacol Biochem Behav 26:483–489.

Bleier R (1969): Retrograde transynaptic cellular degeneration in mammillary and ventral tegmental nuclei following limbic decortication in rabbits of various ages. Brain Res 15:365–393.

Bregman BS (1986): Neural tissue transplants modify central neurons' responses to damage. In Goldberger ME, Gorio A, Murray M (eds): "Development and Plasticity of the Mammalian Spinal Cord." Fidia Research Series, Vol 3, New York: Springer-Verlag, pp 271–290.

Bregman BS (1987): Development of serotonin immunoreactivity in the rat spinal cord and its plasticity after neonatal spinal cord lesions. Dev Brain Res 34:245–263.

Bregman BS, Goldberger ME (1982): Anatomical plasticity and sparing of function after spinal cord damage in neonatal cats. Science 217:553–555.

Bregman BS, Goldberger ME (1983): Infant lesion effect. I. Development of motor behavior following neonatal spinal cord damage in cats. Dev Brain Res 9:103–117.

Briggs I, Barnes JC (1987): Actions of opioids on the dorsal root potential of the isolated spinal cord preparation of the neonate rat. Neuropharmacology 26:-469–475.

Bronstein DM, Mitteldorf P, Sadeghi MM, Kirby K, Lytle LD (1986): Visceral nociception in developing rats. Dev Psychobiol 19:473–487.

Capuano C, Leibowitz SF, Barr GA (1990): The pharmaco-ontogeny of opioid receptors mediating opiate-induced feeding in rats. Neuropharmacology 29:-433–437.

Capuano CA, (1987): The pharmaco-ontogeny of hypothalamic receptor systems mediating independent feeding in the rat. Unpublished doctoral dissertation City University of New York, Dissertation Abst Int. Vol 47:5089B.

Carden SE, Barr GA, Hofer MA (1991): Differential effects of specific opioid receptor agonists on rat pup calls. Dev Brain Res (in press).

Carden SE, Hofer MA (1990a): Socially mediated reduction of isolation distress in rat pups is blocked by naltrexone but not by RO 15-1788. Behav Neurosci 104:-457–463.

Carden SE, Hofer MA (1990b): Independence of benzodiazepine and opiate action in the suppression of isolation distress in rat pups. Behav Neurosci 104:160–166.

Cooper JR, Bloom FE, Roth RH (1986): "The Biochemical Basis of Neuropharmacology." New York: Oxford University Press.

Coyle JT, Campochiaro P (1976): Ontogenesis of dopaminergic-cholinergic interactions in the rat striatum: A neurochemical study. J Neurochem 27:673–678.

Cramer CP, Fite RA, Fanselow MS (1990): Ultrasonic vocalizations as a measure of long-term and short-term tolerance and withdrawal in neonatal rats. Abst Soc Neurosci 16:929.

Cunningham TJ (1982): Naturally occurring neuron death and its regulation by developing neural pathways. Int J Cytol 74:163–184.

Cuomo V, Cagiano R, deSalvia MA, Restani P (1988): Ultrasonic vocalization in rat pups as a marker of behavioral development: An investigation of the effects of drugs influencing brain opioid systems. Neurotoxicol Teratol 10:465–469.

D'Amato CJ, Hicks SP (1968): Normal development and posttraumatic plasticity of corticospinal neurons in rats. Exp Neurol 60:557–569.

Dykstra LA (1985): Behavioral and pharmacological factors in opioid analgesia. In Seiden LS, Balster RL (eds): "Behavioral Pharmacology: The Current Status." New York: Alan R. Liss, pp 111–129.

Ellis S, Axt K, Epstein AN (1983): The arousal of ingestive behaviors by chemical injection into the brain of the suckling rat. J Neurosci 4:945–955.

Finlay BL, Wikler KC, Senglaub DR (1987): Regressive events in brain development and scenarios for vertebrate brain evolution. Brain Behav Evol 30:102–117.

Fitzgerald M (1987): Pain and analgesia in neonates. TINS 10:344–346.

Fitzgerald M, Koltzenberg M (1986): The functional development of descending inhibitory pathways in the dorsolateral funiculus of the newborn rat spinal cord. Dev Brain Res 24:261–270.

Fitzgerald M, McIntosh N (1989): Pain and analgesia in the newborn. Arch Dis Child 64:441–443.

Gardner CR (1985): Distress vocalization in rat pups. A simple screening method for anxiolytic drugs. J Pharmacol Methods 14:181–187.

Giordano J, Barr GA (1987): Morphine- and ketocyclazocine-induced analgesia in the developing rat: Differences due to type of noxious stimulus and body topography. Dev Brain Res 32:247–253.

Goldberger ME (1986): Autonomous spinal motor function and the infant lesion effect. In Goldberger ME, Gorio A, Murray M (eds): "Development and Plasticity of the Mammalian Spinal Cord." New York: Springer Verlag, pp 363–380.

Goldberger ME, Murray M (1985): Recovery of function and anatomical plasticity after damage to the adult and neonatal spinal cord. In CW Cotman (ed): "Synaptic Plasticity." New York: Guilford, pp 77–110.

Goldman PS (1974): An alternative to developmental plasticity: Heterology of CNS structure in infants and adults. In Stein DG, Rosen JJ, Butters N (eds): "Plasticity and Recovery of Function in the CNS." New York: Academic Press, pp 149–174.

Hall WG (1985): What we know and don't know about the development of independent ingestion in rats. Appetite 6:333–356.

Hebb DO (1949): "The Organization of Behavior; a Neuropsychological Theory." New York: Wiley Sons.

Helmstetter FJ, Calcagnetti DJ, Cramer CP, Fanselow MS (1988): Ethylketocyclazocine and bremazocine analgesia in neonatal rats. Pharmacol Biochem Behav 30:817–821.

Herman BH, Panksepp J (1978): Effects of morphine and naloxone on separation distress and approach: Evidence for opiate mediation of social affect. Pharmacol Biochem Behav 9:213–220.

Hofer MA, Shair H (1987): Isolation distress in 2 week old rats: Influence of home cage, social companions and prior experience with littermates. Dev Psychobiol 20:465–476.

Hökfelt T, Holets VR, Staines W, Meister B, Melander T, Schalling M, Schultzberg M, Freedman J, Björkland H, Olson L, Lindh B, Elfvin LG, Lundberg J, Lindgren JA, Samuelsson B, Terenius L, Post C, Everitt B, Goldstein M (1986): Coexistence of neuronal messengers—an overview. Prog Brain Res 68:33–70.

Hökfelt T, Johansson O, Goldstein M (1984): Chemical anatomy of the brain. Science 225:1326–1334.

Hori Y, Watanabe S (1987): Morphine-sensitive late components of the flexion reflex in the neonatal rat. Neurosci Lett 78:91–96.

Hughes HE (1988): The pharmaco-ontogeny of spinal noradrenergic receptor systems mediating behavioral analgesia in the rat. Unpublished Doctoral Dissertation City University of New York, Dissertation Abst Int. Vol 50:2199B.

Hughes HE, Barr GA (1988): Analgesic effects of intrathecally applied noradrenergic compounds in the developing rat: Differences due to thermal vs mechanical nociception. Dev Brain Res 41:109–120

Hyson RL, Rubel EW (1991): Methods for studying experiential influences on brain development. In Shair H, Barr GA, Hofer MA (eds): "Methods and Concepts in Developmental Psychobiology." New York: Oxford University Press, pp 241–254.

Jackson HC, Sewell RD (1984): The involvement of κ but not δ opioid receptors in the body weight gain of suckling rats. Psychopharmacology 84:143–144.

Jacobson M (1978): "Developmental Neurobiology." New York: Plenum Press.

Jacquet YF, Lajtha A (1974): Paradoxical effects after microinjection of morphine in the periaqueductal gray matter in the rat. Science 185:1055–1057.

James IF, Bettaney J, Perkins MN, Ketchum SB, Dray A (1990): Opioid receptor ligands in the neonatal rat spinal cord: Binding and in vitro depression of the nociceptive responses. Brt J Pharmacol 99:503–508.

Johannesson T, Becker BA (1973): Morphine analgesia in rats at various ages. Acta Pharmacol Toxicol 33:429–441.

Kalin NH, Shelton SE, Barksdale CM (1989): Opiate modulation of separation-induced distress in non-human primates. Brain Res 440:285–292.

Kehoe P, Blass EM (1986a): Central nervous system mediation of positive and negative reinforcement in neonatal albino rats. Dev Brain Res 27:69–75.

Kehoe P, Blass EM (1986b): Opioid-mediation of separation distress in 10-day-old rats: Reversal of stress with maternal stimuli. Dev Psychobiol 19:385–398.

Kehoe P, Boylan C, Shoemaker W (1990): Differential effects of specific endogenous opioid systems on affective behaviors in neonatal rats. Neuroscience Abst 16:211.

Kitchen I, McDowell J (1985): Impairment of ketocyclazocine antinociception in rats by perinatal lead exposure. Toxicol Lett 26:101–105.

Kornblum HI, Hurlbut DE, Leslie FM (1987): Postnatal development of multiple opioid receptors in rat brain. Brain Res 465:21–41.

Kupferberg HJ, Way EL (1963): Pharmacologic basis for the increased sensitivity of the newborn rat to morphine. J Pharmacol Exp Ther 141:105–112.

Kuraishi Y, Harada Y, Aratani S, Satoh M, Takagi H (1983): Separate involvement of spinal noradrenergic and serotonergic systems in morphine analgesia: The differences in mechanical and thermal algesic tests. Brain Res 273:245–252.

Kuraishi Y, Hirota N, Satoh M, Takagi H (1985): Antinociceptive effects of intrathecal opioids, noradrenaline and serotonin in rats: mechanical and thermal algesic tests. Brain Res 326:168–171.

Lal KJ, Sewell RD (1989): Possible role for endogenous opiates in the regulation of food intake in the newborn rat. Arch Int Pharmacodyn Ther 301:91–99.

Leão Borges PC, Coimbra NC, Brandão ML (1988): Independence of aversive and pain mechanisms in the dorsal periaqueductal gray matter of the rat. Braz J Med Biol Res 21:1027–1031.

Lindvall O, Björklund A (1974): The organization of the ascending catecholamine neuron systems in the rat brain as revealed by the glyoxylic acid fluorescence method. Acta Physiol Scand Suppl 412:1–48.

Lorén I, Björklund A, Lindvall O (1976): The catecholaminergic systems in the developing rat brain: Improved visualization by a modified glyoxylic acid-formaldehyde method. Brain Res 117:313–318.

Loughlin SE, Massamiri TR, Kornblum HI, Leslie FM (1985): Postnatal development of opioid systems in rat brain. Neuropeptides 5:469–472.

McDowell J, Kitchen I (1987): Development of opioid systems: Peptides receptors and pharmacology. Brain Res Rev 12:397–421.

McLean PD (1985): Brain evolution relating to family, play, and the separation call. Arch Gen Psychiatry 42:405–417.

Miller MW (1988): Development of projection and local circuits in neocortex. In Jones EG, Peters A (ed): "Cerebral cortex, Vol 7, Development." New York: Plenum, pp 133–175.

Moore KE, Kelly PH (1978): Biochemical pharmacology of mesolimbic and mesocortical dopaminergic neurons. In Lipton MA, DiMascio A, Killam KF (eds): "Psychopharmacology: A Generation of Progress." New York: Plenum, pp 41–98.

Morgan MM, Depaulis A, Liebeskind JC (1987): Diazepam dissociates the analgesic and aversive effects of periaqueductal gray stimulation in the rat. Brain Res 423:395–398.

Morley JE, Levine A, Yim GK, Lowy MT (1983): Opioid modulation of appetite. Neurosci Biobehav Rev 7:281–305.

Nicák A, Kohút A (1978): Development of tolerance to morphine and pethidine in rats is dependent on age. Activit Nerv Super 20:231–235.

O'Leary DDM, Stanfield BB, Cowan WM (1981): Evidence that the early postnatal restriction of the cells of origin of the callosal projection is due to the elimination of axonal collaterals rather than to the death of neurons. Dev Brain Res 1:607–617.

Oliveras JL, Besson JM, Guilbaud G, Liebeskind JC (1987): Behavioral and electrophysiological evidence of pain inhibition from midbrain stimulation in the cat. Exp Brain Res 20:32–44.

Panksepp J, Conner R, Forster PK, Bishop P, Scott JP (1983): Opioid effects on social behavior of kennel dogs. Appl Anim Ethol 10:63–74.

Panksepp J, Herman B, Conner R, Bishop P, Scott JP (1978a): The biology of social attachments: Opiates alleviate separation distress. Biol Psychiatry 13:-607–618.

Panksepp J, Herman BH, Vilberg T, Bishop P, DeEskinazi FG (1980): Endogenous opioids and social behavior. Neurosci Biobehav Rev 4:473–487.

Panksepp J, Normansell L, Siviy S, Rossi III J, Zolovick AJ (1984): Casomorphins reduce separation distress in chicks. Peptides 5:829–831.

Panksepp J, Siviy SM, Normansell LA (1985): Brain opioids and social emotion. In Reite M, Fields T (eds): "The Psychobiology of Attachment and Separation." New York: Academic Press, pp3–49.

Panksepp J, Vilberg T, Bean NJ, Coy H, Kastin AJ (1978b): Reduction of distress vocalization in chicks by opiate-like peptides. Brain Res Bull 3:663–667.

Paredes W, Hughes HE, Giordano J, Barr GA (1990): Methods of injecting drugs directly into the spinal cord of neonatal rats. Lab Animal 19:39–41.

Pasternak GW, Zhang AZ, Tecott L (1980): Developmental differences between high and low affinity opiate binding sites: Their relationship to analgesia and respiratory depression. Life Sci 27:1185–1190.

Petrillo P, Travani A, Verolla D, Robson LE, Kosterlitz HW (1987): Postnatal development of μ-, δ- and κ- opioid binding sites in rat brain. Dev Brain Res 428:53–58.

Phifer CB (1991): The study of early feeding and drinking behaviors. In Shair H, Barr GA, Hofer MA (eds): "Methods and Concepts in Developmental Psychobiology." New York: Oxford University Press, pp 189–205.

Reynolds DV (1969): Surgery in the rat during electrical analgesia induced by focal brain stimulation. Science 164:444–445.

Risling M, Culhein S, Hieldebrand C (1983): Reinnervation of the ventral root L7 from ventral horn neurons following intramedullary axotomy in adult cats. Brain Res 280:15–23.

Robinson DJ, D'Udine B, Olivero A (1985): Naloxone influences ultrasonic calling in young mice. Behav Proc 11:253–255.

Rodriguez-Aendejas AM, Chambert G, Lora-Vilchis MC, Epstein AN, Russek M (1986): Ontogeny of epinephrine-induced anorexia in rats. Am J Physiol 250:R313–317.

Saunders NR, Møllgård K (1984): Development of the blood-brain barrier. J Dev Physiol 6:45–57.

Schmidt RH, Björkland A, Lindvall O, Lorén I (1982): Prefrontal cortex: Dense dopaminergic input in the newborn rat. Dev Brain Res 5:222–228.

Schneider GE (1970): Mechanisms of functional recovery following lesions of visual cortex or superior colliculus in neonate and adult hamsters. Brain Behav Evol 3:295–323.

Schwarz MN, Barr GA (1990): The ontogeny of analgesia induced by intraspinal injection of serotonergic drugs. Abst Soc Neurosci 16:97.

Shide DJ, Blass EM (1989): Opioid-like effects of intraoral infusions of corn oil and polycose on stress reactions in 10-day-old rats. Behav Neurosci 103:1168–1175.

Spain J, Roth B, Coscia C (1985): Differential ontogeny of multiple opioid receptors (μ, δ and κ). J Neurosci 5:584–588.

Spear LP, Enters EK, Aswad EK, Louzan M (1985): Drug and environmentally induced manipulations of the opiate and serotonergic systems alter nociception in neonatal rat pups. Behav Neural Biol 44:1–22.

Spear LP, Ristine LA (1982): Suckling behavior in neonatal rats: Psychopharmacological investigations. J Comp Physiol Psychol 96:244–255.

Stelzner DJ, Ershler WB, Weber ED (1975): Effects of spinal transection in neonatal and weaning rats: Survival of function. Exp Neurol 46:156–177.

Stelzner DJ, Weber ED, BryzGornia WF (1986): Sparing of function in developing spinal cord: Anatomical substrate. In Goldberger ME, Gorio A, Murray M (eds): "Development and Plasticity of the Mammalian Spinal Cord." New York: Springer Verlag, pp 81–99.

Tavani A, Robson LE, Kosterlitz HW (1985): Differential postnatal development of μ-, δ- and κ-opioid receptors in mouse brain. Dev Brain Res 23:306–309.

Tive LA, Barr GA (1988): Differential development of the effects of focal morphine and glutamate administration to the periaqueductal grey of the rat. Neurosci Abst 14:716.

Tsang D, Ng SC, Ho KP (1982): Development of methionine-enkephalin and naloxone binding sites in regions of rat brain. Dev Brain Res 3:637–644.

Ungerstedt U (1974): Brain dopamine neurons and behavior. In Schmitt FO, Worden FG (eds): "The Neurosciences Third Study Program." Cambridge, MA: MIT Press, pp 695–703.

Volterra A, Brunello N, Restani P, Galli CL, Racagni G (1986): Ontogenetic studies on mu delta and kappa opioid receptors in rat brain. Pharmacol Res Commun 18:979–990.

Weber ED, Stelzner DJ (1977): Behavioral effects of spinal cord transection in the developing rat. Brain Res 125:241–255.

Winslow JT, Insel TR (1991): Endogenous opiates: Do they mediate the rat pup's social response to social isolation? Behav Neurosci 103:253–263.

Witelson SF (1987): Neurobiological aspects of language in children. Child Dev 58:653–688.

Yaksh TL (1986): The effects of intrathecally administered opioid and adrenergic agents on spinal function. In Yaksh TL (ed): "Spinal Afferent Processing." New York: Plenum Press, pp 165–195.

Yanagisawa M, Murakoshi T, Tamai S, Otsuka M (1984): Tail-pinch method in vitro and effects of some antinociceptive compounds. Eur J Pharmacol 106:-231–239.

Yaster M (1987): Analgesia and anesthesia in neonates. J Pediatr 111:394–396.

Zadina JE, Kastin AJ (1986): Neonatal peptides affecting developing rats: β-endorpin alters nociception and opiate receptors, corticotropin-releasing factor alters corticosterone. Dev Brain Res 29:21–29.

Zeigler HP (1976): Feeding behavior of the pigeon. Adv Study Behav 7:285–389.

Zhang A-J, Pasternak GW (1981): Ontogeny of opioid pharmacology and receptors: High and low affinity site differences. Eur J Pharmacol 73:29–40.

Development of the Central Nervous System:
Effects of Alcohol and Opiates, pages 255–283
© 1992 Wiley-Liss, Inc.

12
Development of Multiple Opioid Receptors

FRANCES M. LESLIE AND SANDRA E. LOUGHLIN
*Departments of Pharmacology (F.M.L.) and Anatomy and Neurobiology
(S.E.L.), University of California Irvine, Irvine, California*

INTRODUCTION

The early ontogenetic appearance of opioid receptors within the brain has led to speculation that these receptors may modulate basic developmental processes (Kent et al., 1982). The short- and long-term functional changes which result from early pharmacological intervention in opioid systems are consistent with this hypothesis (for review see Zagon and McLaughlin, 1983; McDowell and Kitchen, 1987; see also Chapter 14). A detailed understanding of the role of opioids in the development of the central nervous system, and of the functional consequences of drug abuse, requires a careful study of receptor ontogeny. A powerful approach for such analyses has been the use of radioligand binding in combination with quantitative autoradiography. The present chapter will provide a review of the pharmacology of opioid receptors, and the use of ligand binding techniques to characterize their ontogeny.

PHARMACOLOGICAL CHARACTERIZATION OF MULTIPLE OPIOID RECEPTORS

μ, δ, and κ Receptors

While full characterization of opioid receptor properties awaits the outcome of molecular cloning techniques, radioligand binding and bioassay methodologies have provided substantial evidence for the existence of multiple opioid receptors. An early indication of opioid receptor heterogeneity came from in vivo studies in which morphinan and benzomorphan derivatives were found to exhibit differential behavioral profiles and different sensitivities to antagonism by naloxone and other narcotic antagonists (Gilbert and Martin, 1976; Martin et al., 1976). The existence of two separate opioid receptors [mu (μ), for which the prototypical agonist is morphine, and kappa (κ), for which the prototypical agonist is ketocyclazocine] was further suggested by in vitro analyses of the actions of these drugs on isolated peripheral tissues and by radioligand binding studies (Hutchinson et al., 1975; Lord et al., 1977; Kosterlitz et al., 1981). With the discovery of the endogenous opioid peptides (Hughes et al., 1975), met- and leu-enke-phalin, there soon followed functional and binding evidence for a third type of opioid receptor, the δ receptor (Lord et al., 1977).

A large body of literature has since accumulated which confirms the existence of these three opioid receptor types—μ, δ, and κ (for review see Paterson et al., 1983; Goldstein and James, 1984; Martin, 1984; Zukin and Zukin, 1984; Leslie, 1987). While interpretation of some early studies was complicated by the use of drugs which cross-reacted with more than one receptor type, the subsequent development and use of more selective drugs and radioligand binding conditions have led to a more definitive characterization of the anatomical localization and functional roles of μ, δ, and κ receptors. As illustrated in the autoradiograms in Figure 1 and described in detail below, these three receptors exhibit distinct patterns of distribution in the brain, a finding which suggests that they subserve distinct functional roles.

Other Receptor Types

A number of other opioid receptor types have been proposed, although their existence is more controversial. As described in the behavioral studies of Martin and his colleagues, the psychotomimetic effects of several opioid drugs appear to be mediated by another receptor, which has been termed σ (Gilbert and Martin, 1976; Martin et al., 1976). While this receptor is distinct from μ, κ, or δ, it is not sensitive to antagonism by naloxone or naltrexone (Vaupel, 1983), and has therefore been classified as non-opioid. As such, it is not considered relevant to the present discussion. A low affinity naloxone binding site has been identified in rat brain by Sadee and co-workers, and has been proposed as a distinct λ receptor type (Grevel et al., 1985). While this binding site exhibits a unique anatomical distribution in the brain, there is little literature regarding its pharmacological properties and functional relevance. No ontogenetic studies have been done on this putative opioid receptor type, and it will therefore not be included in the present analysis.

There is some functional and binding evidence to suggest the existence of an ε opioid receptor, which has high affinity and selectivity for the opioid peptide, β-endorphin (Schulz et al., 1979; Change et al., 1984). The existence of this putative opioid receptor has been a subject of some controversy, however. As will be described in a later section, we have undertaken an ontogenetic study to determine whether we can identify a unique ε opioid receptor in rat brain. Our data do not provide evidence for the presence of an ε receptor in this tissue at any point of neural development.

The most recent putative opioid receptor type to be identified is the ζ receptor, which reportedly has high affinity for the endogenous opioid peptide, enkephalin (Zagon et al., 1989). This receptor binding site has been characterized in the S20Y neuroblastoma cell line, a tissue in which enke-phalin is a potent inhibitor of growth. Given this finding, the detailed pharmacological characterization of this receptor type has obvious implications for analysis of opioid effects on central nervous system (CNS) development. As yet, however, the presence of this new receptor type in the brain has not been confirmed. Although a unique developmental profile for

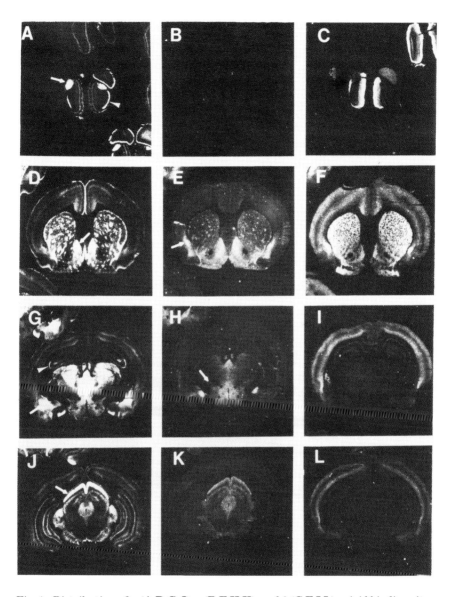

Fig. 1. Distribution of μ (**A,D,G,J**), κ (**B,E,H,K**), and δ (**C,F,I,L**) opioid binding sites in some regions of adult rat brain. Sections were incubated with radioligand and apposed to tritium-sensitive film. The images presented here are printed directly from the resulting autoradiograms. Arrow in A points to the accessory olfactory bulb, while the arrowhead points to the external anterior olfactory nucleus. Arrow in D points to the major island of Calleja (insula magna) at the medial border of the nucleus accumbens. Arrow in E points to the claustrum. Arrowhead in G points to the CA3 layer of the hippocampus, while the arrow points to the basolateral amygdala. Arrow in H points to the zona incerta. Arrow in J points to the superficial gray layer of the superior colliculus. (Reproduced from Kornblum et al., 1987a, with permission.)

[^{3}H]met-enkephalin binding has been characterized in human cerebellum (Zagon et al., 1990), this binding site has a very different pharmacological profile from that described for the ζ receptor in neuroblastoma.

Receptor Subtypes

There are now data to suggest the existence of subtypes of the major classes of opioid receptors. In an early ontogenetic study, Pasternak et al. (1980) demonstrated the differential appearance of high and low affinity morphine binding sites in developing brain. The appearance of these high and low affinity sites correlated with the functional expression of morphine analgesia and respiratory depression, respectively. This finding was interpreted as reflecting the differential ontogeny of two μ receptor subtypes which subserve distinct functional roles. While the existence of μ receptor heterogeneity has not received widespread acceptance, this group and others have provided additional evidence to support the concept (Pasternak and Wood, 1986; Rothman et al., 1989). In this regard, it is of interest to note two recent molecular studies of the properties of brain μ opioid receptors. In one study, the molecular weight of a protein with μ opioid binding properties was shown to change during neural development (McLean et al., 1989). This finding may be interpreted to reflect either the transient expression of a novel μ receptor subtype, as has been reported previously for other receptors (Mishina et al., 1986), or else an ontogenetic change in posttranslational processing of a single receptor protein. A second study has reported the molecular characterization of a protein with opioid binding properties in the brain (Schofield et al., 1989). Although this protein was shown to have many of the pharmacological characteristics of the μ receptor, it did not have the membrane spanning structure predicted of a G-protein linked receptor; nor did its mRNA colocalize with the known distributions of μ or δ receptors in the brain. This protein may have some functional significance in development, however, since it is structurally related to the immunoglobulin family of cell adhesion molecules, as well as to the growth factor tyrosine kinase receptors. Further studies will be needed to clarify the relationship of this interesting protein to the endogenous opioid peptide family and to specify its role, if any, in development.

A number of ligand binding studies have also provided evidence for the existence of heterogeneous κ receptor binding sites (for review see Hurlbut et al., 1991). While there are, as yet, few functional studies available which support these binding data, it seems clear that the pharmacological characterization of κ receptor properties is more complex than originally believed. Current data suggest that there are major species differences in the distribution and properties of κ binding sites. While the CNS of guinea pigs and higher order mammals contain high densities of a κ binding site with high affinity for dynorphin(1-17) and $(5\alpha, 7\alpha, 8\beta)$-(-)-N-methyl-N-[7-(1-pyrrolidinyl)-1-oxaspiro(4,5)-dec-8-yl]benzeneacetamide (U69593) (κ1), this site is present in very low density within rodent CNS (Zukin et al., 1988). The "κ-like" binding site which predominates in rat brain (κ2) has lower affinity for dynorphin(1-17) and little or no affinity for U69593, but does have some affinity for ethylketocyclazocine (EKC) and bremazocine. Since each laboratory uses different labeling conditions, which may label different proportions of these $\kappa 1$ and $\kappa 2$ sites, this may account for some discrepancies in the reported distribution and ontogeny of κ sites in rat brain, as described below.

METHODOLOGICAL CONSIDERATIONS
Radioligand Binding

Radioligand binding is a powerful approach for analysis of receptor ontogeny. Using this technique, a receptor is identified by the unique binding properties of its recognition site. Since this methodology involves the characterization of a binding site rather than a functional end-point, a number of criteria must be fulfilled in order to confirm that the site under investigation is an opioid receptor. These include saturability, stereospecificity, and pharmacological identity (see Leslie, 1987, for review).

A number of methodological issues specifically pertain to the analysis of ontogeny studies.

Have appropriate binding conditions been used? While selective radioligands have recently become available for separate analyses of μ, κ, and δ receptors, the first ontogenetic studies were hampered by the lack of availability of drugs with high selectivity and low cross-reactivity. For example, we have shown that $[^3\text{H}][\text{D-Ala}^2,\text{D-Leu}^5]$enkephalin (DADLE), a radioligand which was initially believed to be δ-selective, has a high affinity for the μ receptor and selectively labels this opioid receptor type at early developmental stages (Leslie et al., 1982; Ilombium et al., 1987a). Although in initial studies such cross-reactivity was frequently overlooked, in later studies experimenters have taken greater precautions to confirm the pharmacological identity of the binding site. Where nonselective radioligands have been used, saturating concentrations of blocking agents are included in the assay buffer to inhibit binding to other receptor types. Alternatively, highly selective radioligands such as $[^3\text{H}][\text{D-Ala}^2, \text{MePhe}^4, \text{Gly-ol}^5]$enkephalin(DAGO), $[^3\text{H}][\text{D-Penicillamine}^2, \text{D-Penicillamine}^5]$enkephalin(DPDPE) and $[^3\text{H}]\text{U69593}$ have been used to label μ, δ, and κ receptors, respectively. It should be noted that since $[^3\text{H}]\text{U69593}$ selectively labels the $\kappa 1$ receptor subtype, this ligand does not label the total population of κ receptors. A comprehensive analysis of the ontogeny of all κ receptor subtypes, using subtype-selective ligands, has not yet been undertaken.

Is the binding site a functional receptor? One critical issue in the analysis of binding data is whether the binding site is functionally coupled. Although some investigators do compare the developmental appearance of binding sites with that of a functional end-point (Milligan et al., 1987; De Vries et al., 1990), this is usually not the case. Rather, most investigators assume that the interaction of a drug or endogenous ligand with the binding site will produce a biological effect. This may not be a valid assumption in view of recent observations of structural differences in the receptor

(McLean et al., 1989) and possible changes in effector coupling throughout ontogeny (Szucs et al., 1986; Szucs and Coscia, 1990). Thus, radioligand binding data can only provide a good starting point from which to examine receptor changes in ontogeny. Ideally, functional studies will be conducted in parallel to confirm the biological significance of the observed changes in opioid binding properties. The recent development of in vitro techniques for analysis of opioid actions on developing brain cells makes this approach more feasible.

Data interpretation. Comparison of the results of a number of laboratories may be hampered by the variety of ways in which the data are expressed. For example, receptor changes may be calculated as either a function of DNA content, protein content, or of tissue wet weight. Depending on which system is used, total opioid receptor number may appear either to increase threefold (as a function of tissue weight) or to remain constant (as a function of protein content) throughout brain development (McDowell and Kitchen, 1987; Petrillo et al., 1987). The use of single concentrations of radioligand to analyze receptor changes may also impede data interpretation, since this approach does not permit determination of whether any observed developmental changes reflect alterations in receptor affinity or density. While most saturation studies have not revealed ontogenetic changes in radioligand K_d values, Spain et al. (1985) have reported a significant increase in δ receptor affinity following the first postnatal week.

Receptor Autoradiography

Quantitative autoradiography (QAR) has proven to be a useful methodology to analyze receptor ontogeny. In this approach, radioligand binding sites are visualized by apposition of brain sections to photographic film and are quantitated by comparison to a set of standards of known radioactivity. Using QAR, temporal changes in receptor localization in discrete brain regions may be more easily assessed than with membrane binding, in which the degree of anatomical resolution is limited by the ability to dissect small brain regions and by a requirement of milligram amounts of tissue for signal detection. Thus, as is described in greater detail below, the developmental appearance of low densities of receptor binding sites may be more readily detected. Regional decreases in binding site density, which may be masked by an overall increase in other brain regions when using membrane binding, may also be quantified. While offering valuable information on receptor ontogeny, a number of issues, in addition to those outlined above, must be considered in interpretation of autoradiographic data. These include:

Tissue quenching. It has been well documented that, when using tritiated radioligands, there is significant quenching of the emitted radioactivity by the underlying tissue (Kuhar and Unnerstall, 1985; Davenport et al., 1989). Because of differences in density, white matter absorbs a greater proportion of the emitted signal than does gray matter. Thus, the process of myelination, which occurs throughout postnatal development, may result in apparent decreases in radioligand binding in certain brain regions. Such artifacts may be avoided by using high energy isotopes, such as ^{125}I, for which quenching does not occur (Kuhar and Unnerstall, 1985). Alternatively, differential quenching of tritiated emissions by gray and white matter may be eliminated by the use of thin tissue sections measuring 10 μ or less (Davenport et al., 1989).

Protein content. Since regional protein content changes throughout ontogeny, it is not appropriate to use protein values obtained in the adult for developmental studies. This difficulty may be circumvented by expressing radioligand binding values as a function of tissue area or wet weight. Alternatively, techniques which have been developed to measure regional protein content in the adult may be applied to map protein content at different developmental stages (Miller et al., 1988).

Transient receptor expression. A number of groups have reported the transient appearance of opioid receptors in certain brain regions, with an apparent loss of binding sites at later developmental stages (Kent et al., 1982; Unnerstall et al., 1983; Kornblum et al., 1987a; see below). While such observations may indicate that receptors are no longer expressed, other possible explanations should also be considered. As described above, tissue myelination may occur, which results in increased signal quenching and an apparent decrease in radioligand binding. Alternatively, apparent receptor decreases may reflect proliferation of other cellular elements, such as glia and afferent projections, or an increase in nonreceptor bearing membrane area or process outgrowth of the cell which expresses the receptor. Finally, it must be remembered that a sufficient tissue section must be collected and carefully analyzed to characterize the heterogeneous distribution of radioligand binding sites within each brain region throughout ontogeny (Recht et al., 1985).

RECEPTOR ONTOGENY
Membrane Binding Studies
Rat brain

The earliest ontogenetic studies used radiolabeled antagonists to characterize the developmental appearance of opioid receptors in rat CNS. Both [³H]naloxone and [³H]naltrexone, which have higher affinity for μ than for κ or δ receptors, were used to analyze opioid receptor ontogeny in the brain. While Coyle and Pert (1976) found no binding detectable prior to gestational day 15 (G15), Clendennin et al. (1976) measured specific labeling of opioid binding sites in whole brain homogenates at G14. Both groups reported that, following this initial appearance, receptor development proceeded in two phases. Clendennin et al. (1976), who reported their data as a function of protein content, found that receptor density increased linearly between G14 and postnatal day 21 (P21), followed by a slower linear increase to adult levels. Coyle and Pert (1976), who reported their data as a function of tissue wet weight, characterized a linear increase in whole brain binding site density until G22, then a plateau phase, followed by another linear increase from P6 to adult. This latter study also showed that there is considerable regional variation in the postnatal expression of opioid binding sites, with minor increases occurring in medulla-pons, striatum, and hypothalamus and greater increases in midbrain/thalamus, cortex, and hippocampus. For further studies in which nonselective ligand binding conditions were used to characterize opioid receptor development in the brain, the reader is referred to an excellent review by McDowell and Kitchen (1987).

Using the nonselective antagonist, [^{3}H]diprenorphine, Kirby (1981) characterized a complex developmental appearance of opioid receptors in spinal cord. Opioid binding sites, which were first detected at G16, exhibited a linear increase in density until G22. A 40% decrease in binding site density then occurred at the time of parturition, followed by a linear increase until P5, after which binding declined to adult levels by P15. In this study, as in those described above, ontogenetic changes were shown to result from differences in maximum binding capacity (B $_{max}$) and not K$_d$.

Recent studies have used more selective binding conditions to analyze the postnatal developmental appearance of μ, δ, and κ receptors in the brain and spinal cord. While differing in some aspects, these studies show general agreement that μ and κ receptors appear early in development, while δ receptors appear later. Using the μ receptor-selective ligand, [^{3}H]DAGO, a decrease in μ opioid receptor density in both whole brain and spinal cord membranes has been characterized during the first postnatal week (Spain et al., 1985; Petrillo et al., 1987; Attali et al., 1990; Fig. 2). During the second and third postnatal weeks, binding site densities increase at a rate slightly above that of overall protein content, then decline to adult levels. These findings correspond well with those of autoradiographic studies (Kent et al., 1982; Unnerstall et al., 1983; Kornblum et al., 1987), which have demonstrated significant declines in μ opioid receptor binding in a number of brain regions during the early postnatal period.

Using nonselective radioligands, under assay conditions in which binding to μ and δ sites is blocked, the postnatal development of κ receptor sites in rat brain has been characterized (Spain et al., 1985; Petrillo et al., 1987). There is overall agreement in these studies that there is a significant density of κ binding sites at birth, and that a small postnatal increase in binding site density occurs at a rate somewhat lower than the overall increase in brain protein content. Using [^{3}H]bremazocine as radioligand, κ receptor development has been shown to be complete by P14 (Petrillo et al., 1987), while studies with [^{3}H]EKC suggest that κ binding sites continue to increase in density until later postnatal stages (Spain et al., 1985). In a recent study in which the more κ-selective ligand [^{3}H]U69593 was used, Kitchen et al. (1990) demonstrated a similar ontogenetic profile to that of [^{3}H]bremazocine (Fig. 2). However, B$_{max}$ values in this study were significantly lower than in studies in which non-selective ligands were used (Spain et al., 1985; Petrillo et al., 1987). Such a finding is consistent with the hypothesis that rat brain contains multiple κ receptor types, one of which is selectively labeled by [^{3}H]U69593. In neonatal spinal cord, there

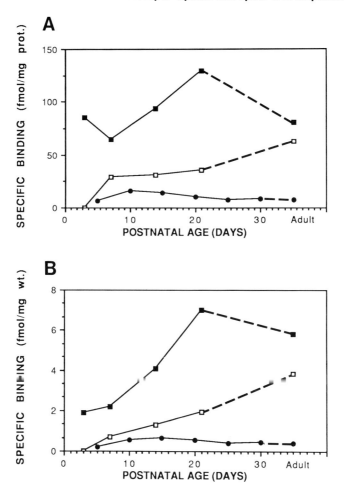

Fig. 2. Development of μ, κ, and δ binding sites in rat whole brain membranes. **A:** Radioligand binding is plotted as fmol/mg of protein. **B:** Binding is expressed as fmol/mg wet tissue weight. Closed squares represent μ binding sites labeled with [3H]DAGO, open squares represent δ binding sites labeled with [3H]DADLE in the presence of μ blockers, and closed circles represent $\kappa 1$ binding sites labeled with [3H]U69593. (Mu and δ binding data are from Petrillo et al., 1987, and κ binding data are from Kitchen et al., 1990.)

is also a significant density of κ binding sites, which appears to consist of a mixed population of $\kappa 1$ and $\kappa 2$ sites (Attali et al., 1990; James et al., 1990). Kappa binding densities in the spinal cord increase significantly during the first 2 postnatal weeks, then decline to adult levels (Allerton et al., 1990; Attali et al., 1990). Functional correlates of this elevated postnatal density of κ binding sites have been noted, including depression of spontaneous and evoked activities of dorsal horn neurons and antinociceptive activity (Allerton et al., 1990; James et al., 1990).

A number of groups have used membrane binding techniques to characterize the postnatal development of δ binding sites (Spain et al., 1985; Szucs et al., 1986; McDowell and Kitchen, 1986; Kornblum et al., 1987; Milligan et al., 1987; Petrillo et al., 1987; Szucs and Coscia, 1990). While some groups have been unable to detect δ binding during the first postnatal week (McDowell and Kitchen, 1986; Petrillo et al., 1987), others have demonstrated a low density of binding sites (Spain et al., 1985; Kornblum et al., 1987a; Milligan et al., 1987; Szucs and Coscia, 1990). Studies using the more sensitive technique of QAR have confirmed the existence of a low density of δ binding sites during the early postnatal period, and have shown that these are discretely localized in a limited number of brain regions (Kornblum et al., 1987a). There is general agreement among all studies that a major increase in δ receptor binding occurs during the second postnatal week, followed by a steady increase which occurs at a rate faster than the overall increase in brain protein content (Fig. 2). Unlike μ and κ binding sites, for which K_d values have consistently been found to remain constant throughout postnatal development, δ sites have been reported to exhibit decreased affinity during the first postnatal week (Spain et al., 1985). While this finding may suggest developmental changes in receptor-effector coupling mechanisms, other groups using [^{3}H]DADLE (with μ binding suppressed) or [^{3}H]DPDPE have not demonstrated any significant differences in K_d values between neonates and adults (Szucs et al., 1986; Kornblum et al., 1987a; Szucs and Coscia, 1990).

Other species

In mouse brain, μ opioid binding sites labeled with [^{3}H]DAGO have reportedly been detected as early as G12.5, 1 day after the initial expression of proopiomelanocortin (Loh, 1991). The ontogenetic profile of opioid receptors in this species is generally similar to that of rat, in that μ and κ receptor sites appear early, while δ binding sites are expressed at later postnatal stages (Tavani et al., 1985). Guinea pig and sheep are altricial species in which the major phase of neural development occurs prenatally. Studies in these animals have indicated that a significant proportion of δ receptor development occurs prenatally, in contrast to rats and mice. Using [^{3}H]diprenorphine in combination with selective inhibitors of μ, δ, or κ binding, Barg et al. (1989) have shown that κ binding site density in guinea pig brain reaches adult levels at G30 and then remains constant, μ binding site density reaches a maximum at G45 (just prior to parturition) and then declines to adult levels, while δ binding levels plateau between G35 and G45 and then increase an additional 50% during the postnatal period. In sheep, a complex developmental pattern has been described (Dunlap et al., 1986). In general, however, both μ and δ binding sites are found to be present in significant densities at mid-gestation. While μ binding levels tend to remain constant throughout subsequent development, δ sites reach peak levels just prior to parturition at G117–G128. The ontogeny of κ binding sites has not been studied in this species.

In fetal human tissue, at an average gestational age of 20 weeks, μ and κ binding sites have been identified, while δ sites have not (Magnan and Tiberi, 1989). Thus, the development of opioid receptors in human brain appears to follow a similar pattern to that of other mammalian species in that μ and κ receptor sites are expressed prior to δ.

The only nonmammalian species in which opioid receptor ontogeny has been studied is chick. Opioid receptor binding sites have been shown to develop prehatch, as early as 4 days of incubation (Gibson and Vernadakis, 1982). Both μ binding sites, labeled with [³H]dihydromorphine, and δ binding sites, labeled with [³H]DADLE, appear to be present at day 5 of incubation (Geladopoulos et al., 1987). These sites appear to be functional prior to hatching (Bronson and Sparber, 1989). These findings suggest that chick may prove to be a useful model in which to study the effects of prenatal manipulation of opioid systems in isolation, without possible confounding effects on the maternal system.

Autoradiography

QAR studies from several laboratories provide general consensus as to the distribution of μ, δ, and κ receptors in adult and developing rat brain, though some minor discrepancies are apparent. The following description of the distributions of opioid receptors in adult brain draws mainly from the studies of Kornblum et al. (1987), Mansour et al. (1987, 1988), and Sharif and Hughes (1989). Developmental data are from Kornblum et al. (1987a), Kent et al. (1982), and Unnerstall et al. (1989). Where discrepancies exist, these are noted. While assay conditions for labeling of κ sites varies considerably between studies, κ1 sites appear to be labeled predominantly in all cases. A detailed study of the distribution and ontogeny of κ2 sites, which appear to represent the majority of κ binding sites in rat brain (Zukin et al., 1988; Hurlbut et al., 1990), has not yet been published.

In general, the findings of autoradiographic studies are in agreement with those of membrane binding studies. The same overall patterns of receptor ontogeny are observed, with μ and κ receptors present in high densities at birth and δ receptors developing later (Figs. 3, 4). At birth, κ receptor densities and distribution are similar to those of the adult, and do not change markedly throughout postnatal development. In contrast, μ receptor binding densities in a number of brain regions are high at birth and decrease throughout postnatal life. This trend is more obvious in autoradiographic studies than in membrane binding studies, where postnatal increases in receptor densities in other brain regions partially mask this loss. Delta receptor binding is very low at birth, and increases throughout postnatal development. While the first appearance of δ receptor binding, as determined by membrane binding, has been a source of controversy (see above), the increased resolution of the autoradiographic method provides evidence for δ receptor labeling of some brain regions during the early postnatal period. The anatomical distribution of the three receptor subtypes in adult and developing rat brain is described in detail below.

Telencephalon

In the anterior forebrain, μ receptors are present in both the main and accessory olfactory bulbs, as well as the accessory olfactory nucleus (Figs. 1, 3). Moderate labeling is present in the glomerulae, external plexiform, and internal layers of the main olfactory bulb, with higher levels of labeling in the accessory olfactory bulb and the accessory olfactory nucleus, especially the pars externa. Delta receptor binding contrasts with μ receptor binding in that densest labeling of δ receptors is in the external plexiform layer, with moderate levels of binding in granule and internal plexiform layers and some binding in accessory olfactory nuclei. Kappa binding is largely absent in the olfactory bulb of the adult.

As in other brain regions, the ontogeny of each receptor type differs. At birth, μ receptor binding is dense in the external plexiform layer and the accessory olfactory bulb (Fig. 3). Binding in the external plexiform layer declines markedly between P2 and P9, and subsequently increases in the glomerular layer. It has been suggested that this reflects either a maturation of the tufted cells, with movement of the receptors to the terminals in the glomerular layer, or the generation of periglomerular cells (Unnerstall et al., 1983). Mu receptor labeling in the internal plexiform layer and the anterior olfactory nucleus is detectable, at close to adult levels, by P9. Delta receptors appear later, between P9 and P13, and increase throughout development. There is virtually no κ binding at any time in the development of olfactory bulb.

In the olfactory tubercle, the distribution of μ receptor binding sites is patchy (Figs. 1, 3). These dense "patch-like" accumulations probably overlie striatal components, including the striatal bridges, and are distributed over sparse background labeling. Kappa and δ receptors are more diffusely distributed, showing moderately high levels of binding. All three receptor types are detectable in this region at birth, with a higher density of μ receptor binding sites than for either κ or δ. The density of μ receptor binding decreases between P2 and P13 (Figs. 3, 4). In contrast, the density of δ binding sites increases throughout development, especially between P9 and P13, while that of κ binding sites remains constant.

In medial nucleus accumbens of the adult, μ receptor binding is dense and homogeneously distributed, whereas the lateral nucleus accumbens is marked by dense patches of μ receptor sites on a lighter background (Figs. 1, 3). Delta and κ receptors are diffusely distributed throughout nucleus accumbens in moderately high concentrations, with κ receptor labeling more dense ventrally and medially. Mu receptor sites are densely localized in medial nucleus accumbens at birth, and decrease in density throughout the first postnatal month (Figs. 3, 4). Some labeling of δ sites is apparent by P2, increasing to near adult levels in medial nucleus accumbens by P20. As in the olfactory tubercle, κ binding site density in nucleus accumbens is high at birth and remains relatively constant throughout development.

Adult striatum shows a particularly striking patchiness in the pattern of μ receptor labeling. These patches are superimposed on a moderately labeled "matrix." Scattered patches are more frequent in anterior caudate putamen, with a large aggregation of μ receptors in the region just beneath the corpus callosum, known as the subcallosal stria (Figs. 1, 3). This lack of homogeneity in the distribution of μ receptor sites corresponds to the patch-matrix organization of rat caudate putamen, which is largely equivalent to the striosomal organization of cat striatum (Graybiel, 1984). A number of neurochemical markers, connectional aspects, and developmental events have been shown to delineate these striatal compartments. Lesion studies indicate that the μ receptors in this region are localized to both striatal neurons and substantia nigra afferents (Sharif and Hughes, 1989). Delta receptor binding in striatum is equal in density overall to that of μ binding, but is not patchy. There is a significant increase in the density of δ binding sites from medial to lateral caudate putamen. Kappa receptor binding is less dense than that of μ or δ, and appears patchy when localized with EKC. Although it has been suggested that these patches may result from insufficient blockade of binding of this nonselective radioligand to μ receptors (Mansour et al., 1987), the differential ontogeny of μ and κ receptor patches which we have observed (Kornblum et al., 1987a) suggests that this is not a valid explanation of this finding. An alternative explanation for this difference between our data and those of others (Mansour et al., 1907, Sharif and Hughes, 1989) is that [³H]EKC may have some affinity for $\kappa 2$ binding sites in rat brain (Zukin et al., 1900, Hurlbut et al. 1990).

The development of opioid receptors in the striatum corresponds to the development of the patch-matrix organization. Mu receptor binding is first seen quite early prenatally, with light labeling in the striatal anlage at G14 (Kent et al., 1982). By G16, diffuse labeling is observed throughout the developing striatum, with this diffuse distribution being apparent until about the day of birth. Although Unnerstall et al. (1983) report diffuse [³H]dihydromorphine labeling of μ receptors at P2, other investigators have shown that [³H]naloxone (Kent et al., 1982), [³H]diprenorphine (Murrin and Ferrer, 1984), and [³H]DAGO (Kornblum et al., 1987a) labeling of the striatum is patchy at P0. The densely labeled patches are superimposed on a moderate background of matrix labeling. These patches of opioid receptor binding correspond to areas of intense catecholamine fluorescence, especially in the dorsal striatum, which reflect the developing dopamine innervation (Murrin and Ferrer, 1984). Throughout the next 2 weeks of development, matrix labeling decreases to nearly undetectable levels and patch binding increases twofold to adult levels (Figs. 3, 4). Kappa binding in striatum differs greatly in its developmental appearance, a finding which supports the conclusion that [³H]EKC labels a site distinct from the μ receptor in this region (Kornblum et al., 1987a). Patches of κ labeling are apparent only after the second postnatal week, while matrix binding is near adult levels at birth and remains relatively stable (Fig. 3).

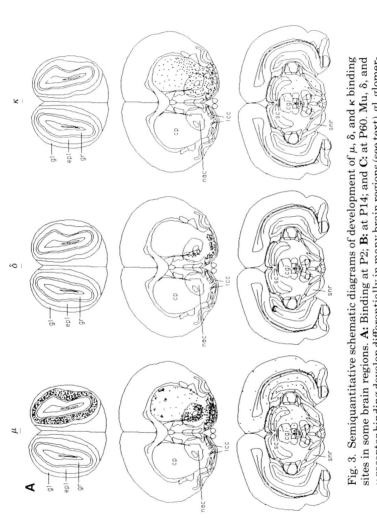

Fig. 3. Semiquantitative schematic diagrams of development of μ, δ, and κ binding sites in some brain regions. **A:** Binding at P2; **B:** at P14; and **C:** at P60. Mu, δ, and κ receptor binding develop differentially in many brain regions (see text). gl, glomerular layer; epl, external plexiform layer; gr, granule cell layer; nac, nucleus accumbens; cp, caudate putamen; icc, islands of Calleja; sc, superior colliculus; snr, substantia nigra pars reticulata; cg, central gray.

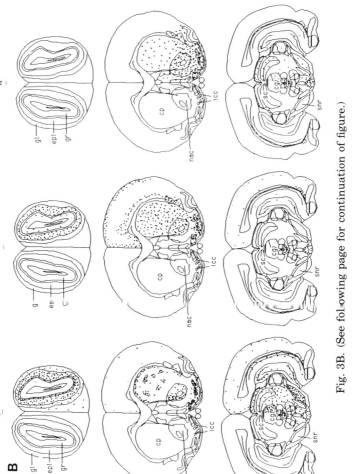

Fig. 3B. (See fol-owing page for continuation of figure.)

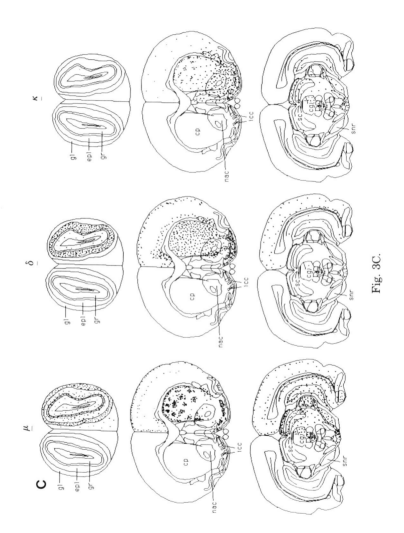

Fig. 3C.

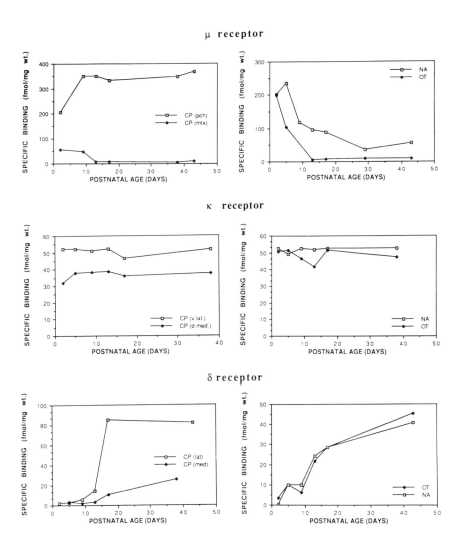

Fig. 4. Quantitative analysis of ontogeny of binding sites in some forebrain regions. Mu, κ, and δ binding develop differentially in different regions. Mu binding in caudate putamen (CP) develops in patch (pch) and matrix (mtx) separately. Mu binding in nucleus accumbens (NA) is measured in medial NA. Olfactory tubercle (OT) binding represents levels in matrix, not striatal bridges. Kappa binding in CP represents matrix levels, not patches, in ventrolateral (v.lat.) and dorsomedial (d.med.)regions. Delta binding in CP also develops differentially in lateral (lat) and medial (med) areas. (Data from Kornblum et al., 1987a, and represent quantitative analysis of autoradiograms.)

Delta receptors in striatum are undetectable until the end of the second postnatal week, and are not patchy at any time in development.

Mu, δ, and κ binding sites are present in very low density in globus pallidus and entopeduncular nucleus, two regions which receive dense projections from opioid peptide-containing neurons (Fallon and Leslie, 1986). Thus, these are areas of apparent ligand-receptor mismatch (Herkenham and McLean, 1986). In the developing animal, however, μ receptors are dense in the globus pallidus throughout the first postnatal week, decreasing 25-fold during the second postnatal week. Kappa receptor binding shows a similar course of development, peaking in the second postnatal week and decreasing to adult levels by P17. Delta receptors differ in that they do not appear until P9, at slightly above adult levels.

In the adult, labeling of all three opioid receptors in the septal nuclei is quite sparse, although moderate μ binding is apparent in medial septum. The nucleus of the diagonal band also exhibits moderate μ and δ labeling, with denser κ binding. There is significant labeling of all three receptor types in the bed nucleus of the stria terminalis. Developmentally, μ receptor binding in the medial septum and the nucleus of the diagonal band is visible at birth, with lateral septum labeling appearing soon after. [³H]naloxone labeling of μ receptors in this region has been detected as early as G16, with little change in density or distribution occurring throughout development.

Mu, δ, and κ receptors are present in cerebral cortex of the adult, exhibiting differences in both laminar and regional distribution (Figs. 1, 3). Mu and δ receptors are moderately dense, with κ binding much less apparent. In many cortical regions, including cingulate cortex, dense μ receptor binding is trilaminar, with increased densities in layers I, III, and IV or V. Delta binding is more diffuse than μ, with two broad bands of moderate binding in deep and superficial cortical layers and a thinner intermediate band of lighter labeling. Kappa binding is quite light in neocortex, with slight elevations in density in deep and superficial layers. Developmentally, μ receptor binding is first detectable at G20, appearing differentially in both cortical laminae and areas. A marked increase occurs in all layers between P13 and 17 (Fig. 3). Delta receptor labeling is first apparent in deeper cortical layers during the first postnatal week, with binding in superficial layers developing during the second postnatal week. Kappa binding in neocortex does not reach significant levels until P12, increasing slightly to adult levels in the next few days. Relatively high levels of κ binding are present in claustrum, endopiriform nucleus, and deep gustatory cortex, and these areas of denser labeling appear earlier than that of other cortical regions.

In adult amygdala there is dense labeling of μ sites in cortical, medial, basolateral, and lateral nuclei, and the intercalated masses. Moderate δ receptor binding is detectable in the same nuclear groups. Kappa receptor binding is moderate in medial nuclei, and present in basolateral nuclei, though less dense than μ and δ binding. The central nucleus contains only κ receptors. Mu binding within amygdala is present at birth, increasing over the next 3 weeks to adult levels. Delta receptor sites are also detectable at birth, increasing gradually to adult levels. Kappa binding sites appear differentially across nuclei, appearing in basolateral nuclei at P5 and at later ages in other nuclei.

In the hippocampus, striking laminar and regional differences in the distributions of μ, δ, and κ receptors also exist (Figs. 1, 3). The density of κ receptors is quite low, though the distribution shows many similarities to that of μ binding. Mu receptors are most dense in the pyramidal layer, especially in the CA3 region, and in the stratum lacunosum moleculare. In the dentate gyrus, the granule cell layer shows dense μ binding, especially ventrally. Delta receptors are present in low concentrations in both the hippocampus and the dentate gyrus, though they show less regional heterogeneity than μ receptors. Mu and κ receptors, and possibly δ receptors, are moderately dense in presubiculum. The distribution of μ receptors in hippocampus is fairly uniform at birth, becoming laminated by the end of the first postnatal week and increasing to near adult levels during the second week (Fig. 3). Kappa and δ receptors are detectable by the end of the second postnatal week.

Diencephalon

Although δ binding sites are present in very low density in diencephalon, there is significant labeling of μ and κ receptors in this region (Fig. 1). Generally, μ receptor binding predominates in thalamus, whereas κ binding is densest in hypothalamus. In both regions, individual nuclei are differentially labeled. Mu binding sites are present throughout much of thalamus in moderate to dense concentrations. Ventroposterior and parafascicular nuclei are largely devoid of μ sites. Thalamic reticular nuclei and zona incerta are also lacking in μ receptor binding but contain significant concentrations of κ receptor sites. Other thalamic nuclei have minor to moderate concentrations of κ receptors. The medial habenula and subfornical organ have dense μ and κ receptor labeling, while the lateral habenula has no opioid binding sites. The development of μ receptor binding in thalamus is essentially postnatal, appearing during the second postnatal week in adult patterns and increasing in density during the third postnatal week to adult levels. Kappa receptors are not detectable until P6 in ventral and midline nuclei and other nuclei until P12. These increase slowly to adult levels by P38.

In hypothalamus, δ receptor binding is largely absent except in the ventromedial nucleus. Kappa binding is dense throughout hypothalamus except for the mammillary nuclei, especially in preoptic area, periventricular, paraventricular, supraoptic, and suprachiasmatic nuclei and median eminence. Mu receptors are most densely localized in the anterior hypothalamic area, suprachiasmatic, dorsomedial, ventromedial and supramammillary nuclei, and the lateral hypothalamic area. The developmental appearance of μ opioid receptors in hypothalamus is earlier than in thalamus, with low concentrations present in most regions at P2. Adult levels are reached by the end of the second postnatal week. Kappa receptors are present in supraoptic and paraventricular nuclei by P12, and in other regions by P17.

Mesencephalon

As in the diencephalon, δ receptor binding is sparse throughout mesencephalon at all stages of development, except for moderate concentrations in the interpeduncular nucleus. Mu and κ receptor labeling predominate, showing very similar distributions if [³H]EKC is used as the radioligand (Kornblum et al., 1987a; Figs. 1, 3), and some differences if low concentrations of [³H]bremazocine (Mansour et al., 1987) or [¹²⁵I]dynorphin 1–8 (Sharif and Hughes, 1989) are used. A striking laminar distribution of μ and κ receptors is present in superior colliculus, with particularly dense labeling in the superficial gray layer. Mu and κ binding sites are homogeneously distributed throughout the superior colliculus during the first postnatal week, increasing in density and becoming laminated over the next 2 weeks. The external nucleus of the inferior colliculus is heavily labeled with both μ and κ binding sites, as is the periaqueductal gray. Very dense concentrations of μ and κ receptor sites are present in the interpeduncular nucleus. In the substantia nigra, μ receptors are present in moderate densities in the pars compacta and the external portion of the pars reticulata. [³H]EKC labels both regions lightly, while [³H]bremazocine or [¹²⁵I]dynorphin 1–8 labels only the pars reticulata. Mu and κ binding sites are detectable early in the postnatal development of the substantia nigra. While the density of κ binding sites (as revealed by [³H]EKC) remains constant, μ receptor density declines twofold (Fig. 3). Portions of the ventral tegmental area also contain μ and κ receptors. Both the medial terminal nucleus and several raphe nuclei have dense μ binding and moderate κ binding.

Pons and medulla

Since little is known of the development of opioid receptors in more caudal brain regions, only a brief review of their localization in the adult will be offered. Mu and κ binding sites are largely parallel in their distributions, with concentrations in a number of brain stem nuclei, including parabrachial, raphe magnus, nucleus tractus solitarius, and spinal trigeminal nucleus. The locus coeruleus also contains μ and κ binding sites. Mu binding sites in locus coeruleus are present by P2. Delta binding sites are largely absent in caudal brain regions, showing significant concentrations only in the nucleus tractus solitarius.

Cerebellum

Both adult and developing rat cerebellum are largely devoid of all three receptor types, as determined by autoradiographic studies.

Spinal cord

In the adult, all three receptor types are localized in the superficial layers of the dorsal horn, the majority of sites being μ, with lower densities of δ and κ sites. Mu binding sites are also detectable in the medial portion of laminae V (Morris and Herz, 1987; Besse et al., 1990). By the second postnatal week, μ binding sites have achieved a density and distribution similar to that of the adult (Allerton et al., 1989). In contrast, κ binding sites have a significantly higher density and more widespread distribution at P9-16 than in the adult (Allerton et al., 1989). The ontogeny of δ receptors in the spinal cord has not yet been examined using QAR.

β-Endorphin Binding

To investigate the distribution of opioid receptors at earlier stages of development, it is useful to use a radioligand of high specific activity. $[^{125}I]\beta$-endorphin has been used to localize μ and δ receptors in prenatal and early postnatal brain (McLean et al., 1989; Kornblum et al., 1989). At P1, cross-linking studies have shown that β-endorphin binds to a 65 kD receptor protein which has the pharmacological properties of a μ receptor (McLean et al., 1989). Beta-endorphin also labels another 55 kD protein, which is present in lower abundance and may represent an immature form of the μ receptor. In adult brain, β-endorphin binds to μ and δ sites. While it has been suggested that β-endorphin also binds to an ϵ receptor (Schultz et al., 1979), neither these biochemical studies nor our autoradiographic studies (Kornblum et al., 1989; Loughlin et al., in preparation) provide evidence that such a site exists in adult or developing rat brain. In the adult, the autoradiographic distribution of β-endorphin sites is equivalent to the combined distribution of μ and δ sites. In developing brain prior to the appearance of δ receptors, the distribution of β-endorphin binding is similar to that of μ-selective ligands. Using this ligand, binding in a few regions is detectable earlier than with tritiated ligands, as in middle layers of cortex. A patchy distribution of receptors in striatum is apparent by P1. Prenatally, binding is detectable by G15 in forebrain. By G15, receptors are present in a number of regions, including the developing striatum and ventral midbrain. Beta-endorphin binding sites appear to be associated with cells of the forebrain germinal zone, suggesting that they may be important in regulation of cellular proliferation.

CONCLUSIONS

Both membrane binding and autoradiographic studies have demonstrated that μ, δ, and κ opioid receptor binding sites develop differentially. In most species, μ and κ sites appear prenatally while δ sites develop later. Some brain regions exhibit transient populations of μ binding sites which decline in early postnatal weeks, while other regions exhibit postnatal increases in μ receptor density. At birth, κ binding sites are present in most regions in adult densities and distributions, and remain relatively constant throughout postnatal development. In contrast, δ sites appear during the first postnatal week in distributions which are quite similar to that of the adult, and increase gradually throughout the remaining developmental period.

The early developmental appearance of μ and κ binding sites suggests that these receptors may modulate developmental processes, while δ receptors are unlikely to play such a role during perinatal development. Binding studies, however, provide no information as to the functional status of receptor populations. In a recent functional study of developing rat striatum and neocortex (De Vries et al., 1990), opioid receptor-mediated inhibition of neurotransmitter release has been detected as early as G17. At this gestational age, strong inhibitory effects of the selective μ-agonist, DAGO, on the electrically stimulated release of [^{3}H]norepinephrine from cortical slices and of the selective κ-agonist, U50488, on the electrically evoked release of [^{3}H]dopamine from striatal slices were found. In contrast, inhibitory effects of the selective δ-agonist, DPDPE, on both striatal [^{3}H]acetylcholine release and adenylate cyclase activity were undetectable until the second postnatal week. These findings, which indicate that functional μ and κ receptors, but not δ receptors, are present during the perinatal period, are consistent with those of binding studies.

As will be reviewed in more detail in Chapter 14, many current studies are directed towards characterizing possible developmental roles of endogenous peptides and their receptors. A number of clinical reports have described somatic growth retardation (Pasto et al., 1989) and behavioral abnormalities (Strauss et al., 1976; Wilson et al., 1981; Rodning et al., 1989) in the children of heroin- and methadone-addicted mothers. Although variables such as malnutrition, poor prenatal care, alcohol consumption, and multiple substance abuse may confound interpretation of human studies, more controlled laboratory studies on experimental animals have confirmed that prenatal exposure to opiates is detrimental to the morphological, neurochemical, and physiological development of the offspring (Zagon and McLaughlin, 1983; Wang et al., 1986; Slotkin, 1988; Hammer et al., 1989; Ricalde and Hammer, 1990). A developmental role of endogenous opioid peptide systems is also suggested by findings that prenatal blockade of opioid receptors influences both morphological development of the brain and behavioral processes (Shepanek et al., 1989). The interpretation of these studies is complicated, however, by the many indirect effects which may occur as the result of alteration of maternal health, circulation, respiration, and behavior by manipulation of opioid systems (Jaffe and Martin, 1985).

Such interpretational difficulties are circumvented in studies in which the developmental effects of postnatal administration of opioid agonists and antagonists are examined. Postnatal administration of opioid agonists has been shown to inhibit a number of basic developmental processes, including DNA synthesis, cellular proliferation, and social and motor development (Vertes et al., 1982; Kornblum et al., 1987b; Najam and Panksepp, 1989). Conversely, administration of high doses of opioid antagonists have been shown to stimulate these developmental parameters (Vertes et al., 1982; Zagon and McLaughlin, 1983, 1986, 1987; Hauser et al., 1987; Najam and Panksepp, 1989; Schmahl et al., 1989). While these findings suggest a developmental role for endogenous opioid peptides and their receptors, the underlying mechanisms cannot be clearly deduced from in vivo studies. Gross developmental changes mediated via alterations of feeding, respiration, hormonal status, and social interaction must be considered and controlled for (Lichtblau and Sparber, 1984). In at least two studies of opioid effects on cellular proliferation, indirect mechanisms have been implicated (Kornblum et al., 1987b; Schmahl et al., 1989).

To determine whether endogenous opioid peptides modulate basic developmental processes, an in vitro approach offers many advantages. Most importantly, it allows the opportunity to manipulate characterized populations of cells or tissue slices in defined conditions. Both neurons and glia, as well as other cell types, have been shown to express opioid peptides and receptors in vitro (Hiller et al., 1978; Hendrickson and Lin, 1980; Knodel and Richelson, 1980; Pearce et al., 1985; Eiden et al., 1988; Maderspach and Solomnia, 1988; Makman et al., 1988; Vilijin et al., 1988; Shinoda et al., 1989; Hauser et al., 1990; Steine-Martin and Hauser, 1990; Vaysse et al., 1990). Whereas one study has reported opioid peptide-induced stimulation of neural development (Ilyinsky et al., 1987), the majority of in vitro studies provide evidence consistent with in vivo data that opioid agonists inhibit growth (Sakellaridis et al., 1986; Zagon et al., 1989; Steine-Martin and Hauser, 1990). However, the effects of opioids in culture may depend on dose and time of exposure. In dissociated mesencephalic neuronal cultures, leu-enkephalin has been shown to modulate process outgrowth of serotonergic neurons, with a complex dose-response profile (Davila-Garcia and Azmitia, 1989), where a single application of leu-enkephalin at the time of plating produced significant stimulation of serotonergic growth, chronic daily administration inhibited serotonergic development.

Although in vitro approaches offer the ability to grow glia or neurons separately, and will be useful in the characterization of these interactions, the nonphysiological conditions of these assay systems must be taken into consideration. For example, much higher levels of proenkephalin expression are detectable in cultured cerebellar astrocytes than in vivo during the first 3 weeks of postnatal development (Hauser et al., 1990). Similar elevated expressions of proopiomelanocortin have been observed in primary cultures of rat hypothalamus (Kapcala, 1989) and spinal cord (Berry and Haynes, 1989) as compared to in vivo. It has been speculated that such abnormal in vitro expression of opioid markers results from the loss of feedback inhibition by an external signal (Rost et al., 1989; Hauser et al., 1990).

Thus, although many studies suggest that endogenous opioid systems play a significant role in pre- and postnatal developmental processes, conclusive evidence is still lacking. Well designed studies, using both in vivo and in vitro approaches, will be necessary to further address this issue. However, regardless of whether opioid peptides and their receptors are found to play a direct modulatory role, studies of their developmental appearance can provide information as to their functional organization and identity, and are thus of inherent value.

REFERENCES

Allerton Ca, Smith JAM, Hunter JC, Hill RG, Hughes J (1990): Correlation of ontogeny with function of [³H]U69593 labelled κ opioid binding sites in the rat spinal cord. Brain Res 502:149–157.

Attali B, Saya D, Vogel Z (1990): Pre- and postnatal development of opiate receptor subtypes in rat spinal cord. Dev Brain Res 53:97–102.

Barg J, Levy R, Simantov R (1989): Expression of the three opioid receptor subtypes μ, δ, and κ in guinea pig and rat brain cell cultures and in vivo. Int J Dev Neurosci 7:173–179.

Berry S, Haynes LW (1989): The opiomelanocortin peptide family: Neuronal expression and modulation of neural cellular development and regeneration in the central nervous system. Comp. Biochem. Physiol 93A:267–272.

Besse D, Lombard MC, Zajac JM, Roques BP, Besson JM (1990): Pre- and postsynaptic distribution of μ, δ and κ opioid receptors in the superficial layers of the cervical dorsal horn of the rat spinal cord. Brain Res 521:15–22.

Bronson ME, Sparber SB (1989): Evidence of single dose opioid dependence in 12- to 14-day-old chicken embryos. Pharmacol Biochem Behav 34:705–709.

Chang KJ, Blanchard SG, Cuatrecasas P (1984): Benzomorphan sites are ligand recognition sites of putative ε-receptors. Mol Pharmacol 26:484–488.

Clendennin NJ, Petraitis M, Simon EJ (1976): Ontological development of opiate receptors in rodent brain. Brain Res 118:157–160.

Coyle JT, Pert CB (1976): Ontogenetic development of [³H]naloxone binding in rat brain. Neuropharmacology 15:555–560.

Davenport AP, Hill RG, Hughes J (1989): Quantitative analysis of autoradiograms. In: Polak JM (ed): "Regulatory Peptides." Berlin:Birkhauser-Verlag, pp 137–153.

Davila-Garcia MI, Azmitia EC (1989): Effects of acute and chronic administration of leu-enkephalin on cultured serotonergic neurons: evidence for opioids as inhibitory neuronal growth factors. Dev Brain Res 49:97–103.

De Vries TJ, Hogenboom F, Mulder AH, Schoffelmeer ANM (1990): Ontogeny of μ-, δ- and κ-opioid receptors mediating inhibition of neurotransmitter release and adenylate cyclase activity in rat brain. Dev Brain Res 54:63–69.

Dunlap CE, Christ GJ III, Rose JC (1986): Characterization of opioid receptor binding in adult and fetal sheep brain regions. Dev Brain Res 24:279–285.

Eiden LE, Siegel RE, Giraud P, Brenneman De (1988): Ontogeny of enkephalin- and VIP-containing neurons in dissociated cultures of embryonic mouse spinal cord and dorsal root ganglia. Dev Brain Res 44:141–150.

Fallon JH, Leslie FM (1986): Distribution of dynorphin and enkephalin peptides in rat brain. J Comp Neurol 249:293–336.

Geladopoulos T, Sakellaridis N, Vernadakis A (1987): Differential maturation of μ and δ opioid receptors in the chick embryonic brain. Neuochem Res 12:279–288.

Gibson DA, Vernadakis A (1982): [³H]etorphine binding activity in early chick embryos: brain and body tissue. Dev Brain Res 4:23–29.

Gilbert PE, Martin WR (1976): The Effects of morphine- and nalorphine-like drugs in the non-dependent, morphine-dependent, and cyclazocine-dependent spinal dog. J Pharmacol Exp Ther 198:66–82.

Goldstein A, James IF (1984): Multiple opioid receptors: criteria for identification and classification. Trends Pharmacol Sci 5:503–505.

Graybiel AM (1984): Correspondence between the dopamine islands and striosomes of the mammalian striatum. Neuroscience 13:1157–1187.

Grevel J, Yu V, Sadee W (1985): Characterization of a labile naloxone binding site (λsite) in rat brain. J Neurochem 44:1647–1656.

Hammer RP Jr, Ricalde AA, Seatriz JV (1989): Effects of opiates on brain development. Neurotoxicology 10:475–484.

Hauser KF, McLaughlin PJ, Zagon IS (1987): Endogenous opioids regulate dendritic growth and spine formation in developing rat brain. Brain Res 416:157–161.

Hauser KF, Osborne JG, Steine-Martin A, Melner MH (1990): Cellular localization of proenkephalin mRNA and enkephalin peptide products in cultured astrocytes. Brain Res 522:347–353.

Hendrickson CM, Lin S (1980): Opiate receptors in highly purified neuronal cell populations isolated in bulk from embryonic chick brain. Neuropharmacology 19:731–739.

Herkenham M, McLean S (1986): Mismatches between receptor and transmitter localizations in the brain. In Boast C, Snowhill EW, Altar CA (eds): "Quantitative Receptor Autoradiography." New York: Alan Liss, pp 131–171.

Hiller JM, Simon EJ, Crain SM, Peterson ER (1978): Opiate receptors in cultures of fetal mouse dorsal root ganglia (DRG) and spinal cord: predominance in DRG neurites. Brain Res 145:396–400.

Hughes J, Smith TW, Kosterlitz HW, Fothergill LA, Morgan BA, Morris HR (1975): Identification of two related pentapeptides from the brain with potent opiate agonist activity. Nature 258:577–579.

Hurlbut DE, Broide RS, Leslie FM (1991): Pharmacological characteristics of non-μ, non-δ opioid binding sites in guinea pig and rat brain. Brain Res (submitted).

Hutchinson M, Kosterlitz HW, Leslie FM, Waterfield AA, Terenius L (1975): Assessment in the guinea-pig ileum and mouse vas deferens of benzomorphans which have strong antinociceptive activity but do not substitute for morphine in the dependent monkey. Br J Pharmcol 55:541–546.

Ilyinsky OB, Kozlova ES, Konrikova ES, Kalentchuk VU, Titov MI, Bespalova ZD (1987): Effects of opioid peptides and naloxone on nervous tissue in culture. Neuroscience 22:719–735.

James IF, Bettaney J, Perkins SB, Dray A (1990): Opioid receptor ligands in the neonatal rat spinal cord: binding and in vitro depression of the nococeptive responses. Br J Pharmacol 99:503–508.

Kapcala LP (1989): Production of immunoreactive adrenocorticotropin and β-endorphin by hypothalamic and extrahypothalamic brain cells. Brain Res 491:253–265.

Kent JL, Pert CB, Herkenham M (1982): Ontogeny of opiate receptors in rat forebrain: visualization by in vitro autoradiography. Dev Brain Res 2:487–504.

Kirby ML (1981): Development of opiate receptor binding in rat spinal cord. Brain Res 205:400–404.

Kitchen I, Kelly M, Viveros PM (1990): Ontogenesis of κ-opioid receptors in rat brain using [^{3}H]U-69593 as a binding ligand. Eur J Pharmacol 175:93–96.

Knodel EI, Richelson E (1980): Methionine-enkephalin immunoreactivity in fetal rat brain cells in aggregating culture and in mouse neuroblastoma cells. Brain Res 197:565–570.

Kornblum HI, Hurlbut DE, Leslie FM (1987a): Postnatal development of multiple opioid receptors in rat brain. Dev Brain Res 37:21–41.

Kornblum HI, Loughlin SE, Fallon JH, Leslie FM (1989): Developmental appearance of opioid receptors in embryonic and neonatal rat brain using [^{125}I]β-endorphin: an autoradiography study. Adv Biosci 75:277–280.

Kornblum HI, Loughlin SE, Leslie FM (1987b): Effects of morphine on DNA synthesis in neonatal rat brain. Dev Brain Res 31:45–52.

Kosterlitz HW, Paterson SJ, Robson LE (1981): Characterization of the κ-subtype of the opiate receptor. Br J Pharmacol 73:939–949.

Kuhar MJ, Unnerstall JR (1985): Quantitative receptor mapping by autoradiography: some current technical problems. Trends Neurosci 8:49–53.

Leslie FM (1987): Methods used for the study of opioid receptors. Pharmacol Rev 39:197–249.

Leslie FM, Tso S, Hurlbut DE (1982): Differential appearance of opioid receptor subtypes in neonatal rat brain. Life Sci 31:1393–1396.

Lichtblau L, Sparber SB (1984): Opioids and development: a perspective on experimental models and methods. Neurobehavtoxicol Teratol 6:3–8.

Loh YP (1991): Prenatal expression of pro-opiomelanocortin (POMC) mRNA, POMC-derived peptides and μ opiate receptors in the mouse embryo. In "Molecular Approaches to Drug Abuse Research." Bethesda, MD: NIDA, in press.

Lord JAH, Waterfield AA, Hughes J, Kosterlitz HW (1977): Endogenous opioid peptides: multiple agonists and receptors. Nature 267:495–499.

Maderspach K, Solomnia R (1988): Glial and neuronal opioid receptors: apparent positive cooperativity observed in intact cultured cells. Brain Res 441:41–47.

Magnan J, Tiberi M (1989): Evidence for the presence of μ- and κ- but not of δ-opioid sites in the human fetal brain. Dev Brain Res 45:275–281.

Makman MH, Dvorkin B, Crain SM (1988): Modulation of adenylate cyclase activity of mouse spinal cord-ganglion explants by opioids, serotonin and pertussis toxin. Brain Res 445:303–313.

Mansour A, Khachaturian H, Lewis ME, Akil H, Watson SJ (1988): Anatomy of CNS opioid receptors. Trends Neurosci 11:308–314.

Mansour A, Khachaturian H, Lewis ME, Akil H, Watson SJ (1987): Autoradiographic differentiation of mu, delta, and kappa opioid receptors in the rat forebrain and midbrain. J Neurosci 7:2445–2464.

Martin WR (1984): Pharmacology of opioids. Pharmacol Rev 35:283–318.

Martin WR, Eades CG, Thompson JA, Huppler RE, Gilbert PE (1976): The effects of morphine- and nalorphine-like drugs in non-dependent and morphine-dependent chronic spinal dogs. J Pharmacol Exp Ther 197:517–532.

McDowell J, Kitchen I (1986): Ontogenesis of δ opioid receptors in rat brain using [^{3}H]D-Pen^{2}, D-Pen^{5}]enkephalin as a binding ligand. Eur J Pharmacol 128:287–289.

McDowell J, Kitchen I (1987): Development of opioid systems: peptides, receptors and pharmacology. Brain Res 12:397–421.

McLean S, Rothman RB, Chuang D-M, Rice KC, Spain JW, Coscia CJ, Roth BL (1989): Cross-linking of [^{125}I]β-endorphin to μ-opioid receptors during development. Dev Brain Res 45:283–289.

Miller JA, Curella P, Zahniser NR (1988): A new densitometric procedure to measure protein levels in tissue slices used in quantitative autoradiography. Brain Res 447:60–66.

Milligan G, Streaty RA, Gierschik P, Spiegel AM, Klee WA (1987): Development of opiate receptors and GTP-binding regulatory proteins in neonatal rat brain. J Biol Chem 262:8626–8630.

Mishina M, Takai T, Imoto K, Noda M, Takahashi T, Numa S, Methfessel C, Sakmann B (1986): Molecular distinction between fetal and adult forms of muscle acetylcholine receptor. Nature 321:406–411.

Morris BJ, Herz A (1987): Distinct distribution of opioid receptor types in rat lumbosacral spinal cord. Naunyn Schmiedebergs Arch Pharmacol 336:240–243.

Murrin LC, Ferrer JR (1984): Ontogeny of the rat striatum: Correspondence of dopamine terminals, opiate receptors and acetylcholinesterase. Neurosci Lett 47:155–160.

Najam N, Panksepp J (1989): Effect of chronic neonatal morphine and naloxone on sensorimotor and social development of young rats. Pharmacol Biochem Behav 33:539–544.

Pasternak GW, Zhong-Zhang A, Tecott L (1980): Developmental differences between low and high affinity opiate binding sites: their relationship to analgesia and respiratory depression. Life Sci 27:1185–1190.

Pasternak GW, Wood PJ (1986): Multiple mu opiate receptors. Life Sci 10:183–193.

Pasto ME, Ehrlich S, Kattenbach K, Graziani LJ, Kurtz A, Goldberg B, Finnegan LP (1989): Cerebral sonographic characteristics and maternal and neonatal risk factors of opiate-dependent mothers.Ann. NY Acad Sci 562:355–357.

Paterson SJ, Robson LE, Kosterlitz HW (1983): Classification of opioid receptors. Dr Med Bull 39.31–36.

Pearce I, Cambray-Deakin M, Murphy S (1985): Astrocyte opioid receptors: activation modifies the noradrenaline-evoked increase in 2-[^{14}C]deoxyglucose incorporation into glycogen. Neurosci Lett 55:157–160.

Petrillo P, Tavani A, Verotta D, Robson LE, Kosterlitz HW (1987): Differential postnatal development of μ-, δ- and κ-opioid binding sites in rat brain. Dev Brain Res 31:53–58.

Recht LD, Kent J, Pasternak GW (1985): Quantitative autoradiography of the development of μ opiate binding sites in rat brain. Cell Mol Neurobiol 5:223–229.

Ricalde AA, Hammer RP Jr (1990): Perinatal opiate treatment delays growth of cortical dendrites. Neurosci Lett 115:137–143.

Rodning C, Beckwith L, Howard J (1989): Prenatal exposure to drugs: behavioral distortions reflecting CNS impairment? Neurotoxicology 10:634–639.

Rost N, Chaffanet M, Nissou MF, Chauvin C, Foote AM, Laine M, Benabid AL (1989): Expression of the proenkephalin A gene in tumor cells and brain glioma: a Northern and in situ hybridization study. Neuropeptides 13:133–138.

Rothman RB, Bykov V, Hong JB, Brady LS, Jacobson AE, Rice KC, Holady JW (1989): Chronic administration of morphine and naltrexone up-regulate μ-opioid binding sites labeled by [^{3}H][D-Ala^2, Me Phe^4, Gly-ol^5] enkephalin: further evidence for two μ binding sites. Eur J Pharmacol 160:71–82.

Sakellaridis N, Mangoura D, Vernadakis A (1986): Effects of opiates on the growth of neuron-enriched cultures from chick embryonic brain. Int J Dev Neurosci 4:293–302.

Schmahl W, Funk R, Miaskowski U, Plendl J (1989): Long-lasting effects of naltrexone, an opioid receptor antagonist, on cell proliferation in developing rat forebrain. Brain Res 486:297–300.

Schofield PR, McFarland KC, Hayflick JS, Wilcox JN, Cho TM, Roy S, Lee NM, Loh HH, Seeburg PH (1989): Molecular characterization of a new immunoglobulin protein with potential roles in opioid binding and cell contact. EMBO J 8:489–495.

Schulz R, Faase E, Wuster M, Herz A (1979): Selective receptors for β-endorphin on the rat vas deferens. Life Sci 24:843–850.

Sharif NA, Hughes J (1989): Discrete mapping of brain mu and delta opioid receptors using selective peptides: quantitative autoradiography, species differences and comparison with kappa receptors. Peptides 10:499–522.

Shepanek NA, Smith RF, Tyer Z, Royall D, Allen K (1989): Developmental, behavioral and structural effects of prenatal opiate receptor blockade. Ann NY Acad Sci 562:377–379.

Shinoda H, Marini AM, Cosi C, Schwartz JP (1989): Brain region and gene specificity of neuropeptide gene expression in cultured astrocytes. Science 245:415–417.

Slotkin TA (1988): Perinatal exposure to methadone: how do early biochemical alterations cause neurofunctional disturbances? In Boer GJ, Feenstra MGP, Mirmiran M, Swaab DF, Van Haaren (eds): "Progress in Brain Research, Vol. 73." Amsterdam: Elsevier Science Publishers, pp 265–279.

Spain JW, Roth BL, Coscia CJ (1985): Differential ontogeny of multiple opioid receptors (μ, δ, and κ). J Neurosci 5:584–588.

Steine-Martin A, Hauser KF (1990): Opioid-dependent growth of glial cultures: suppression of astrocyte DNA synthesis by met-enkephalin. Life Sci 46:91–98.

Strauss ME, Starr RH, Oslrea EM, Chavez CJ, Strylar JC (1976): Behavioral concommitants of prenatal addiction to narcotics. J Pediatr 89:842–846.

Szucs M, Coscia CJ (1990): Evidence for δ-opioid binding and GTP regulatory proteins in 5-day-old rat brain membranes. J Neurochem 54:1425–1491.

Szucs M, Oetting GM, Coscia CJ (1986): Unique characteristics of early neonatal δ-opioid-binding sites. Biochem Soc Tran. 14:1156–1157.

Tavani A, Robson LE, Kosterlitz HW (1985): Differential postnatal development of μ-, δ- and κ-opioid binding sites in mouse brain. Dev Brain Res 23:306–309.

Unnerstall JR, Molliver ME, Kuhar JM, Palacios JM (1983): Ontogeny of opiate binding sites in the hippocampus, olfactory bulb and other regions of the rat forebrain by autoradiographic methods. Dev Brain Res 7:157–169.

Vaupel DB (1983): Naltrexone fails to antagonize the sigma effects of PCP and SKF 10,1047 in the dog. Eur J Pharmacol 92:269–274.

Vaysse PJ-J, Zukin RS, Fields KL, Kessler JA (1990): Characterization of opioid receptors in cultured neurons. J Neurochem 55:624–631.

Vertes Z, Melgh G, Vertes M, Kovacs S (1982): Effect of naloxone and D-Met^2-D-Pro^5-enkephalinamide treatment on the DNA synthesis in the developing rat brain. Life Sci 31:119–126.

Vilijin M-H, Vaysse PJ-J, Zukin RS, Kessler JA (1988): Expression of proenkephalin mRNA by cultured astrocytes and neurons. Proc Natl Acad Sci USA 85:6551–6555.

Wang C, Pasulka P, Perry B, Pizzi WJ, Schnoll SH (1986): Effect of perinatal exposure to methadone on brain opioid and alpha-2 adrenergic receptors. Neurotoxicol Teratol 8:399–402.

Wilson GS, Desmond MM, Wait RB (1981): Follow-up of methadone-treated and untreated narcotic-dependent women and their infants: health, development and social implications. J Pediatr 98:716–722.

Zagon IS, Gibo DM, McLaughlin PJ (1990): Adult and developing cerebella exhibit different profiles of opioid binding sites. Brain Res 523:62–68.

Zagon IS, Goodman SR, McLaughlin PJ (1989): Characterization of zeta (ζ): a new opioid receptor involved in growth. Brain Res 482:297–305.

Zagon IS, McLaughlin PJ (1983): Behavioral effects of prenatal exposure to opiates. Monogr Neural Sci 9:159–168.

Zagon IS, McLaughlin PJ (1986): Opioid antagonist-induced modulation of cerebral and hippocampal development: histological and morphometric studies. Dev Brain Res 28:233–246.

Zagon IS, McLaughlin PJ (1987): Endogenous opioid systems regulate cell proliferation in the developing rat brain. Brain Res 412:68–72.

Zukin RS, Eghbali M, Olive D, Unterwald EM, Tempel A (1988): Characterization and visualization of rat and guinea-pig brain kappa-opioid receptors: evidence for $kappa_1$ and $kappa_2$ opioid receptors. Proc Natl Acad Sci USA 85:4061–4065.

Zukin RS, Zukin SR (1984): The case for multiple opiate receptors. Trends Neurosci 7:160–163.

Development of the Central Nervous System:
Effects of Alcohol and Opiates, pages 285–318

13

Regulation of the Opioid System by Exogenous Drug Administration

ANN TEMPEL

Department of Psychiatry, Hillside Hospital, Long Island Jewish Medical Center, Glen Oaks, New York

INTRODUCTION
History of Substance Abuse

Description in the medical literature of human neonates undergoing withdrawal following opioid abuse during pregnancy date back to the latter part of the 19th century (Goodfriend et al., 1956). Methadone was first synthesized by the Germans during World War II. Following favorable preliminary findings by Dole and Nyswander (1965), wide-scale use in heroin addiction drug treatment programs followed (for review see Hutchings, 1985a). By 1975, there were some 70,000–80,000 female heroin addicts in methadone maintenance programs throughout the country and a signif icant proportion of these women were of childbearing age. At the time, it was estimated that in the New York City metropolitan area alone, 10,000–12,000 such women were enrolled in methadone programs, yet little was known of possible risk to the fetus and the newborn. With the advent of methadone maintenance as an experimental treatment for heroin addiction in the early 1970s, attention turned to the questions of reproductive hazards and developmental toxicity. There are confounding variables in clinical experiments such as women coming from low socioeconomic levels, long histories of drug abuse, poor diets, heavy smokers, use of marijuana, cocaine, barbiturates, tranquilizers or alcohol (for review see Householder et al., 1982; Hutchings and Fifer, 1986).

Infants with "chronic opium intoxication" are reported to exhibit excessive nervousness, rapid breathing and convulsive movements right after birth, with death occurring within the first week of life (Terry and Pellens, 1970). The type of opioid abused has changed over the years. Until the 1950s, morphine appeared to be the drug of choice, with the 1956 report by Goodfriend et al., signaling a change to heroin usage. Following Dole and Nyswander's (1965) advocation of the methadone maintenance treatment program as an alternative to heroin dependency, numerous reports have documented methadone-dependent offspring. Paralleling the change from morphine to utilization of heroin and methadone in the 1950s, a marked increase in the number of births to opioid-dependent women has been recorded. In one municipal hospital in New York City, for example, only 22 infants were born to heroin-dependent mothers from 1955–1959, but 26 infants were delivered during 1960 (Zelson, 1975). In this same hospital, over a six-fold increase in drug-dependent babies was recorded between 1960 (1 in 164 births) and 1972 (1 in 27 births). Recent estimates (Carr, 1975) place the birth rate of heroin- and methadone-addicted mothers at 3,000/year in New York City alone; given that New York City has one-third to one-half of the total number of chronic heroin and methadone users in the United States (Carr, 1975; Salerno, 1977), one could extrapolate 6,000–9,000 births/year to opioid-consuming women. Carr also reports that, as of 1975, 115,000 children of mothers dependent on illegal opioids and methadone maintenance were in the New York City area. Assuming again that this number for New York City is representative of one-third to one-half of the entire United States population, one can estimate that at least 250,000 infants, children, and young adults have already been born to females consuming opioids such as methadone or heroin. Placed within the context of the average number of births in the United States every year (roughly 3.3 million), one can calculate that at least 1 in 1,000 births is by a mother using heroin or methadone. Assuming the population of the United States is 230 million, and given a population of 230,000 children already exposed perinatally to opioids, 1 in 1,000 people in the United States have been subjected to opioids in early life. By themselves, these numbers are significant. However, unreported use of opioids by pregnant women and the possible influence exerted by paternal opioid consumption may indicate an error of underestimation.

Development of Animal Models

As a result, in the mid 1970s, several laboratories attempted to develop animal models of prenatal methadone exposure. Laboratory environments would provide controlled experiments minimizing the confounding variables in the clinical studies. However, there are a host of methodological and interpretive problems in animal studies as well (for a comprehensive bibliography see Zagon et al., 1982; Sparber and Lichtblau, 1985).

Though it is not clear whether methadone ever went through any currently standard preclinical screening for teratogenicity, its wide-scale use for the treatment of heroin addiction began in the late 1960s. By the early 1970s only one or two animal studies had been published and it was still unknown whether methadone produced damage in the developing central nervous system (CNS), with concomitant neurobehavioral deficits. This was one of the major issues addressed by the animal studies. Confounding variables in these studies pointed to issues of dose-response, fostering, and toxicity during pregnancy (Hutchings and Fifer, 1986) as factors influencing experimental results. Although most laboratories have used the rat, procedures have differed with respect to strain, dose level, dosing regimen, route of administration, gestational age at treatment, and fostering techniques. These factors make it difficult to compare results from one laboratory with another.

I will briefly describe these important confounding variables in developmental toxicology research because of their importance in interpretation of data and conclusions drawn.

Surrogate fostering

The evidence is sufficiently convincing that prenatal manipulations of the pregnant dam can alter maternal behavior and the mother-infant dyad to produce effects in her offspring, even when treatment is terminated before the last week or so of gestation. Daily drug treatment can disrupt circadian rhythms, cause acute nutritional deficits, and either inhibit or interfere with hormones that mediate maternal behavior (Hofer, 1984). Recent studies demonstrate the mother's integral role as a regulator of a host of developmental parameters in her offspring that include activity level, sleep-wake states, milk ingestion, heart rate, oxygen consumption, and growth hormone (for review see Hofer, 1984). If not included, interpretation of the data will be compromised in that one cannot rule out with any degree of confidence, that offspring effects have not been maternally mediated during the postnatal period.

Dose-response relationships

Prenatal drug studies involve two mutually interacting biological systems—the pregnant dam and fetoplacental unit. Dose-response relationships are very complex and involve interactive, pharmacological, and toxic effects in the mother and offspring (Hutchings, 1985a). The general principle is as dose is increased from subpharmacological levels through the pharmacological range of the compound, there is a corresponding increase in toxicity culminating in death. For example, thalidomide at subtoxic, pharmacological levels in the pregnant dam is highly embryotoxic, causing morphogenesis. Another compound with the same sort of profile and embryotoxic response in humans is the vitamin A derivative, isotretinoin (Hutchings, 1985a). In animal studies, what is frequently seen is that within the pharmacological range of the compound, and at levels that are not toxic to the dam, there is no embryotoxic response. Embryotoxicity is seen only at levels that produce toxicity in the pregnant dam (for review see Hutchings, 1985b). One example in the rat is phencyclidine (PCP), which has been shown to be teratogenic, but only at doses that are highly toxic to the pregnant dam. In the case of PCP, Hutchings (1985b) administered two doses that were pharmacologically potent as measured by behavioral effects in the dam (5 or 10 mg/kg), but of relatively low toxicity based on weight gain. Yet they observed normal birth weights and no postnatal behavioral effects on two independent behavioral measures (Hutchings et al., 1984).

Dose-response relationships, though complex, are critical for a meaningful description and understanding of effects. It is helpful that every study include some measure of pregnant dam dose-response. This is of particular importance when embryotoxicity is found only at doses that produce toxicity in the pregnant dam. Under these circumstances, it is important to determine whether the effects produced in the offspring are primary effects of the compound or secondary to toxicity to the pregnant dam.

Comparison of Effects in Humans and Animals

Prenatal exposure to alcohol, the opioids heroin and methadone, and their neurobehavioral effects have been reviewed extensively elsewhere (e.g., Hutchings, 1983, 1985 a,b,c; Hutchings and Fifer, 1986; Meyer and Riley, 1986; Streissguth, 1986; see also Chapters 2, 3, and 11). The most serious and debilitating neuropsychiatric effects associated with prenatal drug exposure are the generalized cognitive deficits collectively referred to as mental retardation. This disorder typically includes markedly delayed developmental milestones, significantly below average intellectual functioning with limited speech, and inability to comprehend abstract questions. Associated problems include impaired adaptive functioning, particularly in areas of learning and social interactions. Of several prenatally administered compounds that can produce mental retardation, alcohol has been the most thoroughly studied. These data are summarized in a separate chapter in this book (Chapter 2).

The more recent prenatal alcohol studies with animals have clearly demonstrated that prenatal administration of alcohol is developmentally toxic, producing, as in humans, both dysmorphogenesis and long-term neurobehavioral impairment (Meyer and Riley, 1986). Moreover, the behavioral effects described in the offspring resemble effects observed clinically in affected children: developmental delays, hyperactivity, and inhibitory deficits.

Heroin and methadone provide particularly interesting comparisons because unlike alcohol, neither appears to be teratogenic; that is, the combined animal and human data indicate that none of these opioids produce dysmorphogenesis. They do, however, produce in humans a neonatal abstinence syndrome that appears to reflect a nonspecific increase in CNS arousal characterized by hyperactivity, hyperexcitability, hyperacusis, sleeplessness, tremors, and prolonged high-pitched crying. Though these acute symptoms subside within 3–6 weeks, they are followed by a secondary or subacute withdrawal that persists for 4–6 months and includes restlessness, agitation, tremors, and sleep disturbance. Long-term follow-up studies of children who were exposed prenatally to methadone tend to find that on developmental scales, they score within the normal range and at 4 years of age, no consistent differences were found on several standard measures of cognitive performance. Studies do suggest, however, that these children are at risk for developing an attention deficit disorder accompanied by impaired fine motor coordination. And though they are described as being restless and impulsive when performing structured tasks, they are not, by contemporary diagnostic criteria, hyperactive. Although not definitive or complete by any means, studies on behavioral and neurobehavioral effects as a result of prenatal opioid exposure are informative and meaningful. However, biochemical, cellular, and molecular studies examining these systems' alterations as a result of prenatal opioid exposure are just beginning to emerge in animal studies. This chapter will attempt to review the animal studies in this emerging field of research.

IN VIVO ANIMAL STUDIES

Laboratory studies offer an animal model to study the influences of opioids on development. Laboratory models allow us to study the effects of opioids in postnatally developing animals. Several factors such as routes of administration, drug dosages, and schedules of treatment vary from one experiment to another. Some reports of the effects of exposure to opioids have shown little effect on the estrous cycle, fertility, length of gestation, and parturition (Zagon and McLaughlin 1977a, b, c), although difficulties with conception and a protraction of the gestational period (Buchenauer et al., 1974) as well as positional malformations of the fetus (Chandler et al., 1975) have been recorded. Several toxic effects have been noted such as a reduction in the dam's body weight during pregnancy (McGinty and Ford 1976; White et al., 1978; Seidler et al., 1982; Zagon and McLaughlin, 1977a). In general, gestational exposure to morphine and methadone does not have a detrimental influence on litter size (Davis and Lin, 1972; Zagon and McLaughlin, 1977b, d), although some decreases in litter size with higher doses of methadone have been noted (Middaugh and Simpson, 1980). Teratogenicity appears to be associated with high drug dosages administered acutely or over a short time period (Geber and Schramm, 1975), but not with lower dosages administered chronically. Some increase in stillborns has been observed with high drug dosages (Freeman, 1980; Sobrian, 1977), while other studies reveal little problem in this area (Davis and Lin, 1972).

Behavioral Manifestations

The effect of transplacental exposure to opioids on rat pup viability is determined by drug dosage and whether or not the neonates continue to receive opioids postnatally (i.e., breast milk, direct injection). Opioids are known to accumulate in the brain and nervous tissues of fetal rats (Peters et al., 1972) and preweaning rats (Shah and Donald, 1979), presumably because developing organisms have an increased permeability of the blood-brain barrier. Neonates that do not continue to receive opioids often may be hypersensitive to stimuli and experience tremors at birth, with notable infant mortality found in the first few days of life for those pups exposed to morphine, heroin, and methadone (Davis and Lin, 1972; Zagon and McLaughlin, 1977d; Freeman, 1980). Delays in physical characteristics (e.g., eye opening), spontaneous motor physical characteristics (e.g., walking), and reflexive tests (e.g., visual orientation) have all been noted. Interestingly, animals exposed only prenatally to opioids (i.e., allowed to go through withdrawal at birth and not receive drug postnatally) exhibit the greatest number of delays in attaining behavioral capacities and physical characteristics. Those animals receiving a drug prenatally and postnatally (a situation somewhat comparable to that in humans when therapeutic intervention prevents withdrawal) are often closest to the normal timetable of maturation.

In the rat, behavior in the period shortly after weaning (postnatal days 21–44) has generally been characterized by a reduction in activity and a decreased emotionality relative to control offspring (Freeman, 1980; Grove et all, 1979; Zagon et al., 1979). Zagon and McLaughlin (1981b) have also found an abnormally high incidence of wet-dog-shake and head-shake behaviors during this period that resemble drug withdrawal. In contrast to the reduced activity levels in opioid-treated pups at weaning, young adults (postnatal days 45–89) generally were hyperactive and more emotional (Davis and Lin, 1972; Grove et al., 1979; Zagon et al., 1979; Zagon and McLaughlin, 1984a). Once again, methadone-exposed pups often exhibited head-shake and wet-dog-shake behaviors, suggesting a protracted phase of withdrawal. Peters (1978) has also accumulated pilot data showing learning disabilities in methadone- and morphine-exposed rats at this age.

Effects on Cell Proliferation and Maturation

In regard to other anatomical, physiological, and biochemical correlates to opioid exposure in early life, a number of important observations have been made. This work is reviewed in detail in Chapter 14, so I will only briefly touch on this topic. Somatic growth retardation (e.g., McLaughlin and Zagon, 1980; McLaughlin et al., 1978; Slotkin et al., 1976, 1980), smaller brain dimensions (Zagon and McLaughlin 1977b, 1978), and deficits in organ weights (McLaughlin and Zagon, 1980; McLaughlin et al., 1978) have been reported. Physiological dysfunction in regard to thermoregulation (Thompson and Zagon, 1981; Thompson et al., 1979), nociceptive thresholds (Zagon and McLaughlin, 1980; 1981, 1982b), and aberrant response to opioids and non-opioid drugs (Zagon and McLaughlin, 1981a, 1984b) has also been recorded. Opioid-exposed offspring, particularly those subjected to drugs only prenatally, often exhibit deficits in brain cell number, as well as alterations in brain RNA and protein concentrations and content (Zagon and McLaughlin, 1978). Changes in polyamine metabolism (Slotkin et al., 1976, 1979) and in the ontogeny of catecholaminergic systems, as well as a retardation in the synaptic development of 5-hydroxytryptamine, dopamine (DA), and epinephrine neurons in the nervous system, have been cited (McGinty and Ford, 1980; Rech et al., 1980; Slotkin et al., 1982). The timetable of neurogenesis is delayed with drug exposure (Zagon and McLaughlin, 1982b). Prenatal exposure to opioids for duration of the gestation period causes reductions in cortical thickness and number of cells in the neocortex (Ford and Rhines, 1979). It does not appear that either undernutrition of the pregnant rat or inadequate nutrition of the offspring forms the etiological basis for opioid-related problems (e.g., Ford and Rhines, 1979; Zagon and McLaughlin, 1982a; McLaughlin and Zagon, 1980; Seidler et al., 1982; White et al., 1978; Raye et al., 1977; Smith et al., 1977). Moreover, hypoxia due to opioid consumption does not appear to be responsible for the sequelae recorded (White and Zagon, 1979).

Effects on Growth

The endogenous opioid systems seem to be involved in the trophic regulation of CNS growth and development. Exogenously applied opioids (such as morphine, heroin, and methadone) inhibit both somatic and neurobiological development of humans (Wilson et al., 1973), laboratory animals (Smith et al., 1977; Zagon and McLaughlin, 1977), and growth of cell cultures (Zagon and McLaughlin, 1984a). Naltrexone (opioid antagonist) administration to preweaning rats produces a dual dose-dependent effect on body and brain development, being stimulatory at high doses and inhibitory at low doses (Zagon and McLaughlin, 1984b). In drug paradigms where the dam is treated during all of pregnancy, morphine treatment produces a significant decrease in body weight in postnatal day 30 relative to controls (DiGiulio et al., 1988). The developmental pattern of met-enkephalin containing neurons is also affected by morphine administration. There is little change in early stages of development. However, the effect is magnified with growth. There is a significant increase in the opioid peptide concentrations in the pons-medulla beginning 12 days postnatal and continuing through 30 days postnatal. It is not clear whether the effect on met-enkephalin is a direct consequence of the drug interaction with the opioid receptor or an indirect response to the chronic morphine exposure. When a drug is administered to the pregnant organism, the effects on the fetus could be mediated either directly by the drug which has crossed the placenta and/or by the drug's effects on the homeostasis of the dam or placenta, which in turn influences fetal development. Thus, in the interpretation of drug effects on fetal growth, the unit formed by the pregnant dam, the placenta and the fetus must be taken into consideration.

In Ovo Studies

To eliminate the influence of the pregnant dam and of placental factors in drug effects on fetal brain growth, some researchers have used the chick embryo as an animal model (Vernadakis and Gibson, 1985) as well as neural tissue culture (Sakellaridis and Vernadakis, 1987). The major disadvantages are that these systems do not simulate the in vivo environment. Thus, extrapolation of results to in vivo situations must be done with caution. The narcotic drug L-α-acetylmethadol (LAAM) has been used clinically as a substitute for methadone maintenance of heroin addicts. LAAM is more potent and longer-acting than methadone and therefore offers advantages for therapeutic use. The effects of LAAM on the developing organism, however, are still in the stages of animal investigation.

In studies in which the developing chick embryo was exposed to LAAM at specific periods of development, the toxicity of LAAM was determined as measured by viability, hatchability, maximum number of [^{3}H] etorphine binding sites (B_{max}), and affinity (K_d) of binding in the chick brain (Gibson and Vernadakis, 1983; Vernadakis et al., 1982). Chick embryos were treated at either 7–10 days of embryonic age, or at 15–17 days. Data show that during the first 6 days of embryonic development the chick is especially sensitive to LAAM. LAAM consistently changed the B_{max} and the K_d of (^{3}H) etorphine binding. LAAM also decreased the B_{max} and increased the K_d in neuron-enriched cultures.

IN VITRO SYSTEMS

Effects on Other Neurotransmitter Systems

Ornithine decarboxylase (ODC) reflects immature cells (Slotkin et al., 1980), and this author reports higher levels of ODC in methadone-treated cultures and concludes, therefore, that methadone may retard neuronal differentiation. Numerous studies have confirmed that CNS drugs given to the pregnant organism exert variable degrees of neurotoxicity on the fetus. It has been generally accepted that the effects of drugs on the developing CNS are dependent on the stage of brain maturation at the time the drug is administered. Thus, drugs relatively safe in the adult organism may exhibit severe neurotoxicity in the developing organism.

It is known that infants born to mothers who are addicted to opioids and continue receiving the drugs during their pregnancy exhibit dependency to those drugs immediately after birth as manifested by symptoms of withdrawal. The etiology of this pronounced neurotoxicity remains uncertain despite the numerous studies in this area (for review see Zagon et al., 1982).

The effects of opiates on the maturation of the cholinergic system both in ovo and in culture have been examined by Sakellaridis and Vernadakis (1987). In a series of experiments, they administered either morphine, an opioid agonist, or naloxone, an opioid antagonist, chronically to the chick embryos at embryonic day (E) 1–E3 and examined choline acetyltransferase (ChAT) activity in the whole brain at E4 or E6, or acutely at E1 or E3 and examined at E3 or E6, respectively. ChAT is the synthesizing enzyme of acetylcholine and its presence identifies cholinergic neurons. Consequently, ChAT is a sensitive indicator of the state of development of the cholinergic system.

The striking finding was that during acute administration of morphine or naloxone, the agonist and antagonist had opposing effects: in morphine-treated embryos, ChAT activity was variable (higher, lower, or not changed), whereas in naloxone-treated embryos, ChAT was consistently higher. In contrast to the effects of acute treatment, chronic administration (at E1, E2, or E3) of morphine or naloxone produced a similar effect decreasing ChAT activity. Parallel studies have shown that chronic treatment of chick embryos with morphine did not affect the kinetic properties of opioid binding whereas naloxone did up-regulate the binding. Based on their binding and enzymatic studies, they have put forward the hypothesis that early in development naloxone exerts its effect by blocking the endogenous opioid peptides from their receptor. Supporting evidence for this proposal are the studies of Zagon and McLaughlin (1986) and at the morphological level the studies of Sakellaridis and Vernadakis (1987).

Role of G-Proteins and Second Messenger Systems in
the Development of Tolerance

It has been suggested that opioid receptor density is controlled by either
the inhibition or excitation of the cyclic adenosine monophosphate (cAMP)
system via G-binding proteins (Costa et al., 1988; Sibley and Lefkowitz,
1985; Mayorga et al., 1989). Guanine nucleotide binding regulator proteins
(G-proteins) transduce a variety of extracellular signals across the cell
membranes into changes in the levels of intracellular second messengers
(Gilman, 1987). Members of this protein family are all heterotrimers consisting of α, β and γ subunits. In most biological systems, the GTP-binding
α subunit serves as the transducer of signals between receptors and effec-
tors. In contrast, the role of β-γ is less well understood. The β-γ complex
has been demonstrated to facilitate the interaction of the subunits to recep-
tors (Fung, 1983; Florio and Sternwies, 1985) and to mediate the binding
of α subunit to membranes (Sternweis, 1986). The α subunit of G-protein
exhibits variation in structure classifying it into $G\alpha_s$, $G\alpha_i$, $G\alpha_o$, $G\alpha_t$, and
$G\alpha_z$ (Gilman, 1987; Stryer, 1986; Provost et al., 1988). $G\alpha_s$ can stimulate
the activity of adenylate cyclase, whereas $G\alpha_i$ type inhibits adenylate
cyclase activity. The β-γ complex does not show any variation in structure
and is interchangeable between different $G\alpha$ proteins.

Acute treatment with opioids inhibits adenylate cyclase, and thereby,
decreases cAMP levels. Such changes have been described in cultured
neuroblastoma x glioma hybrid cells (NG108 cells) (Sharma et al., 1975a,b;
Traber et al., 1975) and in brain regions like the locus ceruleus (Duman et
al., 1988; Beitner et al., 1989), neostriatum, and cerebral cortex (Collier and
Roy, 1974; Tsang et al., 1978; Law et al., 1981; Schoffelmeer et al., 1986).
In addition, chronic opioid treatment increases levels of $G_{i\alpha}$ and $G_{o\alpha}$,
adenylate cyclase activity, and cAMP-dependent protein kinase activity in
the locus ceruleus but not in other brain regions (Duman et al., 1988;
Nestler and Tallman, 1988; Guitart and Nestler, 1989, 1990; Nestler et al.,
1989; Guitart et al., 1990). It has been proposed that such an up-regulated
G-protein/cAMP system in the locus ceruleus contributes to opioid tolerance and dependence in the adult CNS (Nestler et al., 1990; Rasmussen et
al., 1990). These results suggest that treatment with opioids alter the G-
protein/cAMP levels in different brain regions; however, a causal relationship between opioid receptor density change and G-protein/cAMP levels
under such conditions has not yet been demonstrated. Sakellaridis and
Vernadakis (1987) have shown in the chick embryo that morphine inhibited forskolin-stimulated adenylate cyclase at E6 and E8, but that morphine had no effect on E10. Naloxone produced the same effect with the
same time schedule. A combination of both morphine and naloxone also
decreased the adenylate cyclase activity. These investigators interpreted
their findings to indicate that the conventional opioid receptor was not
responsible for the observed effects since the inhibitory effects were not
naloxone-reversible and that naloxone itself produced this effect. Studies
investigating the relationship of G-proteins to opiate tolerance are just

beginning to emerge. Results from these studies should elucidate cellular mechanisms underlying opiate addiction.

EFFECTS OF OPIOID ANTAGONISTS ON THE DEVELOPMENT OF OPIOID RECEPTORS

Although opioid receptor supersensitivity has been demonstrated in the CNS of fully mature animals, some evidence indicates that there may be ontogenetic differences in susceptibility to receptor supersensitivity following chronic opioid blockade. The normal developmental pattern of opioid receptors in the CNS has been described in rat (Auguy-Valette et al., 1978; Clendeninn et al., 1976; Coyle and Pert, 1976; Garcin and Coyle, 1976; Kent et al., 1982; Koch et al., 1980; Pasternak et al., 1980; Patey et al., 1980; Wohltmann et al., 1982; Zhong-Zhang and Pasternak, 1981; Tsang et al., 1982; see also Chapter 12). In general, the proliferation in the number of μ receptors in the brain of rat follows a caudal-to-rostral pattern of maturation, with caudal regions exhibiting greater proliferation during the prenatal period and rostral regions exhibiting greater proliferation during the postnatal period (Bardo et al., 1981, 1983a; Kirby, 1981). When naloxone is administered chronically during the prenatal period, the caudal brainstem is more likely than the forebrain to exhibit an increase in opioid receptors (Tsang and Ng, 1980). In contrast, when naloxone is administered chronically during the postnatal period, the rostral brain regions are more likely than the caudal brain regions to exhibit an increase in opioid receptors (Bardo et al., 1982, 1983b). These researchers suggest that opioid receptor systems, which are undergoing rapid ontogenetic proliferation, may be particularly susceptible to receptor supersensitivity following chronic opioid receptor blockade. Rats injected with naloxone during the first 3 postnatal weeks showed significant increase in [^{3}H] naloxone binding in the cortex, striatum, hypothalamus, and spinal cord. Body and brain weights for naloxone and saline-treated rats were similar, indicating that naloxone did not produce a general developmental or nutritional deficit. There were no significant changes in opioid binding 1 week after cessation of naloxone treatment. These results are similar to what was seen in the adult CNS (Tempel et al., 1984, 1985). Naloxone-treated infants displayed an enhanced response to the antinociceptive efficacy of morphine which was also seen in adult rats (Tempel et al., 1985).

Previous studies have shown that chronic exposure to opioid antagonists early in life may produce profound alterations in various behavioral indices which are essentially permanent. Rats treated perinatally with naloxone subsequently display an acceleration in the righting reflex, swimming performance, and startle development (Vorhees, 1981), as well as permanent alterations in locomotor activity and responsivity to pain when tested as adults (Harry and Rosecrans, 1979; Monder et al., 1980; Sandman et al., 1979). In addition, chronic exposure to opioid antagonists early in life affects later responsiveness to opioid drugs. Immature rats given opioid antagonists display a long-lasting supersensitivity to the antinociceptive effect of morphine (Hetta and Terenius, 1980;

Paul et al., 1978) and a subsensitivity (tolerance) to the anorexic effect of naloxone (Diaz et al., 1978). The ontogeny of endorphin- and enkephalin-containing presynaptic elements has recently been characterized (Bayon et al., 1979; Bloom et al., 1980; Patey et al., 1980), and evidence from adults indicates that these presynaptic elements may be altered in the striatum following opioid blockade (Wüster et al., 1980). It is possible that long-lasting behavioral changes may reflect an alteration in presynaptic neuronal elements; however, the long-lasting behavioral changes which follow chronic opioid blockade during infancy may reflect an alteration in neuroendocrine function (Guidotti and Grandison, 1979; Volavka et al., 1980).

EFFECT OF OPIOID AGONIST TREATMENT

The neonatal rat is an excellent experimental animal for studying the syndrome of drug-induced delay of maturation because it matures quickly and a great deal of information exists concerning its structural and biochemical development. The rat brain is relatively immature at birth and undergoes a period of rapid growth during the first few postnatal weeks. Morphological, neurochemical, and neuroendocrine maturational events follow well known sequences. Although little is known about the effects of morphine on the development of the rat brain, the effects of this drug on the adult rat have been extensively studied.

Behavioral Manifestations

Based on research reports, it is clear that the gestational or neonatal exposure of rats to opioid drugs results in a variety of long-lasting and perhaps permanent effects. Most consistent and reproducible among these long-term effects is a syndrome consisting of impaired growth, altered behavior, and altered neurochemical development. The method of addiction, age, duration of exposure, and drug concentrations all affect the development of the CNS. One method of drug exposure is to treat the pups rather than the mother to be sure of the amount of morphine the pup receives as well as to avoid aberrant maternal behavior. Rat pups injected with morphine show depressed body weights (Zimmermann et al., 1974, 1977; Zimmerman and Sonderegger, 1980), delayed eye opening, and early vaginal openings. Both sexes show impaired behavioral responses to the analgesic action of morphine in the hot plate test on day 80. Morphine-treated animals show a reduced steroid response to a challenge dose of morphine on day 96. This early work suggests that a variety of prolonged, possibly permanent, morphine-induced alterations of neurochemical processes subserve neuroendocrine and nociceptive brain mechanisms. In addition, several studies have shown that the effects of early drug treatment may appear in the second generation as well (Friedler, 1972; Joffee et al., 1976; Zimmermann et al., 1977). These studies show that certain behavioral aspects of opioid-induced developmental alterations may be transmitted to subsequent generations.

Opioid Effects on Cell Development

Both DA and norepinephrine (NA) cell bodies can be distinguished using fluorescent methods by day 15 of gestation (Coyle, 1976). NA concentrations reach adult levels by 4 weeks postnatal, whereas DA concentrations reach adult levels as late as 5–6 weeks postpartum (Coyle, 1976). Ultimately, the entire neocortex is innervated by the locus ceruleus.

In contrast to the organization of the noradrenergic system, dopaminergic systems have a more precise topography and organization (Moore and Bloom, 1979). The tubero-hypophyseal DA system appears to participate in regulating the production and release of hypothalamic and pituitary hormones (Bakke et al., 1973). Exposure of the developing organism to drugs which affect catecholamine (CA) systems maturing at different rates could be expected to produce different effects, depending on the stage of development. Such effects may help explain the long-lasting neuroendocrine changes seen following morphine administration (Holt et al., 1978). Body weight depression is a common and reliable response in young mammals exposed to opioids early in life, both in rats (Bakke et al., 1973; Bannerjee, 1974) and humans (Wilson et al., 1973). Again, the magnitude and duration of growth impairments appear to be related to age at the time of drug exposure as well as the dose and duration of the exposure.

In a comparable cross-generational study (Sonderegger et al., 1979), 19 male rats (implanted neonatally on postnatal day 5 or 11 with morphine or placebo pellets) were bred to nulliparous females, producing a total of 245 pups. Again, neither litter size, birth weights, nor sex ratios differed among progeny from sires of different neonatal treatment groups. On the other hand, significant body weight depressions appeared by postnatal day 35 in both the male and female untreated progeny of the morphine 11 males. Significant reduction in body weight persisted until postnatal day 126 in the female, but not in the male offspring. The growth impairment was not observed in the progeny of the 5 morphine-treated males. A sex-related growth impairment was found in the offspring of the males, but no alterations were found in behavioral testing (open-field, activity wheel, and the hot plate test) or in neuroendocrine responsivity. Cross-generational body weight depressions in the offspring of animals treated with morphine (Friedler, 1972) or methadone (Smith et al., 1977; Joffee et al., 1976) have also been found in other laboratories.

The mechanisms responsible for protracted growth, behavioral, and neuroendocrine deficits observed in the morphine syndrome are not known, but most certainly these mechanisms involve altered development of neurochemical processes. Drugs that affect neurotransmitter metabolism in the mature CNS of the rat can alter behavior in later life (Weiner, 1974). Modification of developing neurotransmitter systems by early exposure to morphine is one possible cause of the alterations in developmental patterns.

It is now well known that rapid changes in the amounts of CA and of the enzymes in their metabolic pathways as well as rapid morphological development of the monoaminergic systems occur during the pre- and early postnatal periods. These developing systems are particularly vulnerable to drug manipulations. Morphine administration to adult rats induces changes in the content and rate of turnover of CA in the brain (Clouet, 1977). Both DA and NA levels are reportedly reduced after acute opioid administration (Takagi and Nakama, 1968). Moreover, there is a sharp rise in DA biosynthesis in the striatum after a single dose of morphine (Clouet and Ratner, 1970). Tolerance to these phenomena occurs with repeated morphine administration (Smith et al., 1972).

CA changes have also been demonstrated in perinatally addicted rats, but the changes were different than those seen in the adults, i.e., the CA levels and the activity of the rate limiting step in their biosynthesis, dopamine-β-hydroxylase, were reduced (Slotkin and Anderson, 1975). It is interesting that the time course of the adrenomedullary function of the methadone-addicted rats was significantly delayed in this study. We know from the careful work of Parvez et al. (1979) that adrenocortical functioning is also important to the postnatal development of the CA system.

In summary, a variety of drug-induced deficits have been observed in developing rats neonatally addicted to morphine which persist into adulthood and even into the untreated second generation. In general, these deficits include impaired growth and behavioral and neuroendocrine responses. This spectrum of drug-related developmental deficits may be a general pattern found in the young animal exposed to neurotropic drugs early in life. Neurotropic drugs such as morphine alter both the levels and the biosynthesis of the CA and such effects may be the neurochemical basis of the alterations and deficits in development. Chronic increase or decrease of central adrenergic activity could lead to increased or decreased levels of the relevant biosynthetic enzymes tyrosine hydroxylase and dopamine-β-hydroxylase, and thus, produce protracted effects via processes that have been described as "biochemical hypertrophy or atrophy" (Weiner, 1974). An exaggerated drug-induced surge or inhibition in the release of CA might result from pharmacological or physiological stimuli. Such altered responses may interact with sensitive feedback mechanisms in the developing CNS systems and induce the growth of compensatory neurochemical pathways. Although one must move cautiously in making cause and effect statements about drug exposure early in life and related neurochemical changes, research along these lines may provide valuable insight into the diagnosis and treatment of drug-related effects observed in children born to addicted mothers (Zimmermann and Sonderegger, 1980).

Effects on Opioid Receptors

A major unresolved issue is whether opioid agonist-induced tolerance and dependence in vivo and desensitization in vitro are associated with altered receptor numbers. It has been reported that chronic administration of morphine produces either no significant change in the adult CNS in opioid receptor number (Pert et al., 1973; Klee and Streaty, 1974; Hitzemann et al., 1974; Simon and Hiller, 1978; Bardo et al., 1982; Holaday et al., 1982; Perry et al., 1982) or a modest receptor up-regulation (Brady et al., 1989, Rothman et al., 1986). In contrast, chronic etorphine produces down-regulation of μ and δ receptors in vivo (Tao et al., 1988) and chronic enkephalin produces down-regulation of δ receptors in vivo (Tao et al., 1988; Steece et al., 1986) and in neurotumor cells (Hazum et al., 1981; Chang et al., 1982; Blanchard et al., 1983). Only in the 1-week-old rat pup, however, is there a correlation between morphine-induced receptor down-regulation and the development of tolerance (Tempel et al., 1988).

Antagonist-induced opioid supersensitivity and opioid receptor up-regulation are well correlated in the adult CNS. Long-term in vivo administration of the opioid antagonist naloxone or naltrexone results in enhanced morphine-induced analgesia (Tang and Collins, 1978; Lahti and Collins, 1978; Tempel et al., 1985; Yoburn et al., 1985) and enhanced effects of morphine on neurons of the locus ceruleus (Bardo et al., 1983) and the myenteric plexus (Schulz et al., 1979). This functional supersensitivity reflects both an increased number of μ and δ opioid receptors (Zukin et al., 1982; Brunello et all, 1984; Tempel et al., 1985; Danks et al., 1988; Millan et al., 1988; Yoburn et al., 1989a,b) and an increased coupling of receptor to the inhibitory guanyl nucleotide binding protein G_i (Zukin et al., 1982; Tempel et al., 1985). The changes in opioid receptor density vary heterogeneously throughout the brain; highest increases in μ receptor density occur in the nucleus accumbens, amygdala, striatum, layers I and III of the neocortex, and the periaqueductal gray region (Tempel et al., 1984).

Up-regulation of μ opioid receptors has also been observed in vitro using explant cultures of fetal mouse spinal cord with attached dorsal root ganglia (DRG) (Tempel et al., 1986). Long-term exposure of the explant cultures to naloxone produces an increase in μ opioid receptor density relative to control cultures, even in the presence of the protein synthesis inhibitor cycloheximide at a concentration that blocks > 95% protein synthesis. This finding suggests that antagonist-induced opioid receptor up-regulation does not require the synthesis of new receptor molecules.

A variety of studies in the adult CNS have documented that chronic opioid drugs regulate opioid peptide levels and that this regulation occurs at the level of gene expression. Chronic naltrexone treatment increases met-enkephalin-like immunoreactivity in the striatum and nucleus accumbens (Tempel et al., 1984). Chronic naltrexone also increases substance P immunoreactivity in the striatum (Tempel et al., 1990) and decreases β-endorphin immunoreactivity in the hypothalamus, thalamus, and amygdala (Ragavan et al., 1983). In an effort to determine the mechanism by which opioid antagonists stimulate enkephalin and substance P production, we examined the effects of naltrexone on the mRNA levels of preproenkephalin (PPE) and preprotachykinin (PPT; Tempel et al., 1990). Our study indicated that long-term blockade of opioid receptors by naltrexone leads to large increases in both PPE and PPT mRNA in the striatum. Chronic morphine treatment, on the other hand, decreases striatal PPE mRNA levels (Uhl et al., 1988). These findings suggest that activation or blockade of opioid receptors influence PPE and PPT gene expression.

How does naltrexone treatment lead to stimulation of PPE gene expression? Although the transsynaptic regulation of PPE transcription by specific neurotransmitters and drugs is well documented, only recently have some of the mechanisms underlying this regulation been revealed. A major pathway linking signals at the synapse to the PPE gene involves activation of G-protein linked receptors, leading to altered levels of cAMP, products of the inositol triphosphate pathway, and/or calcium. It is now well established that cAMP (and phorbol esters) can induce PPE gene expression by the activation of transcription factors that bind within the 5'-flanking region of the PPE gene (Comb et al., 1986; Angel et al., 1987). Recent studies (Comb et al., 1988; Hyman et al., 1988) have elucidated the detailed features of a portion of this enhancer region. Two functionally distinct elements, ENKCRE-1 and -2, have been identified and have been shown to activate transcription in a synergistic fashion. Four distinct proteins (or transcription factors) have been identified that bind to overlapping (but non-identical) sites in the region spanning the enhancer. These are ENKTF-1, a novel nuclear factor, which binds to the ENKCRE-1 element; AP-4 and AP-1, which bind to overlapping sites spanning the ENKCRE-2 element; and AP-2, which binds to a site downstream and adjacent to ENKCRE-2. The AP-1 factor is of particular interest because it is known to be a heterodimer comprised of the products of the c-*jun* and c-*fos* oncogenes, immediate-early genes or third messengers involved in the activation of gene transcription in response to neuronal cell stimulation (Gentz et al., 1989; Rauscher et al., 1988; Turner and Tijan, 1989). The c-*fos* oncogene is well known to be highly responsive to changes in levels of neural activity (Curran and Morgan, 1985). The formation of functional synapses during ontogeny requires the expression of opioid receptors in the appropriate postsynaptic neurons. Although the first appearance of opioid binding sites in the rat occurs prior to E14, their neuroanatomical distribution is different from that of adult brain (Clendeninn et al., 1976; Coyle and Pert, 1976; Young and Kuhar, 1979; Herkenham and Pert, 1981; Chapter 12). The different opioid receptor types are expressed at different times during brain development, although in each case the largest increases are observed between 3 and 15 days after birth (Petrillo et al., 1987). Mu opioid receptors are present in the mouse and rat brain at the time of birth and receptor density increases rapidly postnatally (Tavani et al., 1985; Petrillo et al., 1987). By contrast, δ receptors are not detectable until 7–10 days after birth (Tavani et al., 1985; Petrillo et al., 1987; Kent et al., 1982; Leslie et al., 1982; Spain et al., 1985; Tempel et al., 1988), and by 15 days after birth they have reached 50% of adult levels (Tavani et al., 1985). Kappa receptors are present at birth and their density reaches adult levels 1 week after birth (Leslie et al., 1982; Spain et al., 1985; Barr et al., 1986; Loughlin et al., 1985). These diverse patterns of development suggest that different mechanisms may regulate the expression of the various opioid receptor types.

Little is known about the mechanisms regulating the initial expression of opioid receptors. However, receptor development may be influenced quantitatively by a variety of factors in the neuronal environment. Antenatal or perinatal exposure to opioid agonists or antagonists (Bardo et al., 1983a,b) alters the apparent number of opioid receptors in the brain with concomitant changes in antinociceptive responses (Tempel et al., 1988; Handelmann and Quirion, 1983). In addition, stress, pain, and a variety of drugs and toxins alter receptor number (Torda, 1978; Kirby et al., 1982; Watanabe et al., 1983; Moon, 1984); however, the intracellular factors that regulate opioid receptor synthesis, insertion, and degradation are unknown.

Opioid analgesics are well known to produce tolerance and dependence in vivo and desensitization in vitro. Although the mechanisms for these phenomena are not clear, it has been postulated that chronic opioid treatment causes internalization of receptors followed by down-regulation. The majority of studies, however, have failed to show any systematic change in receptor number in adult rats following chronic opioid agonist treatment in vivo (Bardo et al., 1982; Hitzemann et al., 1974; Klee and Streaty, 1974; Perry et al., 1982; Pert et al., 1973; Simon and Hiller, 1978). Some investigators (Holaday et al., 1982), however, have reported an increase in opioid receptor density following chronic morphine treatment in adult rats. Others (Rogers and El-Fakahany, 1986) have shown that it is possible to induce an up- or down-regulation depending on the buffer system or tissue preparation used. Receptor down-regulation has been observed in neurotumor cell lives after chronic exposure to opioid peptides (Blanchard et a., 1983; Chang et al., 1982; Hazum et al., 1981; Simon and Hiller, 1978), but not to opioid alkaloids (Chang et al., 1982).

The ontogenesis of the opioid system is sensitive to pre- and postnatal exposure to drugs. Results from these studies are contradictory and complicated apparently due to differences in exposure time, dose and route of administration, and the age at which animals are tested. In some studies, morphine administration to pups increases μ ligand binding in the striatum and nucleus accumbens (Handelmann and Quirion, 1983), whereas other studies have failed to find any effect on binding following chronic prenatal morphine treatment (Bardo et al., 1982; Coyle and Pert, 1976). Morphine administration to the dam during pregnancy has also been reported to decrease binding during the first week of life (Kirby and Aronstam, 1983) and increase binding later in life (Iyengar and Rabii, 1982; Tsang and Ng, 1980). Chronic administration of opioid agonists during pre and/or postnatal development may alter opioid receptor ontogeny, and concomitantly, sensitivity to opioid drugs. Recently, down-regulation of opioid receptors was demonstrated in whole brain homogenates following chronic morphine treatment (Tempel et al., 1988). One week of prenatal morphine treatment via the dam produced a statistically significant 35% decrease in brain μ opioid receptors of offspring, on the day of birth. There was no significant change in the affinity. Interestingly, this down-regulation was no longer evident by postnatal day 14. Table I illustrates the time course of the down-regulation of brain μ opioid receptors following chronic prenatal treatment with morphine.

Protein values for both morphine-treated animals and saline control animals were not significantly different from one another for each age group, and thus, they do not account for the differences in receptor density seen between the two groups (Tempel et al., 1988). In a separate group of animals, the effects of chronic prenatal morphine treatment on GABA receptors were determined. There were no significant changes in GABA receptors following chronic morphine treatment, illustrating the specificity of the agonist-induced response on opioid receptors (Tempel et al., 1988).

Four days of daily postnatal (days 1–4) morphine treatment produced a significant 30% decrease in brain μ opioid receptors (Tempel et al., 1988). No change in δ or κ receptors was observed. Further treatment with morphine fails to result in any significant changes in μ opioid receptors relative to saline-treated (control) animals. In fact, the degree of μ opioid receptor down-regulation diminished over time (Table II) with the age of the animal. At postnatal day 14, there was no statistically significant difference in receptor density between brains of control and morphine-treated pups, as is observed in adult animals. When rat pups were chronically treated (for 7 or 14 days) with morphine beginning on postnatal day 14 and assayed on either postnatal day 22 or day 29, no significant differences in opioid receptors were detected relative to saline-treated (control) animals (Tempel et al., 1988). Thus, morphine-induced receptor down-regulation appears to occur only during the first week of life.

To visualize the neuroanatomical pattern of opiate receptor changes in specific brain regions, light microscopy receptor autoradiography was carried out on rat brain sections from control and chronic morphine-treated pups (Tempel, submitted). Four days of early postnatal morphine treat-

TABLE I. Changes in Brain μ Opioid Receptor Densities of Infant Rats Following Chronic Prenatal Treatment With Morphine

	[³H] DAGO binding[a]		
Postnatal day	Control (fmol/mg protein)	Morphine-treated (fmol/mg protein)	Change (%)
0	(4) 77 ± 2.3	(4) 50 ± 3.5	−35*
5	(4) 81 ± 4.3	(4) 59 ± 5.3	−27
14	(3) 81 ± 4.1	(3) 83 ± 4.7	↓2
28	(4) 132 ± 12.5	(4) 129 ± 11.7	−2

[a]DAGO, [D-Ala², MePhe⁴, Gly-ol⁵] enkephalin.
*Statistically significant difference (two-tailed t-test, $P < 0.05$). Pregnant female rats were exposed to morphine. Rat pups were sacrificed by decapitation on the day of parturition (day zero), and 5, 14, and 28 days postnatal. Values were generated by computer-assisted linear regression analysis. Receptor density values are reported as means ± S.E.M. from a minimum of three independent experiments. The number of animals per group for each time point are indicated in parentheses. (Reproduced from Tempel et al., 1988, with permission.)

TABLE II. Changes in Brain μ Opioid Receptor Densities of Infant Rats Following Chronic Postnatal Treatment With Morphine

Duration of treatment postparturition	[³H] DAGO binding		Change (%)
	Control (fmol/mg protein)	Morphine-treated (fmol/mg protein)	
4 days	(6) 81 ± 3.8	(6) 57 ± 3.3	−30*
8 days	(6) 74 ± 8.5	(6) 61 ± 11.5	−18
14 days	(4) 156 ± 5.7	(4) 135 ± 10.4	−13
28 days	(3) 132 ± 16.5	(3) 128 ± 8.4	−3

*Statistically significant difference (two-tailed t-test, $P < 0.05$). Neonatal rats were each given one daily subcutaneous injection of morphine or saline beginning on postnatal day 1. Rat pups were sacrificed by decapitation at the times indicated. Values were generated by computer-assisted linear regression analysis. Receptor density values are reported as means $\pm$ S.E.M. from a miimum of three experiments. The number of animals per group for each time point are indicated in parentheses. (Reproduced from Tempel et al., 1988, with permission.)

ment decreased μ opioid receptors by 44% in striosomes in caudate putamen. There was no significant change in the surrounding area. Mu binding in the nucleus accumbens was also significantly decreased following morphine treatment. These results are summarized in Table III. In contrast to what is seen following 4 days of morphine treatment (postnatal 1–4), 8 days of postnatal (postnatal 1–8) morphine treatment does not produce a significant loss in striatal μ opioid receptors. Thus, during a brief period of development, there is a unique plasticity of the immature opioid receptor system that is lost with maturation, however, the significance of these findings are unclear at this time and remain to be elucidated by further studies.

Several hypothesis can be proposed to explain our developmental results relative to adult rat CNS data. For this, we reference work from other

TABLE III. Changes in Striatal Opiate Receptor Densities Following Chronic Morphine Treatment[a]

Region	Control (fmol/mg protein)	Morphine-treated (fmol/mg protein)	Change (%)
Striatum			
patches	231 ± 9	129 ± 6	−44
matrix	80 ± 4	83 ± 3	+4
Nucleus accumbens	173 ± 5	122 ± 3	−29

[a]Receptor density values are reported as means $\pm$ S.E.M. of averaged values from the corresponding sections of a minimum of three rats.

neurotransmitter systems. In the adrenergic system, it has been shown that agonists produce down-regulation of β-adrenergic receptors. This down-regulation was shown to be associated with an internalization mechanism (Chung and Costa, 1979). Conversely, chronic treatment with β-adrenergic antagonists leads to up-regulation or an increase in β-adrenergic receptor number in adult animals (Galant et al., 1978) and in humans (Glaubiger and Lefkowitz, 1977). More recently, several laboratories working with the opioid system have shown that long-term exposure of neurotumor cell lines (Blanchard et al., 1983; Chang et al., 1982; Hazum et al., 1981; Simantov et al., 1982) and adult rats (Steece et al., 1986) to enkephalin results in a decrease in δ receptor density. Studies of [^{3}H][D-Ala^2, D-Leu^5]enkephalin (DADLE) uptake by N4TG1 cells (Blanchard et al., 1983; Chang et al., 1982; Hazum et al., 1981; Simantov et al., 1982) suggest that enkephalin is internalized via receptor-mediated endocytosis. One hypothesis to explain our findings is that long-term exposure of the system to opioid agonists or peptides leads to coupling of the receptors to cyclase, followed by internalization. As active receptors disappear from the membrane surface, they would be replaced by inactive or spare receptors. Three possibilities then exist. 1) If the rate of internalization exceeded reactivation, an apparent down-regulation in receptor density would be observed. 2) If the rate of reactivation paralleled internalization, no apparent change in receptor density would be observed. 3) If down-regulation involves internalization, degradation of receptors, and recycling or reactivation, it is possible that the internalization process is developed by birth but that the recycling process is not fully developed until 2–3 weeks postnatal. When the recycling process is developed, down-regulation is no longer seen because recycling takes place as quickly as internalization; therefore no difference in receptor number is observed.

Another possibility is that opioids affect second messenger systems. It is well known that opioids in the adult are coupled to adenylate cyclase in an inhibitory fashion via a guanyl nucleotide binding protein (referred to as G_i or N_i) (Stadel and Lefkowitz, 1981), however, whether this system is functional at an early age is not known. There may also be a different second messenger system operative in the developing CNS than in adults. In addition, recent electrophysiological studies of opioid effects on sensory DRG neurons in culture have shown that specific μ, δ, and κ opioid receptor agonists can evoke prolongation of the action potential in many cells especially when applied at low concentrations (1–10 nM) (Shen and Crain, 1989; Chen et al., 1988; Crain and Shen, 1990). This is in direct contrast to the shortening of action potentials generally observed at higher concentrations (~1 μM) (Chalazonitis and Crain, 1986). Although this evidence is indirect, the observation of opioid-induced prolongation of action potentials has been interpreted as evidence of excitatory effects of opioids on DRG neuron perikarya (Shen and Crain, 1989; Chen et al., 1988; Crain et al., 1988). This prolongation can be blocked by the opioid antagonists naloxone and diprenorphine at low concentrations (1–10 nM). In addition, opioid-induced prolongation is selectively blocked by cholera toxin A (Crain and Shen, 1990) which has been shown to adenosine diphosphate (ADP)-ribosylate G_s (Gill and Meren, 1978) and attenuate ligand activation of associated receptors (Stadel and Lefkowitz, 1981). In contrast, opioid-induced shortening is blocked by pertussis toxin (Shen and Crain, 1989) which ADP-ribosylates G_i and G_o and interferes with inhibitory receptor functions. These data suggest that excitatory effects of opioids on these neurons are mediated by opioid receptors that are positively coupled via a G_s-like protein to adenyl cyclase (Jones and Reed, 1989) resembling β-adrenoceptors. Inhibitory effects are mediated by opioid receptors linked to G_i/G_o resembling α_2-adrenoceptors (for review see Crain and Shen, 1990). In a separate series of experiments Crain and coworkers investigated the effects of opioid treatment on action potential duration. These researchers showed that chronic opioid exposure of DRG neurons produce a net increase in excitatory opioid receptor-mediated functions (i.e., adenyl cyclase activity and cAMP levels) (Shen and Crain, 1989; Crain and Shen, 1990). They suggest that some mechanisms underlying the development of tolerance and addiction may involve opioid receptor linkage to a G_s-binding protein.

In the developing CNS, it is not yet known which of the G-proteins are present, what proportions they are present in, and whether or not their interaction with the receptor and/or cyclase system is operational. All of these factors may be important in elucidating the mechanisms underlying addiction in the developing CNS in comparison to adult CNS tolerance.

Changes in Opioid Peptide Synthesis

A few clinical studies have examined the effects of prolonged opioid use on enkephalin levels in the newborn of opioid-dependent mothers. Endogenous opioid peptide levels in plasma of newborns of morphine and methadone-dependent mothers have been reported to remain elevated after birth for at least 40 days in the absence of withdrawal signs (Genazzani et al., 1986; Panerai et al., 1983). In contrast, there have been no reports of behavioral abnormalities in newborns exposed in utero to opioids (Bauman and Levine, 1986; Deren, 1986; Lesser-Katz, 1982).

Numerous studies have investigated the effects of chronic opioid treatment on brain enkephalin levels, but they have produced conflicting results. Implantation of morphine pellets in mature rats has been reported to reduce brain enkephalin levels after 3 days (Shani et al., 1979) or 11 days (Bergstrom and Terenius, 1983), but to have no effect after 5 days (Childers et al., 1977; Fratta et al., 1977) or 21 days (Shani et al., 1979). Some studies report marked decreases in β-endorphin as well as enkephalin in several discrete areas of the rat brain following treatment in adults with morphine pellets for 30 days (Holt et al., 1978; Przewlocki et al., 1979). Reduced met-enkephalin levels have also been reported in the hippocampus of the monkey after 10 days of morphine treatment (Elsworth et al., 1986).

In studies of the adult rat CNS, researchers have failed to detect any significant change in opioid peptide levels (Fratta et al., 1977; Wesche et al., 1977; Childers et al., 1977; Shani et al., 1979) in the brain following chronic morphine treatment. Little is known about the molecular alterations in the functioning of endogenous brain opioid peptide systems as a result of chronic exogenous opioid administration. Neither brain opioid receptors, second messenger systems, nor opioid peptide levels have been shown to vary consistently as a result of drug treatment (Akil et al., 1984; Collier, 1985; Redmond and Krystal, 1984; Rothman et al., 1986; Wüster et al., 1983). In a recent study by Uhl et al. (1988), the effect of chronic morphine treatment on opioid peptide gene expression in adult CNS was examined. These researchers demonstrated that rats made tolerant to morphine via subcutaneous implantation of pellets displayed a significant decrease in striatal PPE mRNA that persisted during the withdrawal period. In contrast, levels of met-enkephalin were normal at the end of opioid treatment that reduced after withdrawal.

In an effort to gain more insight into these mechanisms some researchers have turned to clonal cell lines in which to study these phenomena (Schwartz, 1988). In the NG108-15 neuroblastoma-glioma hybrid cell line, it has been demonstrated that enkephalin peptide content increases following exposure to cAMP (Braas et al., 1983; Yoshikawa and Sabol, 1986). The opioid receptor is known to be linked to adenylate cyclase in an inhibitory fashion (Sharma et al., 1975b). Tolerance and dependence that are produced in animals by chronic exposure to morphine can be reproduced in cells (Sharma et al., 1975a, 1977). Schwartz (1988) has shown that opioid agonists stimulate proenkephalin synthesis with increases seen in mRNA, precursor forms, and enkephalin peptides. However, these effects appear to occur independent of changes in adenylate cyclase activity or cAMP content. It is suggested that proenkephalin synthesis in NG108 cells can be regulated by two different mechanisms, one involving cAMP, while the other regulated by the opioid receptor, is yet to be determined.

In the developing CNS, the data become even more complicated to interpret, but there is also very little data in this new and emerging area of interest. In a preliminary study, Tempel et al. (unpublished) have found significant and contrasting effects of morphine treatment on preproenkephalin mRNA levels. Four days of postnatal (postnatal 1–4) morphine treatment produced a 24% *increase* in striatal proenkephalin mRNA levels. Interestingly, longer treatments with morphine (postnatal 1–14) *decreased* striatal PPE mRNA levels by 39%. This decrease is similar to what was observed in the adult striatum following chronic morphine treatment (Uhl et al., 1988). Interestingly, chronic naltrexone treatment produced the exact opposite affect. Four days of postnatal (postnatal 1–4) naltrexone treatment induced a 33% *decrease* in proenkephalin mRNA levels in striatal tissue whereas 8 days of treatment (postnatal 1–8) produced an *increase* (+23%) in opioid peptide gene expression (Table IV). The increase in gene expression is in the same direction, but smaller than that observed in the adult striatum (Tempel et al., 1990). These data suggest that the mechanisms underlying opioid addiction and withdrawal in the developing CNS differ from those in the adult brain. These differences may be due to the opioid receptor system's interaction with the G-protein/cAMP system.

Alternatively, a different second messenger system may be operative in the neonatal brain which could account for the difference seen in adult

TABLE IV. Changes in Striatal Proenkephalin mRNA Levels Following Chronic Naltrexone Treatment[a]

Duration of treatment postparturition	Control (PPE/1B15 mRNA)	Naltrexone-treated (PPE/1B15 mRNA)	Change (%)
4 days (3)	1.20	0.81	−33
8 days (4)	0.95	1.17	+23

[a]mRNA levels for PPE mRNA were normalized to 1B15 mRNA. Ratio values from control animals were compared to those of naltrexone-treated animals to calculate changes in mRNA levels. Alterations are expressed as percentage of control values.

versus neonatal brain following exogenous opiate administration. Future research along these lines will provide valuable information into the mechanisms of addiction and tolerance which will in turn provide insight into the diagnosis and treatment of drug-related effects observed in children born to addicted mothers. Moreover, such studies offer a unique view into the function of the opiate system in normal animals.

REFERENCES

Akil H, Watson SJ, Young E, Lewis ME, Khachaturian H, Walker JM (1984): Endogenous opioids: Biology and function. Ann Rev Neurosci 7:223–255.

Angel P, Imagawa M, Chiu R, Stein B, Imbra RJ, Rahmsdorf HJ, Jonat C, Herrlich P, Karin M (1987): Phorbol ester-inducible genes contain a common cis element recognized by a TPA-modulated trans-acting factor. Cell 49:729–739.

Auguy-Valette A, Cros J, Gouarderes C, Gout R, Pontonnier G (1978): Morphine analgesia and cerebral opiate receptors: A developmental study. Br J Pharmacol 63:303–308.

Bakke JL, Lawrence N, Bennerr J (1973): Late endocrine effects of administering monosodium glutamate to neonatal rats. Biol Neonate 23:59–77.

Bannerjee U (1974): Programmed self-administration of potentially addictive drugs in young rats and its effects on learning. Psychopharmacologia (Berlin) 38:111–124.

Bardo MT, Bhatnager RK, Gebhart GF (1981): Opiate receptor ontogeny and morphine induced effects: Influence of chronic footshock stress in preweanling rats. Dev Brain Res 1:487–495.

Bardo MT, Bhatnagar KP, Gebhart FF (1982): Differential effects of chronic morphine and naloxone on opiate receptors, monoamines and morphine-induced behaviors in preweanling rats. Dev Brain Res 4:139–147.

Bardo MT, Bhatnagar RK, Gebhart GF (1983a): Age-related differences in the effect of chronic administration of naloxone on opiate binding in rat brain. Neuropharmacology 22:453–461.

Bardo MT, Bhatnagar RK, Gebhart GF (1983b): Chronic naltrexone increases opiate binding in brain and produces supersensitivity to morphine in the locus coeruleus of the rat. Brain Res 289:223–234.

Barr GA, Paredes W, Erickson KL, Zukin RS (1986): κ-opioid receptor-mediated analgesia in the developing rat. Dev Brain Res 28:145–152.

Bauman PS, Levine SA (1986): The development of children of drug addicts. Int J Addict 21:849–863.

Bayon A, Shoemaker WJ, Bloom FE, Mauss A, Guillemin R (1979): Perinatal development of the endorphin- and enkephalin-containing systems in the rat brain. Brain Res 179:93–101.

Beitner DB, Duman RS, Nestler EJ (1989): A novel action of morphine in the rat locus coeruleus: Persistent decrease in adenylate cyclase. Mol Pharmacol 35:-559–564.

Bergstrom L, Terenius L (1983): Enkephalin levels decrease in rat striatum during morphine abstinence. Eur J Pharmacol 60:349–352.

Blanchard SG, Chang KJ, Cuatrecasas P (1983): Characterization of the association of tritiated enkephalin with neuroblastoma cells under conditions optimal for receptor downregulation. J Biol Chem 258:1092–1097.

Bloom F, Bayon A, Battenberg E, French E, Koda L, Koob G, LeMoal M, Rossier J, Shoemaker W (1980): Endorphins: Developmental, cellular and behavioral aspects. In Costa E, Trabucchi M (eds): "Neural Peptides and Neuronal Communication." New York: Raven Press, pp 619–632.

Braas KA, Childers SR, U'Prichard DC (1983): Induction of differentiation increases Met⁵-enkephalin and leu⁵-enkephalin content in NG108-15 hybrid cells: An immunocytochemical and biochemical analysis. J Neurosci 3:1713–1727.

Brady LS, Herkenham M, Long JB, Rotham RB (1989): Chronic morphine increases μ-opiate receptor binding in rat brain: A quantitative autoradiographic study. Brain Res 477:382–386.

Brunello N, Volterra A, DiGiulio AM, Cuomo V, Racagni G (1984): Modulation of opioid system in C57 mice after repeated treatment with morphine and naloxone: Biochemical and behavioral correlates. Life Sci 34:1669–1678

Buchenauer C, Turnbow M, Peters MA (1974): Effect of chronic methadone administration on pregnant rats and their offspring. J Pharmacol Exp Ther 189:66–71.

Carr JN (1975): Drug patterns among drug-addicted mothers: Incidence, variance in use, and effects on children. Pediatr Ann 4:408–417.

Chalazonitis A, Crain SM (1986): Maturation of opioid sensitivity of fetal mouse dorsal root ganglion neuron perikarya in organotypic cultures: Regulation by spinal cord. Neuroscience 17:1181–1198.

Chandler JM, Robie P, Schoolar J, Desmond MM (1975): The effects of methadone on maternal-fetal interactions in the rat. J Pharmacol Exp Ther 192:549–554.

Chang KJ, Eckel RW, Blanchard SG (1982): Opioid peptides induce reduction of enkephalin receptors in cultured neuroblastoma cells. Nature 296:446–448.

Chen GG, Chalazonitis A, Shen KF, Crain SM (1988): Inhibitor of cyclic AMP-dependent protein kinase blocks opioid-induced prolongation of the action potential of mouse sensory ganglion neurons in dissociated cell cultures. Brain Res 462:372–377.

Childers SR, Simantov R, Snyder SH (1977): Enkephalin: Radioimmunoassay and radioreceptor assay in morphine dependent rats. Eur J Pharmacol 46:289–293.

Chuang DM, Costa E (1979): Evidence for internalization of the recognition site of β-adrenergic receptors during receptor subsensitivity induced by (-)isoproterenol. Proc Natl Acad Sci USA 76:3024–3028.

Clendeninn NJ, Petraitis M, Simon EJ (1976): Ontological development of opiate receptors in rodent brain. Brain Res 118:157–160.

Clouet DH (1977): Drug induced delay following morphine treatment. In Blum K (ed): "Alcohol and Opiates." New York: Academic Press, pp 237–255.

Clouet DH, Ratner M (1970): Catecholamine biosynthesis in brains of rats treated with morphine. Science 168:854–856.

Collier HOJ (1985): A general theory of the genesis of drug dependence by induction of receptors. Nature 205:181–183.

Collier HOJ, Roy AC (1974): Morphine-like drugs inhibit the stimulation of E prostaglandins of cyclic AMP formation by rat brain homogenate. Nature 248:24–27.

Comb M, Birnberg NC, Seasholtz A, Herbert E, Goodman HM (1986): A cyclic AMP- and phorbol ester-inducible DNA element. Nature 323:353–356.

Comb M, Mermod N, Hyman SE, Pearlberg J, Ross ME, Goodman H (1988): Proteins bound at adjacent DNA elements act synergistically to regulate human proenkephalin cAMP inducible transcription. Embo J 7:3793–3805.

Costa T, Klinz FJ, Vachon L, Herz A (1988): Opioid receptors are coupled tightly to G proteins but loosely to adenylate cyclase in NG108-15 cell membranes. Mol Pharmacol 34:744–754.

Coyle JT (1976): Regional studies of catecholamine development in rat brain. In Brazier MAB, Coceani F (eds): "Brain Dysfunction in Infantile Febrile Convulsions." New York: Raven Press, pp 25–39.

Coyle JT, Pert CB (1976): Ontogenetic development of [³H] naloxone binding in rat brain. Neuropharmacology 15:555–560.

Crain SM, Shen KF (1990): Opioids can evoke direct receptor-mediated excitatory effects on sensory neurons. Trends Pharmacol Sci 11:77–81.

Crain SM, Shen KF, Chalazonitis A (1988): Opioids excite rather than inhibit sensory neurons after chronic opioid exposure of spinal cord-ganglion cultures. Brain Res 455:99–109.

Curran T, Morgan JI (1985): Superinduction of c-fos by nerve growth factor in the presence of peripherally active benzodiazepines. Science 229:1265–1268.

Danks JA, Tortella FC, Bykov V, Jacobson AE, Rice J, Holaday W, Rothman RB (1988): Chronic administration of morphine and naltrexone up-regulate [³H]D-Ala2, D-leu⁵-enkephalin binding sites by different mechanisms. Neuropharmacology 27:965–974.

Davis WM, Lin CH (1972): Prenatal morphine effects on survival and behavior of rat offspring. Res Commun Chem Pathol Pharmacol 3:205–214.

Deren S (1986): Children of substance abusers: A review of the literature. J Subst Abuse Treat 3:77–94.

Diaz J, Paul L, Frenk H, Bailey B (1978): Permanent alterations of central opiate systems as a result of chronic opiate antagonism during infancy in rats. Proc West Pharmacol Soc 21:377–379.

DiGiulio AM, Restant P, Galli CL, Tenconi R, LaCroix R, Gorio A (1988): Modified ontogenesis of enkephalin and substance P containing neurons after perinatal exposure to morphine. Toxicology 49:197–201.

Dole VP, Nyswander MA (1965): Medical treatment for diacetyl-morphine (heroin) addiction. JAMA 193:646–650.

Duman RS, Tallman JF, Nestler EJ (1988): Acute and chronic opiate regulation of adenylate cyclase in brain: Specific effects in locus coeruleus. J Pharmacol Exp Ther 246:1033–1039.

Elsworth JD, Redmond Jr DE, Roth RH (1986): Effect of morphine treatment and withdrawal on endogenous methionine- and leucine-enkephalin levels in primate brain. Biochem Pharmacol 35:3415–3417.

Florio VA, Sternwies PC (1985): Reconstitution of resolved muscarinic cholinergic receptors with purified GTP-binding proteins. J Biol Chem 260:3477–3483.

Ford D, Rhines R (1979): Prenatal exposure to methadone HC1 in relationship to body and brain growth in the rat. Acta Neurol Scand 59:248–262.

Fratta W, Yang HYT, Hong J, Costa E (1977): Stability of met-enkephalin content in brain structures of morphine-dependent or foot-shock stressed rats. Nature 268:452–453.

Freeman PR (1980): Methadone exposure in utero: Effects on open-field activity in weanling rats. Int J Neurosci 11:295–300.

Friedler G (1972): Growth retardation in offspring of female rats treated with morphine prior to conception. Science 175:645–655.

Fung BK-K (1983): Characterization of transducin from bovine retinal rod outer segments. I. Separation and reconstitution of the subunits. Biol Chem 258:-10495–10502.

Galant SP, Durisetti L, Underwood S, Insel PA (1978): Decreased β-adrenergic receptors on polymorphonuclear leukocytes after adrenergic therapy. N Engl J Med 299:933–936.

Garcin F, Coyle JT (1976): Ontogenetic development of [3H] naloxone binding and endogenous morphine-like factor in rat brain. In Kosterlitz HW, (ed): "Opiates and Endogenous Opioid Peptides." New York: Elsevier/North Holland Biomedical Press, pp 267–273.

Geber WF, and Schramm LC (1975): Congenital malformations of the central nervous system produced by narcotic analgesics in the hamster. Am J Obstet Gynecol 123:705–713.

Genazzani AR, Petraglia F, Guidetti R, Volpe A, Facchinetti F (1986): Neonatal β-endorphin secretion in babies passively addicted to opiates. Int Congr Ser Excerpta Med 369:379–382.

Gentz R, Rauscher II, Abate FJ, Curran T (1989): Parallel association of Fos and Jun leucine zippers juxtaposes DNA binding domains. Science 010.1050–1099.

Gibson DA, Vernadakis A (1983): Critical period for LAAM in the chick embryo: Toxicity and altered opiate receptor binding. Dev Brain Res 8:61–69.

Gill DM, Meren R (1978): ADP-ribosylation of membrane proteins catalyzed by cholera toxin: Basis of the activation of adenylate cyclase. Proc Natl Acad Sci USA 75:3050–3054.

Gilman AG (1987): G proteins: Transducers of receptor-generated signals. Annu Rev Biochem 56:615–649.

Glaubiger G, Lefkowitz RJ (1977): Elevated β-adrenergic receptor number after chronic propranolol treatment. Biochem Biophys Res Commun 78:720–725.

Goodfriend MJ, Shey IA, Klein MD (1956): The effects of maternal narcotic addiction on the newborn. Am J Obstet Gynecol 71:29–36.

Grove LV, Etkin MK, Rosencrans JA (1979): Behavioral effects of fetal and neonatal exposure to methadone in the rat. Neurobehav Toxicol Teratol 1:87–95.

Guidotti A, Grandison L (1979): Participation of endorphins in the regulation of pituitary function. In Usdin E, Bunney WE, Kline NS (eds): "Endorphins in Mental Health Research." New York: Oxford, pp 416–422.

Guitart X, Nestler EJ (1989): Identification of morphine and cyclic AMP-regulated phosphoproteins (MARPPs) in the locus coeruleus and other regions of rat brain. Regulation by acute and chronic morphine. J Neurosci 9:4371–4387.

Guitart X, Nestler EJ (1990): Identification of MARPP (14–20), morphine-morphine- and cyclic AMP-regulated phosphoproteins of 14-20 kDa, as myelin basic proteins: Evidence for their acute and chronic regulation by morphine in rat brain. Brain Res 516:57–65.

Guitart X, Hayward MD, Nissenbaum LK, Beitner DB, Haycock JW, Nestler EJ (1990): Identification of MARPP-58, a morphine- and cyclic AMP-regulated phosphoprotein of 58 kDa, as tyrosine hydroxylase. J Neurosci 10:2649–2659.

Handelmann GE, Quirion R (1983): Neonatal exposure to morphine increases μ opiate binding in the adult forebrain. Eur J Pharmacol 94:357–358.

Harry GJ, Rosecrans JA (1979): Behavioral effects of perinatal naltrexone exposure: A preliminary investigation. Pharmacol Biochem Behav 11 Suppl:19–22.

Hazum E, Chang KJ, Cuatrecasas P (1981): Receptor redistribution induced by hormones and neurotransmitters: Possible relationship to biological functions. Neuropeptides 1:217–230.

Herkenham M, Pert CB (1981): Mosaic distribution of opiate receptors, parafascicular projections and acetylcholinesterase in rat striatum. Nature 291:415–418.

Hetta J, Terenius L (1980): Prenatal naloxone affects survival and morphine sensitivity of rat offspring. Neurosci Lett 16:323–327.

Hitzemann R, Hitzemann B, Loh H (1974): Binding of [3H] naloxone in the mouse brain: Effect of ions and tolerance development. Life Sci 14:2393–2404.

Hofer MA (1984): Relationships as regulators: A psychobiologic perspective on bereavement. Psychosom Med 46:183–197.

Holaday JW, Hitzemann RJ, Curell J, Tortella FC, Belenky GL (1982): Repeated electroconvulsive shock or chronic morphine treatment increases the number of [³H]D-Ala2 D-Leu⁵-enkephalin binding sites in rat brain membranes. Life Sci 31:2359–2362.

Holt V, Przewlocki R, Herz A (1978): β-Endorphin-like immunoreactivity in plasma, pituitaries and hypothalamus of rats following treatment with opiates. Life Sci 23:1057–1066.

Householder J, Hatcher R, Burns W, Chasnoff I (1982): Infants born to narcotic-addicted mothers. Psychol Bull 92:453–468.

Hutchings DE (1983): Behavioral teratology: A new frontier in behavioral research. In Johnson EM, Kochhar DM (eds): "Teratogenesis and Reproductive Toxicology." Berlin and New York: Springer-Verlag, pp 207–232.

Hutchings DE (1985a): Issues of methodology and interpretation in clinical and animal behavioral teratology studies. Neurobehav Toxicol Teratol 7:639–642.

Hutchings DE (1985b): Prenatal opioid exposure and the problem of casual inference. In Pinkert TM (ed): "Current Research on the Consequences of Maternal Drug Use." National Institute on Drug Abuse Research Series. DHHS Pub. No. (ADM) 85-1400. Washington, DC: US Govt Printing Office, pp 6–9.

Hutchings DE (1985c): "Methadone: A Treatment for Drug Addiction." New York: Chelsea House.

Hutchings DE Bodnarenko SR, Diaz-DeLeon R (1984): Phencyclidine during pregnancy in the rat: Effects on locomotor activity in the offspring. Pharmacol Biochem Behav 20:251–254.

Hutchings DE, Fifer WP (1986): Neurobehavioral effects in human and animal offspring following prenatal exposure to methadone. In Riley EP, Vorhees CV (eds): "Handbook of Behavioral Teratology." New York: Plenum Press, pp 341–367.

Hyman SE, Comb M, Young SL, Pearlberg J, Green MR, Goodman HM (1988): A common transacting factor is involved in transcriptional regulation of neurotransmitter genes by cyclic AMP. Mol Cell Biol 8:4225–4233.

Iyengar S, Rabii J (1982): Effect of prenatal exposure to morphine on the postnatal development of opiate receptors. Fed Proc 41:1354–1357.

Joffee J, Peterson J, Smith D, Soyka L (1976): Sub-lethal effects on offspring of male rats treated with methadone before mating. Res Commun Chem Pathol Pharmacol 13:611–621.

Jones DT, Reed RR (1989): Golf: An olfactory neuron specific-G protein involved in odorant signal transduction. Science 244:790–795.

Kent JL, Pert CB, Herkenham M (1982): Ontogeny of opiate receptors in rat forebrain: Visualization by in vitro autoradiography. Dev Brain Res 2:487–504.

Kirby ML (1981): Development of opiate receptor binding in rat spinal cord. Brain Res 205:400–404.

Kirby ML, Aronstam RS (1983): Levorphanol-sensitive [3H] naloxone binding in developing brainstem following prenatal morphine exposure. Neurosci Lett 35:191–195.

Kirby ML, Gale TF, Mattio TC (1982): Effects of prenatal capsaicin treatment on fetal spontaneous activity, opiate receptor binding, and acid phosphatase in the spinal cord. Exp Neurol 76:298–308.

Klee WA, Streaty RA (1974): Narcotic receptor sites in morphine-dependent rats. Nature 248:61–63.

Koch B, Sakly M, Lutz-Bucher B (1980): Ontogeny of opiate receptor sites in brain: Apparent lack of low affinity sites during early neonatal life. Horm Metab Res 12:342–343.

Lahti RA, Collins RJ (1978): Chronic naloxone results in prolonged increases in opiate binding sites in brain. Eur J Pharmacol 51:185–186.

Law PY, Wu J, Koehler J, Loh HHJ (1981): Demonstration and characterization of opiate inhibition of the striatal adenylate cyclase. J Neurochem 36:1834–1846.

Leslie FM, Tso S, Hurlbut DE (1982): Differential appearance of opiate receptor subtypes in neonatal rat brain. Life Sci 31:1393–1396.

Lesser-Katz M (1982): Some effects of maternal drug addiction on the neonate. Int J Addict 17:887–896.

Loughlin SE, Massamiri T, Kornblum HI, Leslie FM (1985): Postnatal development of opioid systems in rat brain. Neuropeptides 5:469–472.

Mayorga LS, Diaz R, Stahl PD (1989): Regulatory role for GTP-binding proteins in endocytosis. Science 244:1475–1477.

McGinty JF, Ford DH (1976): The effects of maternal morphine or methadone intake on the growth reflex development and maze behavior of rat offspring. In Ford DH, Clouet DH (eds): "Tissue Responses to Addictive Drugs." New York: Spectrum Publications, pp 611–629.

McGinty JF, Ford DH (1980): Effects of prenatal methadone on rat brain catecholamines. Dev Neurosci 3:224–234.

McLaughlin PJ, Zagon IS (1980): Body and organ development of young rats maternally exposed to methadone. Biol Neonate 38:15–26.

McLaughlin PJ, Zagon IS, White WJ (1978): Perinatal methadone exposure in rats: Effects on body and organ development. Biol Neonate 34:48–54.

Meyer SL, Riley EP (1986): Behavioral teratology of alcohol. In Riley E, Vorhees C (eds): "Handbook of Behavioral Teratology." New York: Plenum, pp 709–737.

Middaugh LD, Simpson LW (1980): Prenatal maternal methadone effects on pregnant C57BL/6 mice and their offspring. Neurobehav Toxicol Teratol 2:307–313.

Millan MJ, Morris BJ, Herz A (1988): Antagonist-induced opioid receptor up-regulation. I. Characterization of supersensitivity to selective μ and κ agonists. J Pharmacol Exp Ther 247:721–728.

Monder H, Yasukawa N, Christian JJ (1980): Perinatal ACTH-naloxone treatment: Effects on physical and behavioral development. Horm Behav 14:329–336.

Moon SL (1984): Prenatal haloperidol alters striatal dopamine and opiate receptors. Brain Res 323(1):109–113.

Moore RY, Bloom FE (1979): Central catecholamine neuron systems: Anatomy and physiology of the norepinephrine and epinephrine systems. Ann Rev Neurosci 2:113–168.

Nestler EJ, Beitner DB, Hayward M, Sevarino KA, Terwilliger R (1990): A general role for adaptations in G-proteins and the cyclic AMP system in mediating the chronic actions of morphine and cocaine on brain function. Abs Soc Neurosci 16:928.

Nestler EJ, Erdos JJ, Terwilliger R, Duman RS, Tallman JF (1989): Regulation by chronic morphine of G-proteins in the rat locus coeruleus. Brain Res 476:230–239.

Nestler EJ, Tallman JF (1988): Chronic morphine treatment increases cyclic AMP-dependent protein kinase activity in the rat locus coeruleus. Mol Pharmacol 33:127–132.

Panerai AE, Martini A, DiGiulio AM, Fraioli F, Vegni C, Pardi G, Marini A, Mantegazza P (1983): Plasma β-endorphin, β-lipotropin, and met-enkephalin concentrations during pregnancy in normal and drug-addicted women and their newborn. J Clin Endocrinol Metab 57:537–543.

Parvez H, Gipois D, Parvez S (1979): Maintenance of central and peripheral monoamine oxidase activity in developing rats subjected to disturbed alimentary rhythms and undernutrition. Biol Neonate 35(3–6):279–289.

Pasternak GW, Zhong-Zhang A, Tecott L (1980): Developmental differences between high and low affinity opiate binding studies: Their relationship to analgesia and respiratory depression. Life Sci 27:1185–1190.

Patey G, de la Baume S, Gros C, Schwartz J (1980): Ontogenesis of enkephalinergic systems in rat brain: Postnatal changes in enkephalin levels, receptors and degrading enzyme activities. Life Sci 27:245–252.

Paul L, Diaz J, Bailey B (1978): Behavioral effects of chronic narcotic antagonist administration to infant rats. Neuropharmacology 17:655–657.

Perry DC, Rosenbaum JS, Sadee W (1982): In vitro binding of [³H]etorphine in morphine-dependent rats. Life Sci 31:1405–1408.

Pert CB, Pasternak G, Snyder SH (1973): Opiate agonists and antagonists discriminated by receptor binding in brain. Science 182:1359–1361.

Peters MA (1978): A comparative study on the behavioral response of offspring of female rats chronically treated with methadone and morphine. Proc West Pharmacol Soc 21:411–418.

Peters MA, Turnbow M, Buchenauer D (1972): The distribution of methadone in the nonpregnant, pregnant, and fetal rat after acute methadone treatment. J Pharmacol Exp Ther 181:273–278.

Petrillo P, Tavani A, Verotta D, Robson LE, Kosterlitz HW (1987): Differential postnatal development of μ-, δ- and κ-opioid binding sites in rat brain. Brain Res 428:53–58.

Provost NM, Somers DE, Hurley JB (1988): A *Drosophila melanogaster* G protein α subunit gene is expressed primarily in embryos and pupae. J Biol Chem 263:12070–12076.

Przewlocki R, Hollt V, Duka T, Kleber G, Gransch C, Haarmann I, Herz A (1979): Long-term morphine treatment decreases endorphin levels in rat brain and pituitary. Brain Res 174:357–361.

Ragavan VV, Wardlaw SL, Kreek MJ, Frantz AG (1983): Effect of chronic naltrexone and methadone administration on brain immunoreactive β-endorphin in the rat. Neuroendocrinology 37:266–268.

Rasmussen K, Beitner-Johnson DB, Krystal JH, Aghajanian GK, Nestler EJ (1990): Opiate withdrawal and the rat locus coeruleus: Behavioral, electrophysiological and biochemical correlates. J Neurosci 10:2308–2317.

Rauscher III FJ, Cohen DR, Curran T, Bos TJ, Vogt PK, Bohmann D, Tijan R, Franza Jr BR (1988): Fos-associated protein p39 is the product of the jun proto-oncogene. Science 240:1010–1016.

Raye JR, Dubin JW, Blechner JN (1977): Fetal growth retardation following maternal morphine administration: Nutrition or drug effects? Biol Neonate 32:222–228.

Rech RH, Lomuscio G, Algeri S (1980): Methadone exposure in utero: Effects on brain biogenic amines and behavior. Neurobehav Toxicol Teratol 2:75–78.

Redmond DE, Krystal JH (1984): Multiple mechanisms of withdrawal from opioid drugs. Ann Rev Neurosci 7:443–478.

Rogers NF, El-Fakahany EE (1986): Morphine-induced opioid receptor down-regulation detected in intact adult rat brin cells. Eur J Pharmacol 124:221–230.

Rothman RB, Danks JA, Jacobson AE, Burke TR Jr, Rice KC, Tortella FC, Holaday JW (1986): Morphine tolerance increases μ- noncompetitive β-binding sites. Eur J Pharmacol 124:113–119.

Sakellaridis N, Vernadakis A (1987): The chick embryo vs. neural tissue culture as models for the study of opiate neurotoxicity in development. In Shahar A, Goldberg A (eds): "Model Systems in Neurotoxicology: Alternative Approaches to Animal Testing." New York: Alan R. Liss, pp 85–100.

Salerno LJ (1977): Prenatal care. In Rementeria JL (ed): "Drug Abuse in Prenancy and Neonatal Effects." St. Louis: C.V. Mosby Co, pp 19–29.

Sandman CA, McGivern RF, Berka C, Walker JM, Coy DH, Kastin AJ (1979): Neonatal administration of β-endorphin produces chronic insensitivity to thermal stimuli. Life Sci 25.1755–1760.

Schoffelmeer ANM, Hansen HA, Stoff JC, Mulder AH (1986): Blockade of D-2 dopamine receptors strongly enhances the potency of enkephalins to inhibit dopamine-sensitive adenylate cyclase in rat neostriatum: Involvement of δ- and μ-opioid receptors. J Neurosci 6:2235–2239.

Schulz R, Wuster M, Herz A (1979): Supersensitivity to opioids following the chronic blockade of endorphin action by naloxone. Naunyn Schmiedebergs Arch Pharmacol 306:93–96.

Schwartz JP (1988): Chronic exposure to opiate agonists increases proenkephalin biosynthesis in NG108 cells. Mol Brain Res 3:141–146.

Seidler FJ, Whitmore WL, Slotkin TA (1982): Delays in growth and biochemical development of rat brain caused by maternal methadone administration: Are the alterations in synaptogenesis and cellular maturation independent of reduced maternal food intake? Dev Neurosci 5:13–18.

Shah NS, Donald AG (1979): Pharmacological effects and metabolic fate of levomethadone during post-natal development in rat. J Pharmacol Exp Ther 208:491–497.

Shani J, Azov R, Weissman BA (1979): Enkephalin levels in rat brain after various regimens of morphine administration. Neurosci Lett 12:319–322.

Sharma SK, Klee WA, Nirenberg M (1975a): Dual regulation of adenylate cyclase accounts for narcotic dependence and tolerance. Proc Natl Acad Sci USA 72:3092–3096.

Sharma SK, Klee WA, Nirenberg M (1977): Opiate-dependent modulation of adenylate cyclase. Proc Natl Acad Sci USA 74:3365–3369.

Sharma SK, Nirenberg M, Klee WA (1975b): Morphine receptors as regulators of adenylate cyclase activity. Proc Natl Acad Sci USA 74:3365–3369.

Sharma SK, Nirenberg M, Klee WA (1975a): Dual regulation of adenylate cyclase accounts for narcotic dependence and tolerance. Proc Natl Acad Sci USA 72:590–594.

Shen KF, Crain SM (1989): Dual opioid modulation of the action potential duration of mouse dorsal root ganglion neurons in culture. Brain Res 491:227–242.

Sibley DR, Lefkowitz RJ (1985): Molecular mechanisms of receptor desensitization using the β-adrenergic receptor-coupled adenylate cyclase system as a model. Nature 317:124–129.

Simantov D, Baram D, Levy R, Hadler H (1982): Enkephalins and a-adrenergic receptors: Evidence for both common and differentiable regulatory pathways and down-regmulation of the enkephalin receptor. Life Sci 31:1323–1326.

Simantov R, Levy R, Baram D (1982): Down-regulation of enkephalin δ receptors -demonstration in membrane-bound and solubilized receptors. Biochim Biophys Acta 721:478–484.

Simon EJ, Hiller JM (1978): In vitro studies on opiate receptors and their ligands. Fed Proc 37:141–146.

Slotkin TA, Anderson TR (1975): Sympatho-adrenal development in perinatally addicted rats. Addict Dis Int J 2:293–306.

Slotkin TA, Lau C, Bartolome M (1976): Effects of neonatal or maternal methadone administration on ornithine decarboxylase activity in brain and heart of developing rats. J Pharmacol Exp Ther 199:141–148.

Slotkin TA, Seidler FJ, Whitmore WL (1980): Effects of maternal methadone administration on ornithine decarboxylase in brain and heart of the offspring: relationships of enzyme activity to dose and to growth impairment in the rat. Life Sci 26:861–867.

Slotkin TA, Weigle SJ, Whitmore WL, Seidler FJ (1982): Maternal methadone administration: Deficient in development of α-noradrenergic responses in developing rat brain as assessed by norepinephrine stimulation of ^{33}Pi incorporation into phospholipids in vivo. Biochem Pharmacol 31:1899–1902.

Slotkin TA, Whitmore WL, Salvaggio M, Seidler FJ (1979): Perinatal methadone addiction affects brain synaptic development of biogenic amine systems in the rat. Life Sci 24:1223–1230.

Smith AA, Hui FW, Crofford MJ (1977): Inhibition of growth in young mice treated with d, 1-methadone. Eur J Pharmacol 43:307–314.

Smith CB, Sheldon MI, Bednarczyk HJ, Villarreal J (1972): Inhibition of cell development following prenatal morphine exposure. J Pharmacol Exp Ther 180:547–557.

Sobrian SK (1977): Prenatal morphine administration alters behavioral development in the rat. Pharmacol Biochem Behav 7:285–288.

Sonderegger T, O'Shea S, Zimmermann E (1979): Progeny of a male rats addicted neonatally to morphine. Proc West Pharm Soc 22:137–139.

Spain JW, Roth BL, Coscia CJ (1985): Differential ontogeny of multiple opioid receptors (μ, δ, and κ). J Neurosci 5:584–588.

Sparber SB, Lichtblau LM (1985): Methadone and heroin: A review of behavioral effects in animal offspring. Neurobehav Toxicol Teratol 7:74–96.

Stadel JM, Lefkowitz RJ (1981): Differential effects of cholera toxin on guanine nucleotide regulation of β-adrenergic agonist high affinity binding and adenylate cyclase activation in frog erythrocyte membranes. J Cyclic Nucleotide Res 7:363–374.

Steece KA, DeLeon-Jones FA, Meyerson LR, Lee JM, Fields JZ, Ritzmann RF (1986): In vivo downregulation of rat striatal opioid receptors by chronic enkephalin. Brain Res Bull 17:255–257.

Sternweis PC (1986): The purified α subunits of Go and Gi from bovine brain require β-γ for association with phospholipid vesicles. J Biol Chem 261:631–637.

Stryer L (1986): Cyclic GMP cascade of vision. Ann Rev Neurosci 9:87–119.

Sutcliffe J, Molner R, Shinnick T, Bloom F (1983): Identifying the protein products of brain specific genes with antibodies to chemically synthesized peptides. Cell 33:671–682.

Takagi H, Nakama M (1968): Studies on the mechanism of action of tetrabenazine as a morphine antagonist II. A participation of catecholamine in the antagonism. Jpn J Pharmacol 18:54–58.

Tang AH, Collins RJ (1978): Enhanced analgesic effects of morphine after chronic administration of naloxone in the rat. Eur J Pharmacol 47:173–174.

Tao PL, Chang LR, Law PY, Loh HH (1988): Decrease in δ-receptor density in rat brain after chronic (D-Ala^2, D-Leu^5) enkephalin treatment. Brain Res 462:313–320.

Tavani A, Robson L, Kosterlitz HW (1985): Differential postnatal development of μ, δ, and κ opioid binding sites in mouse brain. Dev Brain Res 23:306–309.

Tempel A, Crain SM, Peterson ER, Simon EJ, Zukin RS (1986): Antagonist-induced opiate receptor upregulation in cultures of fetal mouse spinal cord-ganglion explants. Brain Res 390:287.

Tempel A, Gardner EL, Zukin RS (1984): Visualization of opiate receptor upregulation by light microscopy autoradiography. Proc Natl Acad Sci USA 81:3893–3897.

Tempel A, Gardner EL, Zukin RS (1985): Neurochemical and functional correlates of naltrexone-induced opiate receptor upregulation. J Pharmacol Exp Ther 232:439–444.

Tempel A, Habas J, Paredes W, Barr GA (1988): Morphine-induced downregulation of μ-opioid receptors in neonatal rat brain. Dev Brain Res 41:129–133.

Tempel A, Kessler JA, Zukin RS (1990): Chronic naltrexone treatment increases expression of preproenkephalin and preprotachykin in mRNA in discrete brain regions. J Neurosci 10:741–747.

Terry CE, Pellens M (1970): "The Opium Problem." New Jersey: Patterson Smith (originally published in 1928 by the Bureau of Social Hygiene, Inc.), pp 312–348.

Thompson CI, Zagon IS (1981): Long-term thermoregulatory changes following perinatal methadone exposure in rats. Pharmacol Biochem Behav 14:653–659.

Thompson CI, Zagon IS, McLaughlin PJ (1979): Impaired thermal regulation in juvenile rats following perinatal methadone exposure. Pharmacol Biochem Behav 10:551–556.

Torda C (1978): Effects of recurrent postnatal pain-related stressful events on opiate receptor-endogenous ligand system. Psychoneuroendocrinology 3:85–91.

Traber J, Gullis R, Hamprecht B (1975): Influence of opiates on the levels of adenosine 3':5'-cyclic monophosphate in neuroblastoma X glioma hybrid cells. Life Sci 16:1863–1868.

Tsang D, Ng SC (1980): Effect of antenatal exposure to opiates on the development of opiate receptors in rat brain. Brain Res 188:199–206.

Tsang D, Ng SC, Ho KP (1982): Development of methionine-enkephalin and naloxone binding sites in regions of rat brain. Dev Brain Res 3:637–644.

Tsang D, Tan AT, Henry JL, Lai S (1978): Effect of opioid peptides on L-noradrenaline-stimulated cyclic AMP formation in homogenates of rat cerebral cortex and hypothalamus. Brain Res 152:521–527.

Turner R, Tjian R (1989): Leucine repeats and an adjacent DNA binding domain mediate the formation of functional cFos-cJun heterodimers. Science 243:1689–1694.

Uhl GR, Ryan JP, Schwartz JP (1988): Morphine alters preproenkephalin gene expression. Brain Res 459:391–397.

Vernadakis A, Gibson A (1985): Neurotoxicity of opiates during brain development: in vivo and in vitro studies. In Marois M (ed): "Prevention of Physical and Mental Congenital Defects. Part C. Basic and Medical Science. Education and Future Strategies." New York: Alan R. Liss, pp 245–253.

Vernadakis A, Estin C, Gibson DA, Amott S (1982): Effects of methadone on ornithine decarboxylase and cyclic nucleotide phosphohydrolase in neuronal and glial cultures. J Neurosci Res 7:111–117.

Volavka J, Bauman J, Pevnick J, Reker D, James B, Cho D (1980): Short-term hormonal effects of naloxone in man. Psychoneuroendocrinology 5:225–234.

Vorhees CV (1981): Effects of prenatal naloxone exposure on postnatal behavioral development of rats. Neurobehav Toxicol Teratol 3:295–301.

Watanabe Y, Shibuya T, Salafsky B, Hill HF (1983): Prenatal and postnatal exposure to diazepam: Effects on opioid receptor binding in rat brain cortex. Eur J Pharmacol 96:141–144.

Weiner N (1974): Neurotoxicity of opiates during brain development. In Vernadakis A, Weiner N (eds): "Drugs and the Developing Brain." New York: Plenum Press, pp 215–227.

Wesche D, Hollt V, Herz A (1977): Radioimmunoassay of enkephalins. Regional distribution in rat brain after morphine treatment and hypophysectomy. Naunyn-Schmiedebergs Arch Pharmacol 301:79–82.

White WJ, Zagon IS (1979): Acute and chronic methadone exposure in adult rats: Studies on arterial blood gas concentrations and pH. J Pharmacol Exp Ther 209:451–455.

White WJ, Zagon IS, McLaughlin PJ (1978): Effects of chronic methadone treatment on maternal body weight and food and water consumption in rats. Pharmacology 17:227–232.

Wilson GS, Desmond MM Verniaud WM (1973): Early development of infants of heroin-addicted mothers. Am J Dis Child 126:457–462.

Wohltmann M, Roth BL, Coscia CJ (1982): Differential postnatal development of μ and δ opiate receptors. Dev Brain Res 3:679–684.

Wüster M, Costa T, Gramsch CH (1983): Uncoupling of receptors is essential for opiate-induced desensitization (tolerance) in neuroblastoma x glioma hybrid cells NG108-15. Life Sci 33:341–344.

Wüster M, Schulz R, Herz A (1980): Inquiry into endorphinergic feedback mechanisms during the development of opiate tolerance/dependence. Brain Res 189:403–411.

Yoburn BC, Goodman RG, Cohen AC, Pasternak GW, Inturrisi CE (1985): Increased analgesic potency of morphine and increased brain opioid binding sites in the rat following chronic naltrexone treatment. Life Sci 36:2325–2329.

Yoburn BC, Kreuscher SP, Inturrisi CE, Sierra V (1989a): Opioid receptor upregulation and supersensitivity in mice: Effect of morphine sensitivity. Pharmacol Biochem Behav 32:727–731.

Yoburn BC, Paul D, Azimuddin S, Lutfy K, Sierra V (1989b): Chronic opioid antagonist treatment increases μ and δ receptor-mediated spinal opioid analgesia. Brain Res 485:176–178.

Yoshikawa K, Sabol SL (1986): Glucocorticoids and cyclic AMP synergistically regulate the abundance of preproenkephalin messenger RNA in neuroblastoma-glioma hybrid cells. Biochem Biophys Res Commun 139:1–10.

Young WS, Kuhar MJ (1979): A new method for receptor autoradiography: [^{3}H] opioid receptors in rat brain. Brain Res 179:255–270.

Zagon IS, McLaughlin PJ (1977a): The effect of chronic maternal methadone exposure on perinatal development. Biol Neonate 31:271–282.

Zagon IS, McLaughlin PJ (1977b): The effects of different schedules of methadone treatment on rat brain development. Exp Neurol 56:538–552.

Zagon IS, McLaughlin PJ (1977c): The effect of chronic morphine administration on pregnant rats and their offspring. Pharmacology 15:302–310.

Zagon IS, McLaughlin PJ (1977d): Morphine and brain growth retardation in the rat. Pharmacology 15:276–282.

Zagon IS, McLaughlin PJ (1978): Perinatal methadone exposure and brain development: A biochemical study. J Neurochem 31:49–54.

Zagon IS, McLaughlin PJ (1980): Protracted analgesia in young and adult rats maternally exposed to methadone. Experientia 36:329–330.

Zagon IS, McLaughlin PJ (1981a): Enhanced sensitivity to methadone in adult rats perinatally exposed to methadone. Life Sci 29:1137–1142.

Zagon IS, McLaughlin PJ (1981b): Withdrawal-like symptoms in young and adult rats maternally exposed to methadone. Pharmacol Biochem Behav 15:887–894.

Zagon IS, McLaughlin PJ (1982a): Comparative effects of postnatal undernutrition and methadone exposure on protein and nucleic acid contents of the brain and cerebellum in rats. Dev Neurosci 5:385–393.

Zagon IS, McLaughlin PJ (1982b): Neuronal cell deficits following maternal exposure to methadone in rats. Experientia 38:1214–1216.

Zagon IS, McLaughlin PJ (1984a): Prenatal exposure of rats to methadone alters sensitivity to drugs in adulthood. Neurobehav Toxicol Teratol 6:314–319.

Zagon IS, McLaughlin PJ (1984b): Duration of opiate receptor blockade determines tumorigenic responses in mice with neuroblastoma: A role for endogenous opioid systems in cancer. Life Sci 35:409–416.

Zagon IS, McLaughlin PJ (1986): Opioid antagonist (naltrexone) modulation of cerebellar development: histological and morphometric studies. J Neurosci 6:1424–1432.

Zagon IS, McLaughlin PJ, Thompson CI (1979): Development of motor activity in young rats following perinatal methadone exposure. Pharmacol Biochem Behav 10:743–749.

Zagon IS, McLaughlin PJ, Weaver DJ, Zagon E (1982): Opiates, endorphins, and the developing organism: A comprehensive bibliography. Neurosci Biobehav Rev 6:439–479.

Zelson C (1975): Acute management of neonatal addiction. Addict Dis 2:159–168.

Zhong-Zhang A, Pasternak GW (1981): Ontogeny of opioid pharmacology and receptors: High and low affinity site differences. Eur J Pharmacol 73:29–40.

Zimmermann E, Sonderegger T (1980): A syndrome of drug-induced delay of maturation. In Parvez H, Parvez S (eds): "Biogenic Amines in Development." New York: Elsevier/North Holland Biomedical Press, pp 591–606.

Zimmermann E, Sonderegger T, Bromley B (1977): Development and adult pituitary-adrenal function in female rats injected with morphine during different postnatal periods. Life Sci 20:639–646.

Zimmermann E, Young J, Branch B, Tyalor AN, Pang CN (1974): Long-lasting effects of prepubertal administration of morphine in adult rats. In Zimmermann E, George R (eds): "Narcotics and the Hypothalamus." New York: Raven Press, pp 183–196.

Zukin RS, Sugarman JR, Fitz-Syaga ML, Gardner EL, Zukin SR, Gintzler AR (1982): Naltrexone-induced opiate receptor supersensitivity. Brain Res 245:285–292.

Development of the Central Nervous System:
Effects of Alcohol and Opiates, pages 319–339
© 1992 Wiley-Liss, Inc.

14

Consequences of Early Exposure to Opioids on Cell Proliferation and Neuronal Morphogenesis

RONALD P. HAMMER, JR., AND KURT F. HAUSER

Department of Anatomy and Reproductive Biology, University of Hawaii School of Medicine, Honolulu, Hawaii (R.P.H.); Department of Anatomy and Neurobiology, University of Kentucky Medical Center, Lexington, Kentucky (K.F.H.)

INTRODUCTION

With the discovery of membrane-bound receptors which bind opiate ligands (Pert and Snyder, 1973; Simon et al., 1973; Terenius et al., 1973), and the subsequent characterization of several types of endogenous opioid peptides (Hughes et al., 1975; Goldstein et al., 1978), the endogenous substrate upon which opiate drugs act in the central nervous system was elucidated. Most studies of endogenous opioid systems have utilized brain tissue derived from the rat brain, and unless otherwise noted, data from this animal model will be described below. The ontogenetic pattern of endogenous opioid systems has been thoroughly described (McDowell and Kitchen, 1987, see also Chapter 12); each peptide and receptor shows a discrete developmental time course. Opioid peptides and their endogenous receptors develop quite early in the rat brain. β-Endorphin (Ng et al., 1984) and the enkephalins (Dahl et al., 1982) have been identified as early as embryonic day 13, while dynorphin tends to be expressed later (Khachaturian et al., 1983). In contrast, the ontogeny of endogenous receptors for these peptides may be quite different from that of the peptides. κ-Receptors are present at low levels at birth in some regions, but have already attained adult levels in others (Spain et al., 1985; Kornblum et al., 1987a). δ-Receptors develop postnatally (Kornblum et al., 1987a), long after the time at which enkephalins are first expressed. μ-Receptors, on the other hand, are present in high levels before birth (Kent et al., 1982; Kornblum et al., 1987a), coincident with the development of β-endorphin in many brain regions.

The mechanism of action and effect of opiates on the developing brain is still unclear; however, it is known that perinatal treatment with opiates or opiate antagonists alters endogenous opioid receptor systems (see Chapter 13). For example, perinatal morphine treatment reportedly down-regulates μ-receptors (Zadina and Kastin, 1986; Tempel et al., 1988; Hammer et al., 1991), while antagonist treatment up-regulates receptors (Bardo et al., 1982). Interestingly, opposite effects of morphine treatment have also been reported during development (Tsang and Ng, 1980; Handelmann and Quirion, 1983) and adulthood (Rothman et al., 1991; Brady et al., 1989), suggesting possible region- and age-specific effects.

Recent evidence suggests that opiates also affect the structure of the developing nervous system, and that endogenous opioid peptides may be involved in the regulation of brain development. Opposite effects on cellular density and differentiation have been described following perinatal treatment with opiate agonists and antagonists in vivo. Additional effects of endogenous opiates on growth-related brain enzymatic activity have also been described (Slotkin et al., 1980; Bartolome et al., 1986, 1987). Moreover, opiate agonists and antagonists affect neuronal and glial differentiation in vitro. The implication of these effects on regulation of neural development will be discussed.

OPIOID ACTION ON THE DEVELOPING NERVOUS SYSTEM
Effects on Cellular Growth

Administration of methadone during development has been shown to affect brain growth (Slotkin et al., 1980; Zagon and McLaughlin, 1977a) and neuronal number (Zagon and McLaughlin, 1982). In addition, neonatal morphine (Kornblum et al., 1987b) and postnatal enkephalinamide (Vertes et al., 1982) or met-enkephalin (Zagon and McLaughlin, 1987) administration inhibit DNA synthesis in the developing rat brain, presumably resulting in decreased cell number. Constant μ-receptor stimulation by subcutaneous osmotic minipump administration of as little as 10 mg/kg/day of morphine from embryonic day 12 to postnatal day 6 in rats results in a significant reduction of neuronal packing density relative to saline vehicle treatment both in preoptic area of the hypothalamus (POA) and primary somatosensory cortex (S_I) (Fig. 1; Hammer et al., 1990). This morphine treatment paradigm also decreases the *thickness* (Fig. 2) and the *number of neurons* (Fig. 3) in S_I, due predominantly to morphine effects on cell-dense layers II–V (Seatriz and Hammer, 1991).

The finding that perinatal morphine treatment reduces the total number of cortical neurons has profound implications. Cortical neurons develop prenatally and migrate from the periventricular, proliferative zones along radial glial fibers to reach the cortical surface (Miller, 1988). Therefore, although some examples of adult neurogenesis of granular neurons in layer IV of rat visual cortex have been described (Kaplan and Hinds, 1977; Kaplan, 1981), additional cortical neurons are not generally added postnatally, especially in primates (Rakic, 1988). Thus, the prognosis for recovery following such a perinatal drug insult is poor, since most neurons in the affected regions originate prenatally. In addition, this effect of morphine occurs in other regions whose neurons originate during the drug treatment period, as morphine also reduces neuronal packing density in

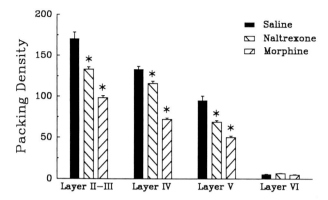

Fig. 1. Effect of perinatal morphine or naltrexone exposure on neuronal packing density in layers of rat primary somatosensory cortex (number of cells/mm² X 10^{-5}). * $P \leq 0.01$ by analysis of variance (ANOVA). (Reproduced from Seatriz and Hammer, 1991, with permission.)

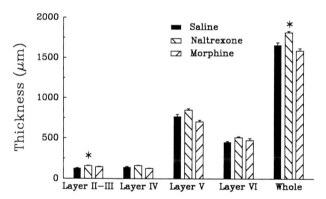

Fig. 2. Effect of perinatal morphine or naltrexone exposure on thickness of rat primary somatosensory cortex by layer. * $P \leq 0.01$ by ANOVA. (Reproduced from Seatriz and Hammer, 1991, with permission.)

the POA (Hammer et al., 1990), in which neurons are generated prenatally (Bayer and Altman, 1987). Perhaps, the magnitude of this effect is due to the extent of the treatment period, which includes both pre- and postnatal treatment. Because the blood-brain barrier is not intact until embryonic day 14, early treatment may produce higher fetal brain morphine levels, resulting in effects on neurogenesis and/or migration.

The trophic effect of perinatal morphine treatment suggests that endogenous opioid peptides may be involved in regulation of neuronal development. In fact, it has been suggested that β-endorphin (Berry and Haynes, 1989) and enkephalins (Zagon et al., 1985) have such a role. Administration of β-endorphin or N-acetyl-β-endorphin, the product of posttranslational

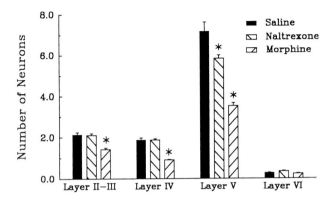

Fig. 3. Effect of perinatal morphine or naltrexone exposure on absolute number of neurons per unit depth in layers of rat primary somatosensory cortex. * $P \leq 0.01$ by ANOVA. (Reproduced from Seatriz and Hammer, 1991, with permission.)

acetylation, alters the activity of ornithine decarboxylase, a growth-related enzyme, in perinatal, but not adult rats (Bartolome et al., 1986, 1987). Furthermore, perinatal β-endorphin treatment decreases DNA synthesis (Bartolome et al., 1989), suggesting a critical role of this peptide in regulation of cell growth. Perhaps the strongest evidence thus far comes from those studies which illustrate the effect of administration of opiate receptor antagonists in doses which induce prolonged inhibition of endogenous opioid peptide binding (Zagon and McLaughlin, 1986a, b). Acute postnatal naltrexone administration increases the proportion of developing cerebellar cells incorporating [³H]thymidine, suggesting that opioid receptor blockade stimulates cell proliferation (Zagon and McLaughlin, 1987). Total receptor blockade using single daily doses of 50 mg/kg naltrexone administered postnatally increases granule cell number in the cerebellum (Zagon and McLaughlin, 1986a) and dentate gyrus (Zagon and McLaughlin, 1986b), without altering the ultrastructural characteristics of these cells (Hess and Zagon, 1988). Neuronal packing density is *reduced,* but cortical thickness is increased in S_I by such daily naltrexone treatment (Zagon and McLaughlin, 1986b). Constant perinatal administration of 10 mg/kg/day naltrexone by subcutaneous osmotic minipump also reduces S_I neuronal packing density and increases cortical thickness (Figs. 1, 2; Seatriz and Hammer, 1991). However, perinatal naltrexone treatment does not affect the number of neurons (neurons per unit area X laminar area) in any cortical layer except layer V (Fig. 3; Seatriz and Hammer, 1991). Thus, perinatal inhibition of endogenous opioid function increases cortical thickness assessed postnatally without affecting neuronal number. This suggests that the pattern of cerebral cortical neurogenesis and neuronal migration is unaffected by endogenous opioids; rather, neuronal differentiation and subsequent neuropil development are altered.

The effect of opioid administration or receptor blockade on glial development appears to be region-dependent. Neither morphine administration nor total opiate receptor blockade has any effect on glial number in S_I (Hammer et al., 1990; Zagon and McLaughlin, 1986b), but perinatal morphine administration increases glial packing density in the POA (Hammer et al., 1990), and postnatal naltrexone administration has the same effect in the cerebellum (Zagon and McLaughlin, 1986a).

The effect of opioids on neuronal development could be region-dependent, with different brain regions manifesting different effects, or opioid peptide-dependent, with different peptides eliciting different responses. Alternatively, the effect of endogenous opioid peptides on neuronal number could be greatest in regions where postnatal neurogenesis occurs (e.g., cerebellum and dentate gyrus), due to putative differential influences of late-developing opioid systems (e.g., δ-receptors; Kornblum et al., 1987a) or transient expression of opioid peptides (enkephalin; Zagon et al., 1985) in these regions. In any case, the morphological effects of exogenous opiate administration during development appear to be more severe and, potentially, sustained than those of endogenous opioid peptide blockade.

Effects on Neuronal Structure

The result of perinatal naltrexone administration, which increases cortical volume without affecting the number of cortical neurons, suggests that the volume of the neuropil and/or extracellular space is likely increased following opiate receptor blockade. Therefore, one might expect to find increased neuronal connectivity and/or dendritic branching following naltrexone treatment. In fact, endogenous opioids have been shown to regulate dendritic growth and spine formation in the developing rat brain (Hauser et al., 1987b, 1989). Postnatal naltrexone-induced opiate receptor blockade increases the total dendritic length in layer III pyramidal neurons of S_I, hippocampal pyramidal neurons, and cerebellar Purkinje neurons by 49%, 52%, and 66%, respectively, at postnatal day 10 (Table I; Hauser et al., 1987b). The greatest effect is observed during the early postnatal period; subsequent treatment results in no increase in dendritic length by postnatal day 21 (Hauser et al., 1989). Camera lucida drawings of Golgi-impregnated hippocampal pyramidal neurons and Purkinje neurons from postnatal vehicle- or naltrexone-treated rats are shown in Figure 4 A, C. Clearly, postnatal blockade of endogenous opioid peptide action has trophic effects, inducing an increase in dendritic branching and length of dendrites in both regions. Moreover, dendritic spine density in layer III pyramidal neurons of S_I, hippocampal pyramidal neurons (Fig. 4B), and granule cells of the dentate gyrus increases following 10 days of postnatal naltrexone treatment, and this effect is sustained until at least postnatal day 21 in hippocampal neurons (Hauser et al., 1989).

These data suggest that, at least during the first postnatal week, endogenous opioid peptides tonically modulate dendritic growth in the cortex and cerebellum. This hypothesis has been tested by administering morphine during pre- and postnatal development and quantitatively reconstructing

TABLE I. Dendritic Length Estimates (Mean Number of Intersections $\pm$ S.E.M.) of Neurons From 10-day-old Rats Treated Daily Since Birth With 50 mg/kg Naltrexone or Water Vehicle[a]

Brain region	Control group	Naltrexone group
Cerebral cortex	25 ± 2	59 ± 3*
Oblique dendrites of pyramidal neurons		
Hippocampus	190 ± 29	287 ± 24**
Basilar dendrites of pyramidal neurons		
Cerebellum	143 ± 15	235 ± 20*
Spiny Purkinje branchlets		

[a]Modified from Hauser et al., 1987b.
*$P \leq 0.01$.
**$P \leq 0.05$.

dendritic arborizations of layer III pyramidal neurons in S_I (Ricalde and Hammer, 1991). Morphine treatment reduces the total dendritic length of basilar dendrites by 49%, and the major locus of this effect is the terminal dendritic branches, which are reduced in length by 20%, in contrast to primary (root) or internode branches, which are unaffected by drug treatment (Table II). When naltrexone was coadministered with morphine, all treatment effects are eliminated. Thus, morphine-induced dendritic growth retardation is opiate receptor-mediated. Given that layer III–IV μ-receptors develop in the affected region during the first postnatal week (Kent et al., 1982), and morphine demonstrates high affinity for μ-receptors (Paterson et al., 1983), it appears likely that these trophic effects of morphine are mediated via μ-receptors.

In the above study, although morphine was administered both pre- and postnatally from embryonic day 12 to postnatal day 6, its major effect was manifested during postnatal development, when terminal basilar dendritic branches of S_I pyramidal neurons are formed (Petit et al., 1988; Wise et al., 1979). This is the same period during which naltrexone increased den-

Fig. 4. Camera lucida drawings (A,C) and photomicrographs (B) of Golgi-Kopsch-stained neurons from 10-day-old rats receiving sterile water (control) or 50 mg/kg/day naltrexone postnatally. **A:** Pyramidal neurons from CA_1 of the hippocampus in naltrexone-treated rats had increased dendritic arborizations. **B:** Basilar and oblique dendrites had more spines (arrow) following naltrexone treatment. **C:** Purkinje neurons in the cerebellum (lobule VIII) exhibited larger dendritic expanse and more complex branching following naltrexone treatment. Bars: A = 50 μm; B = 5 μm; C = 25 μm. (Reproduced from Hauser et al., 1987b, with permission.)

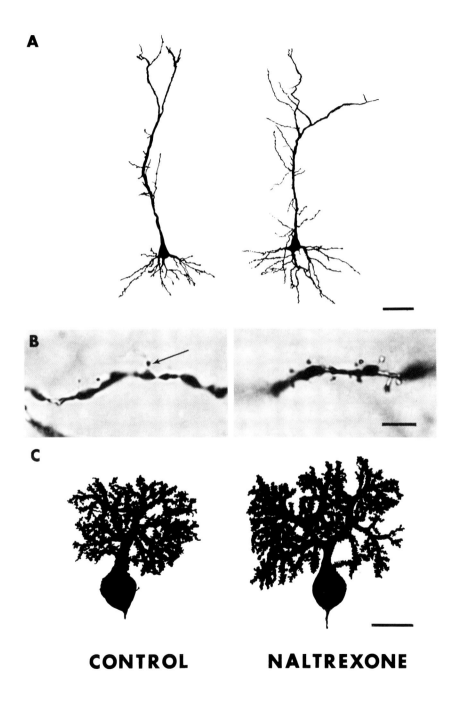

CONTROL   NALTREXONE

TABLE II. Dendritic Length (Mean μm + S.E.M.) by Order of Basilar Dendrites of Layer III Pyramidal Neurons in Primary Somatosensory Cortex From 6-day-old Rats Treated Since Gestation Day 12 With 10 mg/kg/day Morphine, 10 mg/kg/day Naltrexone, or Saline Vehicle[a]

Branch order	Control group	Morphine group	Morphine/Naltrexone group
Root branch	18.4 ± 1.7	18.2 ± 2.5	14.0 ± 1.5
Internode branch	15.5 ± 1.1	15.3 ± 2.0	13.2 ± 0.5
Terminal branch	54.7 ± 1.5	43.7 ± 5.6*	52.7 ± 1.9
Total dendrites	537.7 ± 28.3	274.6 ± 11.0*	466.6 ± 14.7

[a]Modified from Ricalde and Hammer, 1991.
*$P \leq 0.01$.

dritic length and spine counts in neurons located in the same brain region (Hauser et al., 1989). Since afferent fiber input has a major influence on both development of terminal dendrites and dendritic spines located thereon (Wise et al., 1979), it is possible that morphine retards thalamocortical and/or intracortical fiber development and connectivity. If so, then opioid receptor blockade during this period could increase fiber development, which could explain the observed increase of argyrophilic fiber staining in the cortex of naltrexone-treated animals (Zagon and McLaughlin, 1986b). Whether the mechanism of opiate effects on cortical neuronal growth is direct or indirect, the deleterious effect of exogenous opiate drugs on neuronal development is unmistakable. Moreover, a regulatory role for endogenous opioid peptides in the development of neuronal processes and connectivity is clearly established. Further support is derived from in vitro studies of opiate effects on cell growth.

TARGETS FOR OPIOID ACTION

In vitro studies have helped to identify cellular targets of opioid action during development. Emerging evidence suggests that opioids selectively influence specific cell types as well as unique developmental events.

Opioid Effects on Neurons

Ilyinsky et al. (1985, 1986, 1987) report 2- to 3-fold increases of neurite outgrowth in explant cultures of rat spinal cord, dorsal root ganglia, or sympathetic ganglia following 1 week of treatment with opioid peptides. In these studies, opioid-dependent changes in neurite outgrowth were demonstrated to be dose-dependent and dependent on the specific opioid peptide used. Maximal increases in neurite elaboration were found to occur at dosages of 10^{-10}–10^{-14} M. Different opioid peptides yield different magnitudes of response; β-endorphin causes the greatest increase in outgrowth followed by γ-endorphin, met-enkephalin, and leu-enkephalin, all of which significantly increase outgrowth compared with control values. These authors also report that endogenous opioids and opioid antagonists both increase growth rate. However, morphine reportedly inhibits neurite out-growth in neuron-enriched cultures from 6-day-old chick embryos (Sakel-laridis et al., 1986). These variable results might be due in part to the particular nutrient culture medium used in these studies. For example, fetal bovine serum typically contains approximately 10^{-10} M met-enke-phalin (Hauser and Van Loon, unpublished); Ilyinsky et al. (1987) use as much as 50% fetal bovine serum in their nutrient medium, but report trophic effects when as little as 10^{-14} M met-enkephalin is added to their cultures. Alternatively, another source of opioid peptides might be the explants themselves. Spinal cord explants cultured in Maximow double coverslip assemblies, as used by Ilyinsky et al. (1987), reportedly produce enkephalin, especially in the presence of dorsal root ganglia (Chalazonitis et al., 1984). Also β-endorphin-like immunoreactivity is normally present in a subset of motoneurons during development (Haynes et al., 1982; Berry and Haynes, 1989). Despite these concerns, Ilyinsky et al. (1987) provide the first strong evidence that growth of primary neural cells in culture can be directly affected by opioids.

Immature neurons express opioids in culture

In the rat cerebellum, enkephalin-like immunoreactivity transiently appears in germinative cells of the external granular layer (EGL) (Zagon et al., 1985). EGL cells are the progenitors that give rise to granule, stellate and basket neurons, but not glia, of the mature cerebellum (Altman, 1972), but enkephalin products are not observed in these neurons at maturity. Similarly, EGL cells in developing rat cerebellar explant cultures show enkephalin-like immunoreactivity, which is apparently lost with progres-sive maturation (Osborne and Hauser, 1989). This suggests that the matu-rational factors governing the transient appearance of enkephalin-like immunoreactivity in EGL cells are regulated by intrinsic mechanisms present within the developing cerebellum.

Other opioid gene products apparently show increased expression in vitro compared with in vivo. For example, increased expression of proopi-omelanocortin (POMC) mRNA has been observed in primary cultures of the rat hypothalamus (Kapcala, 1989) and spinal cord (Chalazonitis et al., 1984). The reasons for increased gene expression in vitro compared with in vivo are uncertain. It has been suggested that the mRNA may be more stable in vitro in some systems (Greenberg, 1972). However, additional evidence suggests that opioid genes are specifically repressed by external factors. For example, POMC mRNA is expressed by motoneurons during development (Haynes et al., 1982; Berry and Haynes, 1989), but only fol-lowing axotomy in adult motoneurons (Hughes and Smith, 1986; Berry and Haynes, 1989). Similarly, β-endorphin-like immunoreactivity is present only within the germinative cells lining the hypothalamic third ventricle in fetal rats (Loughlin et al., 1985), while large numbers of fetal hypotha-lamic neurons display β-endorphin-like immunoreactivity in culture (Kap-cala, 1989). This has prompted speculation that POMC expression is inhibited by factors which increase progressively with maturation, such as those which might be provided by afferent and/or efferent synaptic connections (Berry and Haynes, 1989). Similarly, expression (derepression) of proenkephalin mRNA by rat C6 glioma cells in vitro (Yoshikawa and Sabol, 1986), which could result from amplification of the proenkephalin gene during malignant transformation, is instead postulated to be due to the loss of externally-signaled feed-back inhibition (Rost et al., 1989). Thus, the presence of increased levels of enkephalin-like immunoreactivity in vitro appears to be the result of an intrinsic property of some populations of neuroblasts, and suggests that the presence of opioid peptides in immature cells is important during growth.

Opioid Effects on Glial Cells

It may be inferred from the work of several investigators that neuroglia are targets for opioid action during development. Chronic treatment with the opioid antagonist, naltrexone, during the first 3 weeks of postnatal development in rodents reportedly alters glial cell number in the cerebellar medullary layer (Zagon and McLaughlin, 1986a). The generation of neurons throughout the central nervous system is essentially complete at birth with the exception of the formation of interneurons of the olfactory bulbs, the dentate gyrus, and the cerebellar cortex (e.g., Altman and Das, 1966; Altman, 1972; Hertz et al., 1985). Therefore, data suggesting that whole brain DNA synthesis is affected by opiate agonists administered postnatally (Vertes et al., 1982; Kornblum et al., 1987b), or by opioid antagonists in older rats (Schmahl et al., 1989) likely reflects altered gliogenesis. This hypothesis is supported by the finding that astrocyte growth is directly inhibited by met-enkephalin in glial cell cultures (Stiene-Martin and Hauser, 1990) and increased by morphine in mixed cell cultures (Sakellaridis et al., 1986). However, these effects, too, may be region-dependent, since perinatal morphine exposure increases glial packing density in hypothalamus, but not in cerebral cortex (Hammer et al., 1990).

Astrocytes in culture are known to express both opioid peptides and receptors. Several investigators have suggested that opioid receptors are present on glial cells (Rougon et al., 1983; Pearce et al., 1985; Maderspach and Solomonia, 1988). Astrocyte-enriched cultures express proenkephalin mRNA and enkephalin peptide products or enkephalin-like immunoreactivity (Vilijn et al., 1988; Shinoda et al., 1989). This suggests that astrocytes are a potential source for endogenous opioids in vivo, and that they are likely to be an important component in the mechanism of opioid action during development. Furthermore, pituicytes in the posterior pituitary, which have some similarities to astrocytes, also exhibit opioid receptors in vivo (Bunn et al., 1985; Herkenham et al., 1986) and in vitro (Bicknell et al., 1989).

DEVELOPMENTAL EVENTS MODIFIED BY OPIOIDS
Cell Proliferation

Opioids are known to modify cell numbers and/or packing density in vivo. Continuous opioid receptor blockade during the first 3 postnatal weeks is known to increase the number and packing density of neurons in the cerebellum (Zagon and McLaughlin, 1986a) and hippocampus (Zagon and McLaughlin, 1986b), and packing density alone in the cerebral cortex (Seatriz and Hammer, 1991; Zagon and McLaughlin, 1986b). While multiple factors normally affect cell density, changes in cell proliferation could underlie such opioid-dependent alteration of cell number. The fact that postnatal opioid receptor blockade increases neuronal number in the cerebellum and dentate gyrus, but not in the cerebral cortex, suggests that opioids affect cell proliferation only in regions in which neurons are generated postnatally, e.g., cerebellum and dentate gyrus. On the other hand, even prenatal opioid blockade cannot enhance neuronal number in cerebral cortex (Fig. 3; Seatriz and Hammer, 1991), wherein neurons are generated prenatally (Miller, 1988). Therefore, the effects of endogenous opioids on the generation of neurons may be age-dependent, occurring during a critical postnatal period.

Met-enkephalin administration decreases the proportion of developing cerebellar neurons which incorporate [^{3}H]thymidine 2 hours later (Zagon and McLaughlin, 1987), and D-met^2-pro^5-enkephalinamide has the same effect in several additional brain regions (Vertes et al., 1982). In contrast, [^{3}H]thymidine incorporation initially increases after naloxone treatment, decreasing several hours later when drug levels are presumably diminished (Vertes et al., 1982). While acute morphine treatment has no affect on [^{3}H]thymidine incorporation in tissues isolated from 1-day-old rats, morphine suppresses [^{3}H]thymidine incorporation in vivo (Kornblum et al., 1987b), suggesting that opioids indirectly inhibit whole brain DNA synthesis. However, studies of glial cultures isolated from newborn mice, wherein suppression of DNA synthesis by 1 μM met-enkephalin was observed after 3 days of treatment, suggest that opioids can have a direct inhibitory effect on the growth of certain glial cells (Stiene-Martin and Hauser, 1990). Obviously, when comparing the above studies, differences in the species/strain, the age and duration of treatment, culture conditions, or ligands used must also be considered.

Additional evidence in support of opioid action on cell proliferation comes from studies which demonstrate that endogenous opioids can modulate the rate of growth of opioid receptor-containing S20Y murine neuroblastoma tumor cells in vitro (Zagon and McLaughlin, 1989). Met-enkephalin inhibits the rate of neuroblastoma cell doubling in a naloxone-reversible manner. Moreover, the expression of the oncogene N-*myc*, assessed by Northern blot analysis in S20Y murine neuroblastoma cells, is also inhibited by met-enkephalin, but is increased in response to naltrexone treatment (Hauser et al., 1987). N-*myc* expression normally varies with mitotic activity in neuroblastoma cells, therefore, these results suggest that fundamental processes associated with growth, such as the timing of events in the cell cycle, may be modified by opioids. It is also noteworthy that neuronally-derived S20Y neuroblastoma cells are reportedly capable of synthesizing opioid peptides, based on cytoplasmic localization of enkephalin-like immunoreactivity in these cells (Zagon and McLaughlin, 1989). Furthermore, if opioid antagonist drugs are added to the culture medium in sufficient quantities to continuously block opioid receptors, neuroblastoma cell number eventually increases. This suggests the potential for an autocrine mechanism of growth regulation by S20Y neuroblastoma cells. However, the presence of opioid peptides in the fetal calf serum-containing nutrient medium used in these studies must also be considered as a confounding variable. Also, by definition, tumor cell lines have altered responsiveness to growth factor regulation. Therefore, the extent to which these data can be generalized to primary neural cells is uncertain.

The total number of cells in primary mixed-glial cultures isolated from 1-day-old mouse cerebral hemispheres is significantly decreased after 6 days of treatment with 1 μM met-enkephalin (Fig. 5; Stiene-Martin and Hauser, 1990). This growth inhibition is naloxone-reversible, and suggests that cell turnover (mitosis and/or survival) can be altered by the action of met-enkephalin on opioid receptors. To determine whether enkephalin might selectively affect the rate of proliferation of individual glial cell types, [^{3}H]thymidine autoradiography was combined with cell-type specific markers. A selective decrease in [^{3}H]thymidine incorporation was noted in glial fibrillary acidic protein (GFAP)-positive flat (type I) astrocytes after 4 and 6 days of enkephalin treatment (Fig. 6). Again, this action of met-enkephalin was reversed by naloxone, and naloxone alone had no effect on [^{3}H]thymidine incorporation. These results suggest that the rate of astrocyte proliferation may be directly modified by opioid action on mixed-glial cultures. Moreover, astrocyte-enriched cultures can express proenkephalin mRNA and/or enkephalin peptide products (Vilijn et al., 1988; Shinoda et al., 1989), suggesting that endogenous opioids might regulate astrocyte growth in vitro via a local (paracrine or autocrine) mechanism.

Thus, in vitro studies suggest that opioids can directly inhibit glial cell proliferation. However, opioid effects on neurogenesis may be region- and age-dependent. Additional studies are needed to examine the mechanism(s) by which endogenous opioids normally influence astrocyte development in vivo, and to determine the extent to which opioid-dependent changes in astrocytes are responsible for the observed opioid-dependent alterations in neuronal development throughout the brain.

Subsequent Developmental Events

Following mitotic division, cells typically migrate from the germinal zone to their final position along radial glial guides, extend dendrites and axons, and form synaptic connections. Since astrocytic proliferation is inhibited by endogenous opioid administration in mixed-glial cultures (Stiene-Martin and Hauser, 1990), the opioid-induced loss or alteration of formative glial guides could disrupt the pattern of neuronal migration. Although neuronal number is reduced following perinatal morphine treatment (Fig. 3), all cell-dense layers are equally affected, suggesting that the amount, but not the timing, of cell proliferation is altered by exogenous opiate administration. The structural or molecular bases for this alteration is unknown.

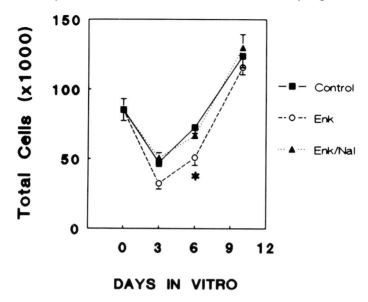

Fig. 5. Effects of met-enkephalin on the absolute numbers of cells in mixed-glial cultures. Cultures were plated at the same density (day 0), and continuously treated with either growth media alone (Control), 1 μM met-enkephalin (Enk), or 1 μM met-enkephalin plus 3 μM naloxone (Enk/Nal). Met-enkephalin caused a significant decrease in cell numbers that was reversed by naloxone treatment. * $P \leq 0.05$. (Reproduced from Stiene-Martin and Hauser, 1990, with permission.)

Abundant evidence suggests that opioids affect the growth of neuronal processes during critical developmental periods. Morphine decreases dendritic growth in cerebral cortex (Ricalde and Hammer, 1991), while chronic postnatal opiate receptor blockade enhances dendritic growth and spine formation in the same brain region (Hauser et al., 1987b, 1989). Moreover, the extension of neuritic processes in vitro is affected by morphine (Sakellaridis et all, 1986) and opioid peptides (Ilyinsky et al., 1987). Postnatal opiate receptor blockade enhances axonal fiber staining in cerebral cortex (Zagon and McLaughlin, 1986b), which may reflect opiatergic regulation of axonal development. However, the extent of opioid effects on axonal growth and targeting is unknown. Presumably, these opioid effects on the growth of neuronal processes result in altered synaptic connectivity, as evidenced by the enhancement of dendritic spine number following postnatal opiate receptor blockade (Hauser et al., 1987b). Furthermore, postnatal naltrexone treatment apparently increases synaptic density and induces precocious synaptogenesis in cerebellum. Naltrexone-induced up-regulation (Bardo et al., 1982) and morphine-induced down-regulation (Tempel et al., 1988; Chapter 12) of opiate receptors in the developing brain may reflect additional opioid-induced activity at synaptic loci.

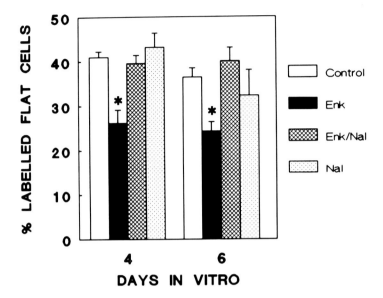

Fig. 6. Effects of met-enkephalin on [³H]thymidine incorporation by GFAP-positive cells (astrocytes) with flat morphology. Cultures were continuously treated with either growth media alone (Control), 1 μM met-enkephalin (Enk), 1 μM met-enkephalin plus 3 μM naloxone (Enk/Nal), or 3 μM naloxone (Nal). The percentage of[³H]thymidine-labelled flat astrocytes was significantly decreased by met-enkephalin after 4 or 6 days in vitro. * $P \leq 0.05$. (Reproduced from Stiene-Martin and Hauser, 1990, with permission.)

PHARMACOLOGICAL MECHANISMS OF OPIOID FUNCTION IN DEVELOPMENT

Opioid effects on development appear to be mediated via opiate receptor interactions. For example, met-enkephalin-induced inhibition of cerebellar (Zagon and McLaughlin, 1987) and cerebral (Stiene-Martin and Hauser, 1990) cell proliferation is blocked by concomitant naloxone administration, and the effect of naloxone on body growth is stereospecific and dependent on the duration of receptor blockade (Zagon and McLaughlin, 1989). These results suggest that opioid effects on cell growth are mediated by specific opiate receptors. The fact that morphine inhibits DNA synthesis (Kornblum et al., 1987b), dendritic growth (Ricalde and Hammer, 1991), and neurite outgrowth (Sakellaridis et al., 1986), and that these effects may be reversed by concomitant naltrexone administration (Ricalde and Hammer, 1991), suggests that these trophic effects are mediated by opioid interactions with a selective population of opiate receptors: μ-receptors. However, while perinatal morphine treatment inhibits brain growth (Zagon and McLaughlin, 1977b) and naltrexone treatment enhances brain growth

(Zagon and McLaughlin, 1983), perinatal administration of β-funaltrexamine (β-FNA), a selective irreversible μ-receptor alkylating agent, has no effect on brain growth (Zagon and McLaughlin, 1986c). Although this suggests that μ-receptors are not involved in growth regulation, μ-receptor involvement cannot be ruled out, because competition studies discriminate two subtypes of μ-receptors, only one of which is β-FNA-sensitive (Rothman et al., 1983).

It is possible that additional opiate receptor types are involved in growth regulation. For example, the inhibition of regional brain DNA synthesis produced by enkephalinamide administration at postnatal day 11 in rat (Vertes et al., 1982) suggests that δ-receptors, to which enkephalinamide binds with high affinity, may be involved. Morphine is incapable of such inhibition of DNA synthesis after postnatal day 4 (Kornblum et al., 1987b), and δ-receptor density begins to increase in the second postnatal week (Kornblum et al., 1987a) coincident with this enkephalinamide effect. Also, met-enkephalin, which demonstrates high affinity for δ-receptors (Paterson et al., 1983), inhibits cerebellar DNA synthesis (Zagon and McLaughlin, 1987). In fact, met-enkephalin appears to be the most potent inhibitor of cerebellar cell proliferation in existence (Cook et al., 1989). The possibility of involvement of other receptors to which these ligands bind should also be considered.

Opioid regulation of brain growth might ultimately involve intermediate and/or second messenger systems, as well. For example, acute morphine administration increases expression of the cellular oncogene, *c-fos*, and its nucleoprotein product, FOS, in the rat striatum (Chang et al., 1988). The naloxone reversibility and selectivity of this effect for μ-receptor-containing brain regions suggests that FOS may act as a signal transducer following morphine-induced μ-receptor activation. The putative expression of c-*fos* during brain injury (Sharp et al., 1989) suggests that it may also provide signal transduction during growth. However, not all opioid effects may be receptor-mediated. Morphine inhibits forskolin-stimulated adenylate cyclase activity in the embryonic chick brain, but this effect is not reversed by naloxone (Sakellaridis and Vernadakis, 1986). This latter effect occurs only during a critical developmental period (embryonic days 6–8), and may represent an unusual mechanism for opioid action. In any case, these studies represent the first investigations into the mechanisms of signal transduction by which opioids may elicit their trophic effects.

CONCLUSIONS

Exogenous and endogenous opioids affect the generation of neurons and glia, the extension of neuronal processes, and formation of connections during critical developmental periods. Maximal effects in vivo seem limited to the early postnatal period; primary effects on neuronal branching are directed at those processes which develop during this period (Ricalde and Hammer, 1991), and cell proliferation is most affected in brain regions in which postnatal cell division occurs (e.g., cerebellum and dentate gyrus of hippocampus) (Zagon and McLaughlin, 1986a, b, 1987). Therefore, a critical postnatal period of opioid trophism, whose boundaries are yet to be determined, may exist.

Perinatal opioid exposure can produce severe alterations of brain morphology, affecting both neuronal and glial cells. However, exogenous opioid administration apparently produces additive effects, both in time and severity. That is, the effect of exogenous opioids is not simply the opposite of that produced by opiate receptor blockade; rather, exogenous and endogenous opioid actions may be additive. For example, perinatal morphine treatment inhibits generation of neurons, neuropil development, and dendritic branching in S_I, while perinatal naltrexone only affects the developing neuropil without affecting neuronal number (Ricalde and Hammer, 1991; Seatriz and Hammer, 1991). The morphological changes produced by morphine occur both pre- and postnatally, whereas natrexone-induced changes probably occur postnatally. Thus, perinatal morphine produces more drastic morphological effects, across a greater developmental time period than does opiate receptor blockade.

While few studies have been conducted which examine the long-term morphological consequences of developmental opioid exposure, one might predict that such severe perinatal effects as reduction of neuronal number (Seatriz and Hammer, 1991; Zagon and McLaughlin, 1987), neurite outgrowth (Sakellaridis et al., 1986), and branching (Ricalde and Hammer, 1991) would produce long-lasting alterations. While considerable plasticity of neuronal structure exists, opioid-induced alteration of neuronal generation, in particular, may be irreversible. Thus, the prognosis for recovery from developmental opioid exposure is poor, particularly if exposure occurs during the critical period for opioid trophism.

In addition to the apparent neurotoxic effects of exogenous opioids in the central nervous system, considerable evidence supports a role for endogenous opioids in growth regulation during normal development. Although numerous studies suggest that enkephalins (Vertes et al., 1982; Zagon and McLaughlin, 1987) and/or β-endorphin (Bartolome et al., 1986) inhibit, while opiate receptor blockade enhances (Zagon and McLaughlin, 1986a, b, 1987) brain growth and cell proliferation, it is inappropriate to view endogenous opioids simply as growth inhibitors. Rather, they appear to act in a complex manner to modulate growth. Such a "negative neurotrophic factor" may be required to promote appropriate cellular growth and neurite targeting (Carboni and Schwab, 1988; Savio and Schwab, 1989) in the central nervous system. Thus, the cellular control of endogenous opioids may provide a mechanism for local neurotrophic modulatory activity during critical developmental periods.

ACKNOWLEDGMENTS

This work was supported by USPHS awards DA04081, NS01161, and GM08125 to R.P.H., and DA06204 and RR05374 to K.F.H.

REFERENCES

Altman J (1972): Postnatal development of the cerebellar cortex in the rat. I. The external germinal layer and the transitional molecular layer. J Comp Neurol 145:353–398.

Altman J, Das GP (1966): Autoradiographic and histological studies of postnatal neurogenesis. I. A longitudinal investigation of the kinetics, migration and transformation of cells incorporating tritiated thymidine in neonatal rats, with special reference to postnatal neurogenesis in some brain regions. J Comp Neurol 126:337–390.

Bardo MT, Bhatnagar RK, Gebhart GF (1982): Differential effects of chronic morphine and naloxone on opiate receptors, monoamines, and morphine-induced behaviors in preweanling rats. Dev Brain Res 4:139–147.

Bartolome JV, Bartolome MB, Daltner LA, Evans CJ, Barchas JD, Kuhn CM, Schanberg SM (1986): Effects of β-endorphin on ornithine decarboxylase in tissues of developing rats: A potential role for this endogenous neuropeptide in the modulation of tissue growth. Life Sci 38:2355–2362.

Bartolome JV, Bartolome MB, Harris EB, Schanberg SM (1987): N-acetyl-β-endorphin stimulates ornithine decarboxylase activity in preweanling rat pups: Opioid- and non-opioid-mediated mechanisms. J Pharmacol Exp Ther 240:895–899.

Bartolome JV, Bartolome MB, Schanberg SM (1989): CNS beta-endorphin as a regulator of DNA synthesis in central and peripheral tissues in preweanling rats. Int Soc Neurochem Abstr 12.

Bayer SA, Altman J (1987): Development of the preoptic area: Time and site of origin, migratory routes, and settling patterns of its neurons. J Comp Neurol 265:65–95.

Berry S, Haynes LW (1989): The opiomelanocortin peptide family: Neuronal expression and modulation of neural cellular development and regeneration in the central nervous system. Comp Biochem Physiol 93A:267–272.

Bicknell RJ, Luckman SM, Inenaga K, Mason WT, Hatton GI (1989): β-adrenergic and opioid receptors on pituicytes cultured from adult rat neurohypophysis: Regulation of cell morphology. Brain Res Bull 22:379–388.

Brady LS, Herkenham M, Long JB, Rothman RB (1989): Chronic morphine increases μ-opiate receptor binding in rat brain: A quantitative autoradiographic study. Brain Res 477:382–386.

Bunn SJ, Hanley MR, Wilkin GP (1985): Evidence for kappa-opioid receptors on pituitary astrocytes: An autoradiographic study. Neurosci Lett 55:317–323.

Carboni P, Schwab ME (1988): Two membrane protein fractions from rat central myelin with inhibitory properties for neurite growth and fibroblast spreading. J Cell Biol 106:1281–1288.

Chalazonitis A, Groth J, Hiller JM, Simon EJ, Crain SM (1984): Development of met-enkephalin immunoreactivity in organotypic explants of fetal mouse spinal cord and attached dorsal root ganglia. Dev Brain Res 12:183–189.

Chang SL, Squinto SP, Harlan RE (1988): Morphine activation of c-fos expression in rat brain. Biochem Biophys Res Commun 157:698–704.

Cook KL, McLaughlin PJ, Zagon, IS (1989): Identification of opioid peptides associated with cell proliferation in the developing brain. Soc Neurosci Abstr 15:145.

Dahl JL, Epstein ML, Silva BL, Lindberg I (1982): Multiple immunoreative forms of met- and leu-enkephalin in fetal and neonatal rat brain and in rat gut. Life Sci 31:1853–1856.

Goldstein A, Tachibana S, Lowney LI, Hunkapiller M, Hood L (1979): Dynorphin-(1-13), an extraordinarily potent opioid peptide. Proc Natl Acad Sci (USA) 76:6666–6670.

Greenberg JR (1972): High stability of messenger RNA in growing cultured cells. Nature 240:102–104.

Hammer RP, Ricalde AA, Seatriz JV (1990): Effects of opiates on brain development. Neurotoxicology 10:475–484.

Hammer RP, Seatriz JV, Ricalde AA (1991): Regional dependence of morphine-induced μ-receptor downregulation in perinatal rat brain. Eur J Pharmacol (in press).

Handelmann GE, Quirion R (1983): Neonatal exposure to morphine increases mu opiate binding in adult forebrain. Eur J Pharmacol 94:357–358.

Hauser KF, Kaysen JH, McLaughlin PJ, Zagon IS (1987a): Endogenous opioids are associated with changes in N-*myc* oncogene mRNA expression. Anat Rec 211:-184.

Hauser KF, McLaughlin PJ, Zagon IS (1987b): Endogenous opioids regulate dendritic growth and spine formation in the developing rat brain. Brain Res 416:-156–171.

Hauser KF, McLaughlin PJ, Zagon IS (1989): Endogenous opioid systems and the regulation of dendritic growth and spine formation. J Comp Neurol 290:13–22.

Haynes LW, Smyth DG, Zakarian S (1982): Immunocytochemical localization of lipoprotein c-fragment (β-endorphin) in the developing rat spinal cord. Brain Res 232:115–128.

Herkenham M, Rice KC, Jacobson AE, Rothman RB (1986): Opiate receptors in rat pituitary are confined to the neural lobe and are exclusively kappa. Brain Res 382:365–371.

Hertz L, Juurlink HJ, Szuchet S (1985): Cell cultures. In Lajtha A (ed): "Handbook of Neurochemistry." New York: Plenum Press, pp 603–661.

Hess GD, Zagon IS (1988): Endogenous opioid systems and neural development: Ultrastructural studies in the cerebellar cortex of infant and weanling rats. Brain Res Bull 20:473–478.

Hughes J, Smith TW, Kosterlitz HW, Fothergill LA, Morgan BA, Morris HR (1975): Identification of two related pentapeptides from the brain with potent opiate agonist activity. Nature 258:577–579.

Hughes S, Smith ME (1986): The expression of proopiomelanocortin peptides in motoneurons of the rat following contralateral nerve section may depend on a transneuronal signal. J Physiol 403:59P.

Ilyinsky OB, Kozlova MV, Kondrikova ES, Kalenchuk VU (1986): Effects of opioid peptides on processes of growth and regeneration of rat nerve tissue. J Evol Biochem Physiol 21:337–342.

Ilyinsky OB, Kozlova MV, Kondrikova ES, Kalentchuk VU, Titov MI, Bespalova ZhD (1987): Effects of opioid peptides and naloxone on nervous tissue in culture. Neuroscience 22:719–735.

Ilyinsky OB, Kozlova MV, Kondrikova ES, Titov MI, Bespalova ZhD, Yarygin KN, Yurchenko NN (1985): Influence of opioid peptides on nerve tissue in vitro. Neurophysiology 17:402–409.

Kapcala LP (1989): Production of immunoreactive adrenocorticotropin and β-endorphin by hypothalamic brain cells. Brain Res 491:253–265.

Kaplan MS (1981): Neurogenesis in the 3-month-old rat visual cortex. J Comp Neurol 195:323–338.

Kaplan MS, Hinds JW (1977): Neurogenesis in the adult rat: Electron microscopic analysis of light radioautographs. Science 197:1092–1094.

Kent JL, Pert CB, Herkenham M (1982): Ontogeny of opiate receptors in rat forebrain: Visualization by in vitro autoradiography. Dev Brain Res 2:487–504.

Khachaturian H, Alessi NE, Munfakh N, Watson SJ (1983): Ontogeny of opioid and related peptides in the rat CNS and pituitary: An immunocytochemical study. Life Sci 33S:61–64.

Kornblum HI, Hurlbut DE, Leslie FM (1987a): Postnatal development of multiple opioid receptors in rat brain. Dev Brain Res 37:21–41.

Kornblum HI, Loughlin SE, Leslie FM (1987b): Effects of morphine on DNA synthesis in neonatal rat brain. Dev Brain Res 31:45–52.

Loughlin SE, Massamiri TR, Kornblum HI, Leslie FM (1985): Postnatal development of opioid systems in rat brain. Neuropeptides 5:469–472.

Low KG, Allen RG, Nielson CP, Saneto RP, Young SL, Melner MH (1989): Regulation of type I astrocyte proenkephalin: transcription, translation, and secretion. Soc Neurosci Abstr 15:983.

Maderspach K, Solomonia R (1988): Glial and neuronal opioid receptors: Apparent positive cooperativity observed in intact cultured cells. Brain Res 441:41–47.

McDowell J, Kitchen I (1987): Development of opioid systems: Peptides, receptors and pharmacology. Brain Res Rev 12:397–421.

Miller M (1988): Development of projection and local circuit neurons in cerebral cortex. In Peters A, Jones EG (eds): "Cerebral Cortex." New York: Plenum Press, Vol. 7, pp 133–175.

Ng TB, Ho WKK, Tam PPL (1984): Brain and pituitary β-endorphin levels at different developmental stages of the rat. Int J Prot Res 24:141–146.

Osborne JG, Hauser KF (1989): Enkephalin immunoreactivity in organotypic cultures of the developing rat cerebellum: Evidence for transient opioid expression in vitro. Soc Neurosci Abstr 15:278.

Paterson SJ, Robson LE, Kosterlitz HW (1983): Classification of opioid receptors. Br Med Bull 39:31–36.

Pearce B, Cambry-Deakin M, Murphy S (1985): Astrocyte opioid receptors: Activation modifies the noradrenaline-evoked increase in 2-[^{14}C]deoxyglucose incorporation in glycogen. Neurosci Lett 305:715–717.

Pert CB, Snyder SH (1973): Opiate receptor: Demonstration in nervous tissue. Science 179:1011–1014.

Petit TL, LeBoutillier JC, Gregorio A, Libstug H (1988): The pattern of dendritic development in the cerebral cortex of the rat. Dev Brain Res 41:209–219.

Rakic P (1988): Specification of cerebral cortical areas. Science 241:170–176.

Ricalde AA, Hammer RP (1991): Perinatal opiate treatment delays growth of cortical dendrites. Neurosci Lett 115:137–143.

Rost N, Chaffanet M, Nissou MF, Chauvin C, Foote AM, Laine M, Benabid AL (1989): Expression of the preproenkephalin A gene in tumor cells and brain glioma: A Northern and in situ hybridization study. Neuropeptides 13:133–138.

Rothman RB, Bowen WD, Schumacher UK, Pert CB (1983): Effect of β-FNA on opiate receptor binding: Evidence for two types of μ-receptors. Eur J Pharmacol 95:147–148.

Rothman RB, Long JB, Bykov V, Xu H, Jacobson AE, Rice KC, Holaday JW (1991): Upregulation of the opioid receptor complex by the chronic administration of morphine: A biochemical marker related to the development of tolerance and dependence. Peptides 12:151–160.

Rougon G, Noble M, Mudge AW (1983): Neuropeptides modulate the β-adrenergic response of purified astrocytes in vitro. Nature 305:715–717.

Sakellaridis N, Mangoura D, Vernadakis A (1986): Effects of opiates on the growth of neuron-enriched cultures from chick embryonic brain. Int J Dev Neurosci 4:293–302.

Sakellaridis N, Vernadakis A (1986): An unconventional response of adenylate cyclase to morphine and naloxone in the chicken during early development. Proc Natl Acad Sci (USA) 83:2738–2742.

Savio T, Schwab ME (1989): Rat CNS white matter, but not gray matter, is nonpermissive for neuronal cell adhesion and fiber outgrowth. J Neurosci 9:1126–1133.

Schmahl W, Funk R, Miaskowski U, Plendl J (1989): Long-lasting effects of naltrexone, an opioid antagonist, on cell proliferation in developing rat forebrain. Brain Res 486:297–300.

Seatriz JV, Hammer RP (1991): Effects of endogenous and exogenous opiates on neuronal development in rat cerebral cortex. Brain Res Bull (in press).

Sharp FR, Gonzalez MF, Hisanaga K, Mobley WC, Sager SM (1989): Induction of the c-fos gene product in the rat forebrain following cortical lesions and NGF injections. Neurosci Lett 100:117–122.

Shinoda H, Marini AM, Cosi C, Schwartz JP (1989): Brain region and gene specificity of neuropeptide gene expression in cultured astrocytes. Science 245:415–475.

Slotkin TA, Seidler FJ, Whitmore WL (1980): Effects of maternal methadone administration on ornithine decarboxylase in brain and heart of the offspring: Relationships of enzyme activity to dose and to growth impairment in the rat. Life Sci 26:861–867.

Spain JW, Roth BL, Coscia CJ (1985): Differential ontogeny of multiple opioid receptor (μ, δ, and κ). J Neurosci 5:584–588.

Stiene-Martin A, Hauser KF (1990): Opioid-dependent growth of glial cultures: Suppression of astrocyte DNA synthesis by met-enkephalin. Life Sci 46:91–98.

Tempel A, Habas J, Paredes W, Barr GA (1988): Morphine-induced downregulation of μ-opiate receptors in neonatal rat brain. Brain Res 469:129–133.

Tsang D, Ng SC (1980): Effect of antenatal exposure to opiates on the development of opiate receptors in the rat brain. Brain Res 188:199–206.

Vernadakis A, Gibson DA, Amott S (1982): Effects of methadone on ornithine decarboxylase and cyclic phosphohydroxylase in neuronal and glial-cell cultures. J Neurochem Res 7:111–117.

Vertes Z, Melegh G, Vertes M, Kovacs S (1982): Effect of naloxone and D-met^2-pro^5-enkephalinamide treatment on the DNA synthesis in the developing rat brain. Life Sci 31:119–126.

Vilijn M-H, Vayasse P-J, Zukin RS, Kessler JA (1988): Expression of preproenkephalin messenger RNA by cultured astrocytes and neurons. Proc Natl Acad Sci (USA) 85:6551–6555.

Wise SP, Flechman JW, Jones EG (1979): Maturation of pyramidal cell form in relation to developing afferent and efferent connections of rat somatic sensory cortex. Neuroscience 4:1275–1297.

Yoshikawa K, Sabol SL (1986): Expression of the enkephalin precursor gene in C6 rat glioma cells: Regulation by β-adrenergic agonists and glucocorticoids. Mol Brain Res 1:75–83.

Zadina JE, Kastin AJ (1986): Neonatal peptides affect developing rats: β-endorphin alters nociception and opiate receptors, corticotropin-releasing factor alters corticosterone. Dev Brain Res 29:21–29.

Zagon IS, McLaughlin PJ (1977a): The effects of different schedules of methadone treatment on rat brain development. Exp Neurol 56:538–552.

Zagon IS, McLaughlin PJ (1977b): Morphine and brain growth retardation in the rat. Pharmacol 15:276–282.

Zagon IS, McLaughlin PJ (1982): Neuronal cell deficits following maternal exposure to methadone in rats. Experentia 38:1214–1216.

Zagon IS, McLaughlin PJ (1983): Increased brain size and cellular content in infant rats treated with an opiate antagonist. Science 221:1179–1180.

Zagon IS, McLaughlin PJ (1986a): Opioid antagonist (naltrexone) modulation of cerebellar development: Histological and morphometric studies. J Neurosci 6:1424–1432.

Zagon IS, McLaughlin PJ (1986b): Opioid antagonist-induced modulation of cerebral and hippocampal development: Histological and morphometric studies. Dev Brain Res 28:233–246.

Zagon IS, McLaughlin PJ (1986c): β-Funaltrexamine (β-FNA) and the regulation of body and brain development in rats. Brain Res Bull 17:5–9.

Zagon IS, McLaughlin PJ (1987): Endogenous opioid systems regulate cell proliferation in the developing rat brain. Brain Res 412:68–72.

Zagon IS, McLaughlin PJ (1989): Endogenous opioid systems regulate growth of neural tumor cells in culture. Brain Res 490:14–25.

Zagon IS, Rhodes RE, McLaughlin PJ (1985): Distribution of enkephalin immunoreactivity in germinative cells of developing rat cerebellum. Science 227:1049–1051.

Development of the Central Nervous System:
Effects of Alcohol and Opiates, pages 341–361
© **1992 Wiley-Liss, Inc.**

15

Effects of Perinatal Opiate Addiction on Neurochemical Development of the Brain

CYNTHIA M. KUHN, ROLF T. WINDH, AND PATRICK J. LITTLE
Department of Pharmacology, Duke University Medical Center, Durham, North Carolina

INTRODUCTION

The purpose of this chapter is to review what is known about the effect of chronic opiate exposure during ontogeny on the neurochemical development of the brain, to synthesize this information into a concise summary, and to discuss gaps in our knowledge which need to be addressed in the future. This review complements other chapters in this volume which cover the normal ontogeny of endogenous opioid systems (Chapter 12), opiate effects on behavioral development (Chapter 11), and the clinical outcome of perinatal opiate addiction (Chapter 3).

A single goal has guided most of the studies reviewed in this chapter: to determine potential mediators of the suppression of growth, perturbations in behavioral development, and (theoretically) potential risk for opioid self administration in adulthood which can result from exposure of infants to opiates in utero. Animal studies provide a tremendous advantage in identifying potential mechanisms of action because the direct impact of opioids on biochemical processes can be understood in the absence of poly-drug use, human immunodeficiency syndrome (HIV) infection, and the tremendous impact of social environment which complicate the interpretation of clinical studies. Despite these strengths, many issues about the precise model of drug exposure can influence the outcome, and so a brief section discussing how such issues guide interpretation of various studies has been included. This is a particularly important issue in integrating the results of many different treatment paradigms which include different test drugs, dose regimens, and most important, periods of drug exposure, throughout a developmental time span when the neural substrate of drug action is changing almost hourly.

It must be emphasized that this chapter has been written with the advantage of hindsight. Many of the studies cited preceded identification of the endogenous opioid peptides and opiate receptors, and so these investigators pursued studies with little knowledge of the neural substrate of drug action. Therefore, many early studies described opiate effects on the then-known neurotransmitter systems, which we now know to be indirect targets of endogenous opioids, distinct neurotransmitters in their own right. In this regard, recent studies of the trophic effects of opioids provide a new perspective for interpreting such effects. In the present review, we will take advantage of this hindsight, and first review what is known about perinatal opiate effects on the ontogeny of the endogenous opioid systems as the most likely target, opioid effects on cell growth and replication, and finally, opiate effects on non-opioid neurotransmitter systems.

Finally, we will discuss briefly the impact of these biochemical changes on brain function in adulthood. There are numerous studies of behavioral development following perinatal opiate exposure (see excellent reviews by Zagon et al., 1982, McDowell and Kitchen, 1987; Zagon et al., 1989b). However, most of these studies focused on opiate effects on spontaneous development, or the normal ontogeny of behavior. Few focused on specific neural substrates of behavior (e.g. catecholamine-mediated behaviors). Those studies which do focus on the function of the endogenous opioid systems suggest that focusing on identified neural substrates by studying agonist-induced behaviors will be particularly fruitful in identifying, and more importantly, predicting the types of central nervous system (CNS) impairment which result from perinatal opiate exposure. Therefore, the discussion of behavioral issues is restricted to published studies of opiate-mediated behaviors.

EXPERIMENTAL DESIGN IN PERINATAL OPIATE RESEARCH

There are several important methodologic issues which must be considered when designing and interpreting studies of perinatal opiate exposure. Many of these issues are inherent to all developmental studies; however, opiate research provides a classic example of the need to establish experimental designs which allow clear experimental results.

The first and major issue which must be addressed is the starting time and duration of exposure to opiates. First, opiate exposure must be considered within the context of the developmental framework for the ontogeny of endogenous opioid systems. As with many developing neural systems, cell bodies are formed during early to midgestation, while functionally-competent systems are first established late in gestation, with a large rise postnatally (Tsang et al., 1982a,b; Alessi and Khachaturian, 1985; Khachaturian et al., 1985; Loughlin et al., 1985). The impact of opiate exposure on these different processes is highly dependent upon the phase of development during which the animal is exposed to opiates. Opiate effects on receptor function might be minimal early in gestation, although trophic effects on opioid cell division will be substantial only during this early phase of development. Furthermore, there is significant divergence among the different opioid systems in ontogeny. For example, met-and leu-enkephalin levels are relatively low at birth and increase to adult levels over the first 4 weeks, while endorphin levels are much higher than enkephalin at midgestation (Bayon et al., 1979). Similarly, there is a divergence in the ontogeny of different opiate receptor types. Functional mu and kappa receptors can be detected at birth, and probably prenatally in rats, while significant numbers of delta receptors only appear during the second and third postnatal weeks (Spain et al., 1985; Kornblum et al., 1987a).

Dosing schedule represents another critical issue in experimental design. In choosing the dosing regimen in experimental studies, it is necessary to choose a dose which is sufficiently large to produce an effect, yet not toxic to the fetus, and within a clinically relevant range. Maternal, fetal, and neonatal pharmacokinetics must be considered carefully in the design of dose, regimens. As the blood-brain barrier changes dramatically postnatally in rats , even to relatively lipid soluble opiates (Kupferberg and Leong-Way, 1963; Auguy-Valette et al., 1978; Shah and Alexander, 1979), the amount of morphine delivered changes. The point at which this issue becomes most relevant is the transition at birth. Maternal administration is necessary to study gestational opiate effects, however at birth, continuing opiate delivery through the dam results in a dramatic decline in opiate dose to the pup. For example, while fetal rats show tissue methadone levels 3–4 fold above that of the dam, a study in humans suggests that so little methadone is excreted into the milk that transfer to the infant is limited to no more than a fraction of the dose received by the mother (Peters et al., 1972; Kreek, 1979). The alternative of treating the pups directly can therefore provide some advantages. Furthermore, substantial drug accumulation can result which makes investigation of precise developmental windows difficult. For example, methadone treatment between day 16 and day 22 of gestation resulted in brain levels of methadone which persisted for several weeks following birth (Levitt et al., 1983). Finally, the issue of opiate tolerance must be considered in the design of treatment paradigms. Two opposite strategies have been used to deal with this issue. To avoid opiate effects on maternal physiology, numerous studies initiated opiate treatment even before mating. While this strategy optimizes maternal physiology, it guarantees that both maternal and probably fetal tissues will be tolerant to many opiate effects by the time critical periods of receptor development during postnatal life are reached. Therefore, the converse strategy of treating with opiates during the "critical period" for cell division, synaptogenesis, receptor development, etc., provides an important alternative. With either scenario, the well known differences in the development of tolerance to various opiate actions must be considered (Jaffe and Martin, 1990).

The age at which animals are tested following opiate treatment can impact interpretation of the studies tremendously. Substantial effects which can be detected at the end of a perinatal treatment regimen often normalize as the animal matures. For example, Temple et al. (1988) report significant down-regulation of opiate receptors early in postnatal life, but these changes proved to be transient. Furthermore, "developmental" effects must meet two criteria. First, they must be measurable in adulthood, not simply at postnatal day 10 or 20. Second, they must be different from similar effects observed after chronic treatment of adult animals. This is an often neglected issue of data interpretation. Chronic opiate administration has marked and persistent effects on the adult nervous system, and part of the outcome of perinatal treatment regimens might simply reflect changes in the brain identical to those produced during treatment of adults.

In addition to the issues of pharmacologic treatment strategies and interpretation raised above, there are other factors which can influence and confound the outcome of perinatal opiate treatment regimens. Opiate-induced changes in maternal physiology can play a central role in determining the physiologic state of the fetus. For example, a decline in maternal, not just fetal, weight gain occurs following chronic gestational methadone treatment (White et al., 1978). It is well established that maternal undernutrition has long-term effects on fetal development (Sparber, 1986). Furthermore, non-nutritional effects on the dam including effects on hormone secretion, placental blood flow, and maternal respiration (and hence blood oxygen content) could contribute to opiate effects on fetal development. Therefore, the popular paradigm of pair-feeding provides a poor approximation of opiate effects on maternal physiology (Raye et al., 1977).

Maternal behavior as well as physiology affects the growth and development of neonates. Endogenous opiate systems may result in the onset and quality of maternal responsiveness in rats (Bridges and Grimm, 1982; Grimm and Bridges, 1983). Thus, maternal opiate treatment during postnatal life can influence pup development through actions on maternal responsiveness to the pups.

Maternal "stress" or "stress" to the offspring is often cited as a mediator of adverse drug effects on development. As endogenous opioids are thought to play a major role in stress responsivity, this argument is justifiable, as prolonged periods of stress might produce changes in the sensitivity of opiate systems independent of direct opiate action. Periodic abstinence has been a particular concern in perinatal opiate studies, as abstinence can lead to an increase in morbidity of neonates (Lichtblau and Sparber, 1981a, 1984), and can be demonstrated to occur even in utero (Umans and Szeto, 1985). This concern has lead to increasing use of continuous infusion paradigms, which avoid peaks and valleys in drug levels.

In summary, design and interpretation of perinatal opiate studies must take into consideration major concerns about opiate pharmacokinetics in developing organisms, opiate actions on maternal physiology, and abstinence-induced stress. However, these problems are not insurmountable. Careful utilization of dose-response strategies, utilization of constant infusion paradigms, and careful timing of opiate exposure in relationship to the parameter under investigation can provide improved experimental control for these issues.

OPIATE EFFECTS ON ENDOGENOUS OPIOID SYSTEMS

Opiate Receptors

Opiate receptors represent the most direct target of opiate treatment. In adults, the ability of opiate antagonists to upregulate receptor number and function is well established (Zukin and Temple, 1986; Zukin et al., 1982), although the ability of opiate agonists to downregulate receptors is unclear, and has been demonstrated unequivocally in vivo in only a few cases (Davis et al., 1979; Dingeldine et al., 1983; Rogers and El-Fakahany, 1986; Steece et al., 1986; Tao et al., 1987). During ontogeny, however, receptor populations are more dynamic. These receptors are regulated potentially not only by agonist occupation, but also by all those mechanisms regulating the development of the postsynaptic cells. Therefore, opiate effects in the adult nervous system are not necessarily good predictors of the outcome of chronic opiate exposure in the developing nervous system.

The most thorough study of opiate receptor numbers in ontogeny is that reported by Temple et al. (1988) (see Chapter 13 for a more extended description of this work). These authors reported that morphine pellet implantation into pregnant or neonatal rats resulted in a significant decrease in mu opiate receptor number in the brain only until postnatal day 8. An identical treatment did not influence receptor number in older pups. Three other studies reported similar findings of a decrease in opiate receptor number after perinatal treatment. In two studies, Kirby and colleagues (Kirby et al., 1982; Kirby and Aronstam, 1983) reported that gestational morphine treatment to pregnant rats decreased naloxone binding in brainstem of offspring at the end of treatment (day 21 of gestation). This decrease had disappeared by adulthood. In addition, Wang et al., (1986) reported that methadone administration during gestation and early postnatal life resulted in a decrease in hypothalamic and cortical mu receptors in adulthood. Zadina and colleagues reported that administration of β-endorphin to pups during the last third of gestation decreased mu and delta receptor binding on postnatal day 14 (Zadina et al., 1985; Zadina and Kastin, 1986). Finally, opiate receptor down-regulation has been observed in fetal brain aggregates (Lenoir et al., 1984). In contrast to the above findings of receptor decreases, Bardo et al. (1982) reported no effect of morphine treatment on days 1–21 on naloxone binding in several brain regions on postnatal day 22 or in adulthood, while Handelman and Quirion (1983) reported that morphine treatment on days 1–7 increased mu receptor binding in adulthood. Whereas most of these studies report receptor number at one or two time points (generally at the end of treatment and in adulthood), the one study which followed opiate receptor binding throughout ontogeny reported that chronic morphine treatment through gestation causes a complex, region-specific *sequence* of changes in the binding of met-enkephalin (Tsang and Ng, 1980). Although receptor number was uniformly suppressed in the brainstem, receptors in forebrain were increased on postnatal days 1–2 followed by a later suppression.

The several studies of opiate receptor number following perinatal administration of opiate antagonists report more consistent findings: an increase in receptor number at the end of treatment. Bardo et al. (1982, 1983) report an increase in naloxone binding after treatment on postnatal days 1–21 in rats. The reported rise is dose-dependent and greater than that following administration of a similar treatment regimen to adults.

Methodologic considerations complicate the integrated interpretation of these studies. These complications include use of different agonists, treatment across various phases of development, and most important, the frequent use of radioligand binding techniques which label multiple opiate receptor populations. Nevertheless, several general conclusions can be drawn. In general, agonist administration decreases and antagonist treatment increases receptor number, and opiate receptor numbers appear more sensitive to perturbation by opiates in the developing nervous system than in the mature nervous system. Rises and falls in response to antagonist and agonist treatment regimens have been reported following treatment of developing animals with paradigms which in adults exert minimal effects. Moreover, receptor changes in ontogeny tend to be even more transient than in adults. Finally, treatment during gestation or the first few days of life consistently results in larger changes in receptor number than treatments during later phases of ontogeny. This last finding suggests that a "critical period" of receptor plasticity exists, although changes induced even during this most sensitive time have proven transient. It is important in interpreting studies of perinatal opiate effects on receptor ontogeny to remember that opiate effects on receptor numbers could result from two general mechanisms: classic up- and down-regulation induced by changes in agonist occupation of receptor, or alteration in the ontogeny of the cell population expressing the receptors. The latter possibility represents a plausible explanation for the complex sequence of changes observed in such studies. Such patterns can reflect a delay or acceleration in differentiation of a target neuron population rather than simple receptor up- or down-regulation.

Endogenous Opioids

Within the CNS, neuronal activity and/or presynaptic mechanisms responsible for the synthesis, storage, and degradation of neurotransmitters frequently are changed in response to chronic agonist or antagonist treatment, presumably through polysynaptic negative feedback pathways. The sparse literature available in adults suggests that similar presynaptic adaptations of endogenous opioid neurons result from chronic opiate agonist treatment. However, the impact of treatment during ontogeny on endogenous opioid synthesis, release, and degradation is just beginning to be elucidated. These few reports suggest that presynaptic mechanisms represent an additional target of perinatal opiate exposure. Gianoulakis (1986) reported that gestational morphine treatment resulted in a slight decrease in hypothalamic and pituitary β-endorphin perinatally, followed by a transient rebound increase on postnatal day 4 and subsequent normalization of peptide levels. Similar findings by Tiong and Olley (1988) suggest that gestational morphine exposure causes a transient decrease in brain enkephalin levels on postnatal day 8. In contrast, Bianchi et al. (1988) reported that chronic morphine throughout gestation increased β-endorphin and met-enkephalin in the hypothalamus throughout gestation, whereas chronic postnatal morphine treatment increased met-enkephalin synthesis in pons-medulla (DiGiulio et al., 1988). Exciting preliminary results from Temple (see Chapter 13) show that changes in both opioid peptide and mRNA for these peptides occur with late gestational and/or early postnatal morphine treatment.

These studies are more difficult to integrate than the receptor studies reported above. No simple pattern of peptide production emerges from them. However, some general conclusions can be reached. As is true for receptor number, changes in peptides resulting from perinatal opiate exposure seem to be transient, and largest following gestational treatments. Similar methodologic limitations are imposed by the different phases of development studied by different laboratories, and the poor anatomic resolution of sampled regions. The recent development of radioimmunoassays for peptide neurotransmitters and methodologies for studying precursor mRNA formation have provided a new approach to this problem. More extensive studies utilizing the well characterized anatomic and biochemical differentiation of the multiple opioid peptide systems will be able to provide considerably more information in the future about the real effects of chronic agonist or antagonist treatment on opioid peptide dynamics in development.

Effects of Opiates on Opioid Neuron Function

The correlations between the effects of perinatal opiate exposure on receptor number, endogenous opioid synthesis, and opiate receptor function as assessed with a response to pharmacologic challenge are poor (see Chapter 12). This inconclusive relationship resembles findings in adults, and remains one of the great challenges of opiate receptor biochemistry. Evaluation of the role of biochemical changes in opioid systems on the behavioral effects of opiates is complicated further by the difficulty of comparing receptor studies conducted in one laboratory using one opiate treatment paradigm, and behavioral studies conducted by another investigator using a different treatment paradigm. One particularly interesting finding emerges from a study that did directly compare behavior and receptor number after gestational or early postnatal morphine pellet implantation. Temple et al. (1988) demonstrated that tolerance to opiate analgesia was observed even after decline in opiate receptors had disappeared. Similar tolerance has been reported after even single doses of opiates to older rat pups (Huidobro and Huidobro, 1973), and in endocrine systems after postnatal methadone or morphine administration (Kuhn and Bartolome, 1984; Kuhn et al., 1987). Careful comparison of opiate analgesia across ages suggests that tolerance is much less robust and more transient after perinatal treatment than after treatment of adults (Fanselow and Cramer,

1988; Windh and Kuhn, 1990; Blass, personal communication). This behavioral finding might represent a correlate to the greater plasticity in opioid receptor function that has been observed in developmental studies.

Changes in sensitivity to opiates after perinatal treatment which persist into adulthood are harder to explain on the basis of reported changes in opioid neuron biochemistry. While effects on pain perception have been reported, results conflict widely. An excellent review of the older literature has been published recently (McDowell and Kitchen, 1987). Zagon and McLaughlin (1980, 1982) found that basal pain thresholds are elevated following pre- and/or postnatal methadone exposure, while opposite effect (hyperalgesia) has been reported following gestational methadone or post- but not prenatal treatment with β-endorphin (Hovious and Peters, 1984; Zadina et al., 1985, 1987). Furthermore, gestational morphine or methadone exposure has been found to either decrease or increase sensitivity to morphine-induced analgesia (Jóhannesson and Becker, 1972; Steele and Johannesson, 1975b; O'Callaghan and Holtzman, 1976; Kirby et al., 1982; Hovious and Peters, 1984). It is important to reiterate that the poor correlation between behavioral effects of opiates and measurable changes in opiate receptor function are not unique to developmental studies, as the same difficulties have plagued studies in adults.

Sexual behavior and control of gonadotropin secretion represent one of the few brain functions in which tonic opioid control can be demonstrated in the adult. Therefore, it is not surprising that several studies report that perinatal opiate treatment influences ongoing sexual behavior as well as opioid modulation of sexual behavior. Beta-endorphin treatment during the early postnatal period in rats changes male copulatory behavior, and perinatal naltrexone administration facilitates sexual behavior in female rats and decreases the effect of morphine on copulatory behavior (Meyerson, 1982, 1985; Meyerson and Berg, 1985; Meyerson et al., 1988). Similarly, opioid modulation of luteinizing hormone (LH) secretion is thought to play an important role in pubertal development, which is delayed at least in male rats by chronic morphine treatment (Cicero et al., 1984) while naloxone has been reported to accelerate puberty in females (Sirinathsinghji et al., 1985). These findings suggest that opioid modulation of reproductive function might provide an extremely useful model function for studying developmental effects of opiates.

Surprisingly, although the clinical importance of perinatal opiate effects on the vulnerability to opiate self administration has been widely discussed, there are few published studies of this issue. Hovious and Peters (1984) did show that methadone exposure through gestation and lactation increased self administration of morphine in offspring. On the other hand, methadone self administration did not change in these animals. A similar increase in morphine self administration has been reported in the offspring of morphine-treated dams (Glick et al., 1977). This finding is difficult to reconcile with the biochemical studies of opiate receptors mentioned above, but the role of conditioning and learning in drug self administration is significant, and can potentially play a role even early in development.

In summary, although persistent effects of perinatal opiate treatment on the function of opiate receptors in adulthood have been reported, no consistent pattern emerges, nor is there a consistent relationship between reported changes in opioid neuron function and receptor number. Both attenuated and augmented responses have been reported. This inconsistency might reflect in part the different developmental periods of drug exposure used in various studies: exposure during a critical period early in ontogeny when opioid neurons are first forming might have quite different consequences than administration later in development. In addition, it is difficult to compare different indices, as tolerance to different opiate actions develops to a varying extent even in adults. Finally, the work of Zagon suggests that the particular treatment paradigm might prove extremely important, as treatment with high doses of long-lasting drugs which produce monophasic actions might produce effects exactly the opposite of those produced by low doses of short-acting agents, which can elicit rebound changes in endogenous opioid release.

OPIATE EFFECTS ON CELL GROWTH AND REPLICATION

Opiate effects on growth have been examined at both the organismic and molecular level, using a variety of opiate compounds, treatment regimens, control groups, and measured indices. Despite differences in these experimental conditions, there is a general consensus that perinatal opiate treatment decreases body weight and brain weight at birth and into adult life. Treating pregnant rats or neonatal rat pups with methadone, morphine, or levo-alpha-acetylmethadol (LAAM) produces these effects (Crofford and Smith, 1973; Hutchings et al., 1976; Smith et al., 1977; Anderson and Slotkin, 1975; Slotkin et al., 1976; McGinty and Ford, 1976; McLaughlin and Zagon, 1978, 1980; Lichtblau and Sparber, 1981b). Studies have shown the perturbations to be dose-dependent, stereoselective, and naloxone-reversible, indicating that specific opiate receptors mediate these responses. Although opiate-induced undernutrition, hypoxia, and withdrawal have been discussed as potential indirect mediators of these responses, the general conclusion which can be reached from the aggregate findings of these studies is that direct opiate effects on growth probably contribute to the observed effects.

Biochemical studies verify that perinatal opiate treatments actually suppress brain growth. Both pre- and postnatal treatment decrease RNA, protein, and in some cases DNA content of developing brain. Prenatal methadone treatment resulted in a decrease in brain RNA and protein at birth. While the second author reported normalization of biochemical indices after the cessation of treatment, the first reported changes persisted into adulthood. Postnatal morphine treatment of mice also has been reported to decrease RNA and protein content and synthesis in brain (Jóhannesson et al., 1972; Hui et al., 1978). An interesting potential mechanism explaining these effects is suggested by the work of Steele and Jóhannesson (1975a). These authors reported that acute morphine treatment to pregnant rats increased the proportion of disomes in fetal brain.

Disomes are thought to form by aggregation of free ribosomes, presumably due to deficits in the interaction of mRNA, tRNA, and nascent poplypeptides that normally inhibit dimerization. These results suggest that morphine directly inhibits RNA synthesis in developing brain.

Although the above studies found no changes in DNA content following prenatal methadone treatment, other studies do report such changes. Zagon and McLaughlin (1978) report that opiate agonists decrease brain DNA content in pups treated prenatally with methadone. The decrease in RNA/DNA and protein/DNA ratios observed in these studies suggests that the effects on DNA exceeded effects on RNA and protein. The findings of DNA decreases are supported by other studies reporting that opiates directly inhibit DNA synthesis in vitro in developing brain (Vértes et al., 1982; Kornblum et al., 1987b). The latter findings are particularly convincing evidence that opiate effects are in part direct, rather than the results of undernutrition, etc.

The most exciting findings relating opiates to cell growth in the brain are the reports of Zagon and McLaughlin (1985, 1987, 1989, 1990a) demonstrating that opiate antagonists have significant effects on cell growth themselves. An extensive series of studies from this laboratory have shown that opiate antagonists actually increase brain weight, cell number, and several anatomic indices of brain maturation (see review of this area in Chapter 14). Large doses of antagonists increase, and small doses decrease brain growth (as well as somatic growth). These authors have concluded that the effects of small doses reflect rebound release of endogenous opioids, that these endogenous opioids actively modulate brain growth in rodents, and that the observed effects of agonists represent supramaximal stimulation of receptors that normally are involved in the regulation of growth and development. More detailed anatomical studies validating the presence of opioids and receptors in germinal zones of developing cerebellum and demonstration that morphine inhibits dendritic growth support these conclusions (Zagon and McLaughlin, 1990a,b; Ricalde and Hammer, 1990).

Modulation of nucleic acid and protein synthesis provides some measure of opiate effects on the subcellular processes occurring in development. The specific mechanism through which opiates influence cell growth and differentiation is unclear, however, opiate effects on ornithine decarboxylase (ODC) provide considerable insight into the path of receptor occupation-signal transduction-gene activation which leads to changes in these processes (Slotkin, 1979). ODC is the rate-limiting enzyme in the synthesis of polyamines putrescine, spermine, and spermidine. Activity of this enzyme is high in tissues which are proliferating rapidly, including brain, and a decline in its activity often signals the end of cell growth (Russell, 1981; Bell and Slotkin, 1988). Furthermore, inhibition of this enzyme inhibits tissue growth, and in brain, slows synaptogenesis (Slotkin et al., 1976, 1980, 1983), demonstrating a direct role for the products of ODC in modulation of brain growth. ODC provides a unique link between cellular receptor occupation and gene activation for two reasons. First, it has an extremely short half life (10 minutes) and so provides a rapidly responding index of stimuli which evoke changes in cell growth. Second, its activity is altered by a large number of hormonal stimuli: the gene for this enzyme is part of the complex of genes including c-*fos* and c-*myc* which respond to trophic signals in brain and other tissues (Kaczmarek and Kaminska, 1989). Therefore, changes in ODC activity provide a measure upstream to nucleic acid synthesis in the cascade of events from receptor activation to growth inhibition.

The acute inhibition of ODC activity by opiates in developing brain provided the first evidence that opiate receptor occupation generates intracellular signals involved in regulating cell growth and differentiation. Butler and Schanberg (1975) first demonstrated that maternal morphine administration decreases ODC activity in neonatal brain. These studies have been expanded recently by Bartolome et al. (1986), who reported that central administration of β-endorphin decreases ODC activity in brain and peripheral tissues. These effects occur only until weaning. Surprisingly, naloxone blocked effects only on brain ODC activity, suggesting that classical mu receptors are involved in the regulation of brain growth, but perhaps not peripheral trophic processes. This conclusion is supported by another finding by Bartolome et al. (1987) demonstrating that the nonopioid peptide N-alpha-acetyl-beta-endorphin increases rather than decreases ODC activity by an action not blocked by naloxone.

Studies of chronic opiate effects on ODC activity provide additional evidence that ODC activity is regulated by opiate receptors. Slotkin and co-workers (Slotkin et al., 1976; Seidler et al., 1982) demonstrated that pre- and postnatal methadone administration delayed the normal postnatal fall in ODC in brain which signals the end of cell growth. This effect was even more pronounced in peripheral tissues than in brain, where effects were more dramatic, and observed at lower doses of methadone.

The specific cellular mechanisms through which opiates inhibit ODC activity, and perhaps other aspects of cell growth, remain unclear. However, recent studies of the mechanism of opiate receptor action suggest a new interpretation for several older studies of opiate action on cyclic nucleotide levels. Acute opiate administration decreases cyclic adenosine monophosphate (cAMP) levels in developing brain, and simultaneously suppress ODC activity (Persitz et al., 1984). Furthermore, opiate-induced declines in AMP-dependent protein kinase, cAMP accumulation, and ODC activity occur simultaneously in cultured neuroblastoma x glioma cells, suggesting that direct cellular actions of opiates mediate these effects (Benalal and Bachrach, 1985). Cyclic AMP functions as an intracellular regulator of ODC activity in many tissues (Byus and Russell, 1974; Baudry et al., 1988; Otani et al., 1990). Therefore, occupation of mu opiate receptors could mediate trophic effects of opioids. In fact, Zagon and co-workers (Zagon et al., 1989a, 1990a,b) have conducted preliminary biochemical characterization of a receptor they postulate mediates the growth suppressing effects of opioids which resembles in many ways the mu opiate receptor, although these authors suggest that these receptors exist within the cell rather than on the cell surface.

Elucidation of the specific chain of intracellular events through which opiates regulate gene expression and cell growth represents one of the exciting directions in perinatal opiate research. Such effects could provide a possible explanation for the retardation of somatic and brain growth, and perhaps, specific effects on non-opioid target neurons, the growth of which might be modulated in this way. The latter topic will be covered in the following pages.

OPIATE EFFECTS ON NON-OPIOID NEUROTRANSMITTER SYSTEMS
Opiates and Catecholamine Systems

The effects of perinatal opiate exposure on the ontogeny of central and peripheral catecholamine systems have been better described than opiate effects on opioid neurons. This research interest is based historically upon the well known effects of opiate agonists on catecholamine neuron function, which predates discovery of the opioids.

The most comprehensive series of studies are those of Slotkin and co-workers, who have characterized perinatal methadone effects on the biochemical development of central and peripheral catecholamine neurons. The earliest of these studies described the effects of maternal methadone administration on the development of the peripheral sympathetic nervous system. In these studies, maternal methadone administration through gestation and suckling resulted in a decrease in catecholamine biosynthetic enzymes in the adrenal medulla whereas administration of methadone to the pups caused an increase in enzyme activity (Slotkin and Anderson, 1975; Lau et al., 1977). These apparently contradictory results were reconciled by later studies which demonstrated that perinatal methadone administration resulted in precocious sympathetic innervation of all peripheral tissues as demonstrated by premature rises in norepinephrine uptake, synaptic vesicle uptake, biosynthetic enzymes, and the appearance of sympathetic reflex activation by insulin (Bareis and Slotkin, 1978, 1980; Slotkin et al., 1980). These studies have been integrated in an elegant review (Slotkin, 1988) which draws on more recent findings from his laboratory. His thesis is that methadone-induced precocious innervation causes a premature cessation of cell growth and differentiation, leading to ultimate deficits in sympathetic neuron function.

The effect of perinatal methadone exposure on the development of central catecholamine systems is quite different. Rather uniformly, these studies suggest that gestational and/or postnatal methadone administration delays and in some cases permanently decreases the function of these systems. Slotkin and co-workers have shown that the same perinatal methadone treatments which accelerate peripheral sympathetic development slow synaptogenesis of central noradrenergic and dopaminergic systems as evidenced by delays in synaptosomal uptake of neurotransmitter, biosynthetic enzymes, and postsynaptic alpha adrenergic receptor function (Slotkin and Anderson, 1975; Lau et al., 1977; Slotkin, 1979; Slotkin et al., 1981,

1982; McGinty and Ford, 1980). Although no changes in whole brain norepinephrine turnover were observed by these authors, they did report a decline in dopamine turnover (Slotkin et al., 1981). Consistent findings from other laboratories include reports that perinatal morphine has no effect on norepinephrine turnover (Bardo et al., 1982) and that methadone treatment through gestation and suckling decreased dopamine turnover in striatum, an effect which persisted into adulthood (Rech et al., 1980). Adrenergic receptor function also may be affected by perinatal opiate exposure, as decreases in both alpha-1 stimulated phospholipid turnover, and alpha-2 receptor number in cortex have been reported (Slotkin et al., 1982; Wang et al., 1986). The finding that gestational and postnatal methadone administration also decrease the normal developmental rise in the catecholamine catabolic enzyme monoamine oxidase (Tsang et al., 1986) further demonstrates that delayed ontogeny of monoaminergic transmission include both pre- and postsynaptic components of the system. These findings emphasize the point raised earlier that all changes in biochemical indices do not reflect the simple up- and down-regulation of synaptic function by agonist occupation.

Opiates and Serotonin

Although endogenous opioid interactions with serotonin neurons have been widely described in the adult CNS, few studies of perinatal opiate effects upon the ontogeny of these systems have been published. Those few that exist suggest that, like catecholamines, the ontogeny of central serotonin neurons is slowed by perinatal opiate treatment. Total brain serotonin content is unchanged by gestational or postnatal morphine administration (Bardo et al., 1982), whereas decrements in presynaptic markers have been reported. Two groups (De Montis et al., 1983; Slotkin et al., 1979) reported that gestational methadone treatment delays the ontogeny of synaptosomal uptake of serotonin, and imipramine binding sites. In the former study, ^{3}H-serotonin binding (presumably reflecting 5HT1 receptors) was unchanged in adult offspring of animals exposed to methadone during gestation. Incubation of fetal serotonin neurons in culture with leu-enkephalin inhibited the development of these neurons as assessed with serotonin uptake by a naloxone sensitive mechanism (Davlia-Garcia and Azmitia, 1989). These exciting results raise the possibility that direct opioid modulation of serotonin neuron maturation might mediate the observed responses.

Opiates and Cholinergic Neurons

There are only sporadic reports of perinatal opiate effects on biochemical indices of cholinergic neuron function. The same report cited above which described delay of serotonin synaptogenesis in the absence of receptor changes also reported that gestational methadone treatment did not influence muscarinic receptor number (De Montis et al., 1983). Another isolated report suggests that brain levels of the catabolic enzyme acetylcholinesteraseare diminished during early postnatal life following gestational methadone treatment (Field et al., 1977).

SUMMARY

The major conclusion which can be drawn from the preceding review is that the impact of opiate exposure during ontogeny on neurochemical ontogeny of the brain is virtually unexplored. This lack of information derives mainly from the recent development of neurochemical tools for characterizing opiate receptors and endogenous opioid dynamics, and from the difficulty of establishing even in adult animals the neural substrates of chronic opiate effects on opioid neuron function.

Nevertheless, several conclusions can be drawn. First, the incomplete but intriguing literature on opioid receptors suggests that chronic agonist or antagonist exposure can have more dramatic effects on developing opioid receptors than similar exposure in adults, although the functional impact of observed changes in receptor number is unclear. Opiate receptors seem to be more labile than presynaptic mechanisms directing opioid synthesis and degradation, although relevant studies are just beginning. Second, a growing body of knowledge suggests that opioids have a dual function in the developing nervous system as neurotransmitters and as trophic agents regulating brain growth. The work of Zagon and others suggests that opioids exist in developing brain in a unique distribution, and possess identifiable effects on indices of growth and development. This work has provided a novel mechanism of opioid effects on CNS development. Third, the work on catecholamine neuron ontogeny suggests that opioids have converse effects on peripheral and central catecholamine systems, accelerating peripheral ontogeny, but delaying, and perhaps permanently altering, the activity of central norepinephrine and dopamine systems. These effects might be explained either by classic opioid synaptic interactions with these systems, or in part by trophic actions of opioids.

Although some positive findings about opiate effects on opiate receptors and catecholamine systems exist, the gaps in our knowledge are tremendous. There is virtually no information available about opiate effects on other synaptic targets of opioid systems. More important, our information about even the normal ontogeny of receptor coupling to transduction systems limits our understanding of how opiate-induced changes in receptor number are translated into postsynaptic effects. As recent studies have focused on normal ontogeny of opioid systems, little new work on chronic opiate exposure in ontogeny has been published in 10 years. Given the incredible advances in methodologic approaches available for studying receptor function as well as presynaptic neurotransmitter dynamics at this time, this field is poised for an explosion of productive research. This work will be critical both in understanding the potential clinical significance of perinatal opiate exposure and the normal development of the brain.

Research into possible mediators of the observed effects of perinatal opiate exposure on neurochemical parameters represents another important area for future research. With the demonstration of trophic actions of opioids, the relative contributions of synaptic actions of opioids upon other neurons and trophic actions, perhaps of non-neuronal opioids, remain to be explored.

Finally, the impact of these biochemical changes on CNS function represent the most important outcome of perinatal opiate addition. As reviewed above, a number of studies suggest that opiate receptor-mediated responses are significantly influenced by perinatal opiate exposure, although these changes correlate poorly with the biochemical responses which have been observed. A few intriguing studies suggest that responses modulated by noradrenergic function are influenced. However, again, the area to be explored remains immense. Two areas of particular importance which have been neglected are the often-speculated vulnerability of perinatally addicted animals to drug self administration. There are virtually no studies of opiate self administration in animals exposed to opiates during development. Similarly, the impact of perinatal opiate exposure on monoamine neuron function has not been explored. Two important areas for exploration include the possible role of noradrenergic neurons in affective behavior, physiologic regulation, and neuronal plasticity.

REFERENCES

Alessi NE, Khachaturian H (1985): Postnatal development of beta-endorphin immunoreactivity in the medulla oblongata of rat. Neuropeptides 5:473–476.

Anderson TR, Slotkin TA (1975): Maturation of the adrenal medulla-IV: Effects of morphine. Biochem Pharmacol 24:1469–1474.

Auguy-Valette A, Cros J, Guoarderes C, Gout R, Pontonnier G (1978): Morphine analgesia and cerebral opiate receptors: A developmental study. Br J Pharmacol 63:303–308.

Bardo MT, Bhatnagar RK, Gebhart GF (1982): Differential effects of chronic morphine and naloxone on opiate receptors, monoamines, and morphine-induced behaviors in preweanling rats. Dev Brain Res 4:139–147.

Bardo MT, Bhatnagar RK, Gebhart GF (1983): Age-related differences in the effect of chronic administration of naloxone on opiate binding in rat brain. Neuropharmacology 22:453–461.

Bareis DL, Slotkin TA (1978): Responses of heart ornithine decarboxylase and adrenal catecholamines to methadone and sympathetic stimulants in developing and adult rats. J Pharmacol Exp Ther 25:164–174.

Bartolome JV, Bartolome MB, Daltner LA, Evans CJ, Barchas JD, Kuhn CM, Schanberg SM (1986): Effects of β-endorphin on ornithine decarboxylase in tissues of developing rats: A potential role for this endogenous neuropeptide in the modulation of tissue growth. Life Sci 38:2355–2362.

Bartolome JV, Bartolome MB, Harris EB, Schanberg SM (1987): Nα-acetyl-β-endorphin stimulates ornithine decarboxylase activity in preweanling rat pups: Opioid- and non-opioid-mediated mechanisms. J Pharmacol Exp Ther 240:895–899.

Baudry M, Shahi K, Gall C (1988): Induction of ornithine decarboxylase in adult rat hippocampal slices. Brain Res 464:313–318.

Bayon A, Shoemaker WJ, Bloom FE, Mauss A, Guillemin R (1979): Perinatal development of the endorphin- and enkephalin-containing systems in the rat brain. Brain Res 179:93–101.

Bell JM, Slotkin TA (1988): Coordination of cell development by the ornithine decarboxylase (ODC)/polyamine pathway as an underlying mechanism in developmental neurotoxic events. Prog Brain Res 73:349–363.

Benalal D, Bachrach U (1985): Opiates and cultured neuroblastoma x glioma cells. J Biochem 227:389–395.

Bianchi M, Marini A, Sacerdote P, Cocco E, Brini A, Panerai AE (1988): Effect of chronic morphine on plasma and brain beta endorphin and methionine enkephalin in pregnant rats and in their fetuses or newborns. Neuroendocrinology 47:89–94.

Bridges RS, Grimm CT (1982): Reversal of orphine disruption of maternal behavior by concurrent treatment with the opiate antagonist naloxone. Science 218:166–168.

Butler SR, Schanberg SM (1975): Effect of maternal morphine administration on neonatal rat brain ornithine decarboxylase (ODC). Biochem Pharmacol 24:1915–1918.

Byus CV, Russell DH (1974): Effects of methyl xanthine derivatives on cyclic AMP levels and ornithine decarboxylase activity in rat tissues. Life Sci 15:1991–1997.

Crofford M, Smith AA (1973): Growth retardation in young mice with d, l-methadone. Science 181:947–949.

Davis ME, Akera T, Brody TM (1979): Reduction of opiate binding to brainstem slices associated with the development of tolerance to morphine in rats. J Pharmacol Exp Ther 211:112–119.

DiGuilio AM, Restani P, Galli CL, Tenconi B, La Croix R, Gorio A (1988): Modified ontogenesis of enkephalin and substance P containing neurons after perinatal exposure to morphine. Toxicology 49:197–201.

Dingledine R, Valentino RJ, Bostock E, King ME, Chang KJ (1983): Down-regulation of ∂ but not μ opioid receptors in the hippocampal slice associated with loss of physiological response. Life Sci 33, Supp. I: 333–336.

Fanselow MS, Cramer CP (1988): The ontogeny of tolerance and withdrawal in infant rats. Pharmacol Biochem Behav 31:431–438.

Field T, McNelly A, Sadava D (1977): Effect of maternal methadone addiction on offspring in rats. Arch Int Pharmacodyn The 228:300–303.

Gianoulakis C (1986): Effect of maternally administered opiates on the development of the β-endorphin system in the offspring. NIDA Res Monogr 75:595–598.

Glick SD, Strumpf AJ, Zimmerberg B (1977): Effect of in utero administration of morphine on subsequent development of self-administration behavior. Brain Res 132:194–196.

Grimm CT, Bridges RS (1983): Opiate regulation of maternal behavior in the rat. Pharmacol Biochem Behav 19:609–616.

Handelmann GE, Quirion R (1983): Neonatal exposure to morphine increases μ opiate binding in the adult forebrain. Eur J Pharmacol 94:357–358.

Hess GD, Zagon IS (1988): Endogenous opioid systems and neural development: Ultrastructural studies in the cerebellar cortex of infant and weanling rats. Brain Res Bull 20:473–478.

Hovious JR, Peters MA (1984): Analgesic effect of opiates in offspring of opiate treated female rats. Pharmacol Biochem Behav 21:555–559.

Hui FW, Krikun E, Smith AA (1978): Inhibition by d,l-methadone of RNA and protein synthesis in neonatal mice: Antagonism by naloxone or naltrexone. Eur J Pharmacol 49:87–93.

Huidobro JP, Huidobro F (1973): Acute morphine tolerance in newborn and young rats. Psychopharmacol 28:27–34.

Hutchings DE, Hunt HF, Towey JP, Rosen TS, Gorinson HS (1976): Methadone during pregnancy in the rat: Dose level effects on maternal and perinatal mortality and growth in the offspring. J Pharmacol Exp Ther 197:171–179.

Jaffe JH, Martin WR (1990): Opioid analgesics and antagonists. In Gilman A G, Rall T W, Nies A S, Taylor P (eds): "The Pharmacological Basis of Therapeutics, 8th Edition." New York: Pergamon Press, pp 485–522.

Jóhannesson T, Becker BA (1972): The effects of maternally administered morphine on rat foetal development and resultant tolerance to the analgesic effect of morphine. Acta Pharmcol Toxicol 31:305–313.

Jóhannesson T, Steele WJ, Becker BA (1972): Infusion of morphine in maternal rats at near-term: Maternal and foetal distribution and effects on analgesia, brain DNA, RNA, and protein. Acta Pharmcol Toxicol 31:353–368.

Kaczmarek L, Kaminska B (1989): Molecular biology of cell activation. Exp Cell Res 183:24–35.

Khachaturian H, Lewis ME, Alessi NE, Watson SJ (1985): Time of origin of opioid peptide-containing neurons in the rat hypothalamus. J Comp Neurol 236:538–546.

Kirby ML, Aronstam RS (1983): Levorphanol-sensitive [³H]naloxone binding in developing brainstem following prenatal morphine exposure. Neurosci Lett 35:191–195.

Kirby ML, De Rossett SE, Holtzman SG (1982): Enhanced analgesic response to morphine in adult rats exposed to morphine prenatally. Pharmacol Biochem Behav 17:1161–1164.

Kornblum HI, Hurlburt DE, Leslie FM (1987a): Postnatal development of multiple opioid receptors in rat brain. Dev Brain Res 37:21–41.

Kornblum HI, Loughlin SE, Leslie FM (1987b): Effects of morphine on DNA synthesis in neonatal rat brain. Dev Brain Res 31:45–52.

Kreek MJ (1979): Methadone disposition during the perinatal period in humans. Pharmacol Biochem Behav 11, Suppl.:7–13.

Kuhn CM, Bartolome M (1984): Effect of chronic methadone administration on neuroendocrine function in developing rats. Dev Pharmacol 7:384–397.

Kuhn CM, Bero L, Ignar D, Lurie S, Field E (1987): Early maturation of mu and kappa opiate control of hormone secretion and effects of perinatal opiate addiction. NIDA Res Monogr 81:71–94.

Kupferberg HJ, Leong-Way E (1963): Pharmacological basis for the increased sensitivity of the newborn rat to morphine. J Pharmacol Exp Ther 141:105–112.

Lau C, Bartolomé M, Slotkin TA (1977): Development of central and peripheral catecholaminergic systems in rats addicted perinatally to methadone. Neuropharmacology 16:473–478.

Lenoir D, Barg J, Simantov R (1984): Characterization and down-regulation of opiate receptors in aggregating fetal rat brain cells. Brain Res 304:285–290.

Levitt M, Hutchings DE, Bodnaarenko SR (1983): Fate of tritium derived from prenatally administered tritiated methadone in dams and neonatal rats. Pharmacol Biochem Behav 19:1051–1053.

Lichtblau L, Sparber SB (1981a): Opiate withdrawal in utero increases neonatal morbidity in the rat. Science 212:943–945.

Lichtblau L, Sparber SB (1981b): Outcome of pregnancy in rats chronically exposed to l-α-acetylmethadol (LAAM). J Pharmacol Exp Ther 218:303–308.

Lichtblau L, Sparber SB (1984): Opioids and development: A perspective on experimental models and methods. Neurobehav Toxicol Teratol 6:3–8.

Loughlin SE, Massamiri TR, Kornblum HI, Leslie FM (1985): Postnatal development of opioid systems in rat brain. Neuropeptides 5:469–472.

McDowell J, Kitchen I (1987): Development of opioid systems: Peptides, receptors and pharmacology. Brain Res Rev 12:397–421.

McGinty JF, Ford DH (1976): The effects of maternal morphine or methadone intake on the growth, reflex development and maze behavior of rat offspring. in Ford, DH, Clouet DH (eds): "Tissue Responses to Addictive Drugs." New York: Spectrum Publishing, pp 611–629.

McGinty JF, Ford DH (1980): Effects of prenatal methadone on rat brain catecholamines. Dev Neurosci 3:224–234.

McLaughlin PJ, Zagon IS (1980): Body and organ development of young rats maternally exposed to methadone. Biol Neonate 38:185–196.

McLaughlin PJ, Zagon IS, White WJ (1978): Perinatal methadone exposure in rats: Effects on body and organ development. Biol Neonate 34:48–54.

Meyerson BJ (1982): Neonatal β-endorphin and sexual behavior. Acta Phys Scand 115:159–160.

Meyerson BJ (1985): Influence of early β-endorphin treatment on the behavior and reaction to β-endorphin in the adult male rat. Psychoendocrinology 10:135–147.

Meyerson BJ, Berg M, Johansson B (1988): Neonatal naltrexone treatment: Effects on sexual and exploratory behavior in male and female rats. Pharmacol Biochem Behav 31:63–67.

O'Callaghan JP, Holtzman SG (1976): Prenatal administration of morphine to the rat: Tolerance to the analgesic effect of morphine in the offspring. J Pharmacol Exp Ther 197:533–544.

Otani S, Matsui-Yuasa I, Goto H, Moriwasa S (1990): Effects of Ca2+ ionophore A23187, 1,2-dioctanoylglycerol, and dibutyryl cAMP on the activity and expression of ornithine decarboxylase in guinea pig lymphocytes. J Biochem 107:526–529.

Persitz E, Benalal D, Bachrach U, No-Yoseph S (1984): Effect of maternal pethidine administration on neonatal brain cyclic AMP levels and ornithine decarboxylase activities. Biochem Pharmacol 33:1816–1818.

Peters MA, Turnbow M, Buchenauer D (1972): The distribution of methadone in nonpregnant, pregnant, and fetal rat after acute methadone treatment. J Pharmacol Exp Ther 181:273–278.

Raye JR, Dubin JW, Blechner JN (1977): Fetal growth retardation following maternal morphine administration: Nutritional or drug effect? Biol Neonate 32:222–228.

Ricalde AA, Hammer RP (1990): Perinatal opiate treatment delays growth of cortical dendrites. Neurosci Lett 115:137–143.

Rogers NF, El-Fakahany EE (1986): Morphine-induced opioid receptor down-regulation detected in intact adult rat brain cells. Eur J Pharmacol 124:221–230.

Russell DH (1981): Ornithine decarboxylase: A key regulatory protein. Med Biol 59:286–295.

Seidler FJ, Whitmore WL, Slotkin TA (1982): Delays in growth and biochemical development of rat brain caused by maternal methadone administration: Are the alterations in synaptogenesis and cellular maturation independent of reduced maternal food intake. Dev Neurosci 5:13–18.

Shah NS, Alexander DG (1979): Pharmacological effects and metabolic fate of levomethadone during postnatal development in rat. J Pharmacol Exp Ther 208:491–497.

Sirinathsinghji DJS, Motta M, Martini L (1985): Induction of precocious puberty in the female rat after chronic naloxone administration during the neonatal period: The opiate 'brake' on prepubertal gonadotrophin secretion. J Endocrinol 104:299–307.

Slotkin TA (1979): Ornithine decarboxylase as a tool in developmental neurobiology. Life Sci 24:1623–1630.

Slotkin TA (1988): Perinatal exposure to methadone: How do early biochemical alterations cause neurofunctional disturbances? Prog Brain Res 73:265–279.

Slotkin TA, Anderson TR (1975): Sympatho-adrenal development in perinatally addicted rats. Addictive Diseases 2:293–306.

Slotkin TA, Lau C, Bartolomé M (1976): Effects of neonatal or maternal methadone administration on ornithine decarboxylase activity in brain and heart of developing rats. J Pharmacol Exp Ther 199:141–148.

Slotkin TA, Seidler FJ, Whitmore WL (1980): Effects of maternal methadone administration on ornithine decarboxylase in brain and heart of the offspring: Relationships of enzyme activity to dose and to growth impairment in the rat. Life Sci 26:861–867.

Slotkin TA, Weigel SJ, Barnes GA, Whitmore WL, Seidler FJ (1981): Alterations in the development of catecholamine turnover induced by perinatal methadone: Differences in central vs. peripheral sympathetic nervous systems. Life Sci 29:2519–2525.

Slotkin TA, Weigel SJ, Whitmore WL, Seidler FJ (1982): Maternal methadone administration: Deficit in development of alpha-noradrenergic responses in developing rat brain as assessed by norepinephrine stimulation of $^{32}P_i$ incorporation into phospholipids in vivo. Biochem Pharmacol 31:1899–1902.

Slotkin TA, Whitmore WL, Salvaggio M, Seidler FJ (1979): Perinatal methadone addiction affects brain synaptic development of biogenic amine systems in the rat. Life Sci 24:1223–1230.

Smith AA, Hui FW, Crofford MJ (1977): Inhibition of growth in young mice treated with d,l-methadone. Eur J Pharmacol 43:307–314.

Spain JW, Roth BL, Coscia CJ (1985): Differential ontogeny of multiple opioid receptors (μ, ∂, and κ). J Neurosci 5:584–588.

Sparber SB (1986): Developmental effects of narcotics. Neurotoxicology 7:335–348.

Steece KA, DeLeon-Jones FA, Meyerson LR, Lee JM, Fields JZ, Ritzmann RF (1986): In vivo down-regulation of rat striatal opioid receptors by chronic enkephalin. Brain Res Bull 17:255–257.

Steele WJ, Jóhannesson T (1975a): Effects of morphine infusion in maternal rats at near-term on ribosome size distribution in foetal and maternal rat brain. Acta Pharmacol Toxicol 36:236–242.

Steele WJ, Jóhannesson T (1975b): Effects of prenatally administered morphine on brain development and resultant tolerance to the analgesic effect of morphine in offspring of morphine treated rats. Acta Pharmacol Toxicol 36:243–256.

Tao PL, Law PY, Loh HH (1987): Decrease in delta and mu opioid receptor binding capacity in rat brain after chronic etorphine treatment. J Pharmacol Exp Ther 240:809–816.

Tempel A, Habas J, Parcdes W, Barr G (1988): Morphine-induced downregulation of μ-opioid receptors in neonatal rat brain. Dev Brain Res 41:129–133.

Tiong GKL, Olley JE (1988): Effects of exposure in utero to methadone and buprenorphine on enkephalin levels in the developing rat brain. Neurosci Lett 93:101–106.

Tsang D, Ho KP, Wen HL (1986): Effect of maternal methadone administration on the development of multiple forms of monoamine oxidase in rat brain and liver. Dev Brain Res 26:187–192.

Tsang D, Ng SC (1980): Effect of antenatal exposure to opiates on the development of opiate receptors in rat brain. Brain Res 188:199–206.

Tsang D, Ng SC, Ho KP (1982a): Development of methionine-enkephalin and naloxone binding sites in regions of rat brain. Dev Brain Res 3:637–644.

Tsang D, Ng SC, Ho KP, Ho WKK (1982b): Ontogenesis of opiate binding sites and radioimmunoassayable β-endorphin and enkephalin in regions of rat brain. Dev Brain Res 5:257–261.

Umans JG, Szeto HH (1985): Precipitated opiate abstinence in utero. Am J Obstet Gynecol 151:441–444.

Vértes Z, Melegh G, Vértes M, Kovács S (1982): Effect of naloxone and D-Met^2-Pro^5-enkephalinamide treatment on the DNA synthesis in the developing rat brain. Life Sci 31:119–126.

Wang C, Pasulka P, Perry B, Pizzi WJ, Schnoll SH (1986): Effect of perinatal exposure to methadone on brain opioid and α_2-adrenergic receptors. Neurobehav Toxicol Teratol 8:399–402.

White WJ, McLaughlin PJ, Zagon IS (1978): Effects of chronic methadone treatment on maternal body weight and food and water consumption in rats. Pharmacology 17:227–232.

Windh RT, Kuhn CM (1990): Mu tolerance in ontogeny: Antinociceptive studies. Soc Neurosci Abstr 16:1028.

Zadina JE, Kastin AJ (1986): Neonatal peptides affect developing rats: β-endorphin alters nociception and opiate receptors, corticotropin-releasing factor alters corticosterone. Dev Brain Res 29:21–29.

Zadina JE, Kastin AJ, Coy DH, Adinoff BA (1985): Developmental, behavioral, and opiate receptor changes after prenatal or postnatal β-endorphin, CRF, or Tyr-MIF-1. Psychoneuroendocrinology 10:367–383.

Zadina JE, Kastin AJ, Manasco PK, Pignatiello MF, Nastiak KL (1987): Long-term hyperalgesia induced by neonatal β-endorphin and morphiceptin is blocked by neonatal Tyr-MIF-1. Brain Res 409:10–19.

Zagon IS, McLaughlin PJ (1978): Perinatal methadone exposure and brain development: A biochemical study. J Neurochem 31:49–54.

Zagon IS, McLaughlin PJ (1980): Protracted analgesia in young and adult rats maternally exposed to methadone. Experimentia 36:329–330.

Zagon IS, McLaughlin PJ (1982): Analgesia in young and old rats perinatally exposed to methadone. Neurobehav Toxicol Teratol 4:455–457.

Zagon IS, McLaughlin PJ (1985): Opioid antagonist-induced regulation of organ development. Physiol Behav 34:507–511.

Zagon IS, McLaughlin PJ (1987): Endogenous opioid systems regulate cell proliferation in the developing rat brain. Brain Res 412:68–72.

Zagon IS, McLaughlin PJ (1989): Naloxone modulates body and organ growth of rats: Dependency on the duration of opioid receptor blockade and stereospecificity. Pharmacol Biochem Behav 33:325–328.

Zagon IS, McLaughlin PJ (1990a): Opioid antagonist (naltrexone) stimulation of cell proliferation in human and animal neuroblastoma and human fibrosarcoma cells in culture. Neuroscience 37:223–226.

Zagon IS, McLaughlin PJ (1990b): Ultrastructural localization of enkephalin-like immunoreactivity in developing rat cerebellum. Neuroscience 34:479–489.

Zagon IS, Gibo DM, McLaughlin PJ (1990a): Adult and developing cerebella exhibit different profiles of opioid binding sites. Brain Res 523:62–68.

Zagon IS, Goodman SR, McLaughlin PJ (1989a): Characterization of zeta: A new opioid receptor involved in growth. Brain Res 482:297–305.

Zagon IS, Goodman SR, McLaughlin PJ (1990b): Demonstration and characterization of zeta, a growth-related opioid receptor, in a neuroblastoma cell line. Brain Res 511: 181–186.

Zagon IS, Zagon E, McLaughlin PJ (1989b): Opioids and the developing organism: A comprehensive bibiography, 1984–1988. Neurosci Biobehav Rev 13:207–235.

Zukin RS, Sugarman JR, Fitz-Syage ML, Gardner EL, Zukin SR, Gintzler AR (1982): Naltrexone-induced opiate receptor supersensitivity. Brain Res. 245:285–292.

Zukin RS, Tempel A (1986): Neurochemical correlates of opiate receptor regulation. Biochem Pharmacol 35:1623–1627.

Development of the Central Nervous System:
Effects of Alcohol and Opiates, pages 363–377

16

Prenatal Ethanol Exposure: Endogenous Opioid Systems, Inappropriate Emotional Responsiveness, and Autism

WILLIAM J. SHOEMAKER, PRISCILLA KEHOE, AND
ROSS A. BAKER
*Department of Psychiatry, University of Connecticut Health Center,
Farmington, Connecticut (W.J.S., R.A.B.); Psychobiology Laboratory,
Trinity College, Hartford, Connecticut (P.K.)*

INTRODUCTION

Prenatal alcohol exposure produces a constellation of behavioral and anatomical alterations in affected offspring termed fetal alcohol syndrome (FAS) (Rosett and Weiner, 1984; West, 1986). A number of studies have been carried out that report neurotransmitter alterations in the central nervous system of experimental animals exposed to ethanol prenatally (Chapter 7). This chapter will deal with the effects of prenatal alcohol on the endogenous opioid systems of the brain, especially β-endorphin.

The pro-opiomelanocortin (POMC) derived peptides, including β-endorphin, may serve as trophic substances in the developing mammalian brain (van Ree et al., 1981; Swaab et al., 1976). β-endorphin can be detected as early as embryonic day 13 in the rat (Bayon et al., 1979; Khachaturian et al., 1983, 1985); the mRNA for POMC can be detected by in situ hybridization on embryonic day 10 in mice (Elkabes et al., 1989). Thus, even before these peptides can function in behaviorally organized neuronal networks, they can play a role in the processes of neuronal genesis, migration, and synapse formation. (Miller, 1988; see also Chapter 4).

This chapter will focus on the postnatal behavioral functions of endogenous opioid systems in animal models and human infants. Such behaviors range from relief from distress or calming to mediating pleasurable sensations and euphoria, possibly leading to addictive behavior. We will discuss some recent studies on the activation of neuronal circuits that result in β-endorphin being released in specific regions of the brain. The discussion will then describe the effects of prenatal alcohol on the activation of opioid peptide systems, which suggest that such exposure produces a system which appears to be *hyporesponsive* when activated. Subsequently, we will expand on that concept by making comparisons to the behavior of FAS children. A second aspect of this chapter will explore the responsivity of prenatally exposed animals to exogenously administered opiate agonists and antagonists. In short, these animals are *hyperresponsive*. It appears that a subset of children with FAS—those with concomitant autism—may also present as being supersensitive to the opiate antagonist, naltrexone. Implicit in this hypothesis is that a major aspect of the pathophysiology in FAS involves the endogenous opioid systems. From such a hypothesis we can derive some ideas about possible therapeutic treatment for all children with FAS.

PRENATAL ALCOHOL'S EFFECTS ON OPIOID PEPTIDES

The endogenous opioid peptide, β-endorphin, is markedly increased in the midbrain and hindbrain (but not forebrain) of newborn (Shoemaker et al., 1983) and adult (Baker and Shoemaker, 1988) rats which were fetally exposed to ethanol (Fig. 1; see Vavrousek-Jakuba et al., 1991, for details of raising rats prenatally exposed to ethanol using liquid diets fed during gestation). In a study using ethanol exposure by inhalation, Nelson et al. (1988) reported that the offspring of exposed dams had increased β-endorphin levels in several brain regions at 21 days of age. Weinberg et al. (1986) confirmed the earlier report of increased levels of β-endorphin at birth using ethanol-containing liquid diets fed to the dams, but found the increases to be present in all brain regions. Nelson et al. (1988) also reported both marked increases and decreases in met-enkephalin, another opioid neuropeptide, depending on ethanol dose and brain region. The increases in met-enkephalin agree with an earlier report by McGivern et al. (1983) in which both leu- and met-enkephalin were increased in rats after prenatal ethanol.

In a recent study, our laboratory has explored whether differences in β-endorphin levels are due to changes in the number of neuronal cell bodies containing β-endorphin, changes in the distribution and density of endorphin-containing nerve terminals, or changes in the physiological responsiveness of this brain system. A quantitative, histological analysis of β-endorphin neurons was performed using immunocytochemical staining with antisera specifically directed against β-endorphin. The results demonstrated that prenatal ethanol exposure does *not* change the number of β-endorphin-containing neurons in the brain (Baker and Shoemaker, 1991a). Our attention then turned to the terminal regions of β-endorphin-containing fibers. We had noticed, both in our own data and those of other's, a great deal of variance within groups of β-endorphin levels in terminal regions (Shoemaker et al., 1983; Perry et al., 1984; Bronstein et al., 1990). Although statistical significance between alcohol-exposed and control groups was frequently achieved, this was due more to the magnitude of the effect than to the tight clustering of values around means of experimental and control groups. The wide variance was seen in alcohol-exposed groups and both control groups (chow pellet

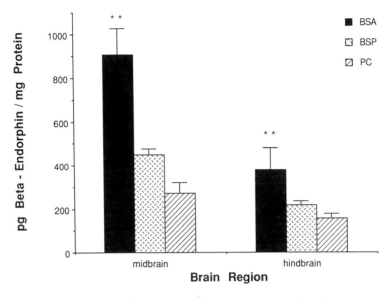

Fig. 1. Levels of β-endorphin in the midbrain (including the diencephalon) and hindbrain (pons and medulla) of prenatally ethanol-exposed adult rats and their controls. Data are expressed as mean $\pm$ SEM concentration of β-endorphin as determined by radioimmunoassay. BSA (n = 6, black bar) represents adult offspring of dams fed 5% ethanol (vol) in a liquid diet from embryonic day 7 through parturition. BSP (n = 17, stippled bar) represents adult offspring of dams pair-fed the same liquid diet as BSA, except maltose/dextrin is substituted isocalorically for ethanol. PC (n = 7, lined bar) represents offspring of dams fed a standard laboratory rat chow throughout gestation. For a detailed description of diet composition and administration, see Vavrousek-Jakuba et al., 1991. Asterisks indicate that the mean level of β-endorphin is significantly higher (ANOVA, $P < 0.01$) in adult rats exposed to ethanol during gestation than in control rats unexposed to ethanol.

controls as well as liquid diet without alcohol controls). Several investigators have reported that footshock stress alters brain β-endorphin levels (Rossier et al., 1977; Millan et al., 1981; Vendite et al., 1985). This indicated that the widespread assumption of steady-state levels of the opioid peptides may need to be re-evaluated. We then devised a study to measure brain β-endorphin in treated and control rats under conditions where stress, handling, and arousal were held to a minimum. Under these tightly controlled conditions, levels of β-endorphin in offspring of ethanol-treated dams were not significantly different from pair-fed and chow pellet controls (Fig. 2). This finding has been replicated several times now; the conclusion is clear—when the animals are in a non-stressed, non-aroused condition, levels of β-endorphin are not altered by prenatal ethanol exposure. These data led to the conclusion that prenatal ethanol alters neither the number of β-endorphin neurons nor the steady-state levels of the neuropeptide in cell body regions or in terminal regions. It appears that the previously reported dramatic increases in β-endorphin in alcohol-exposed pups and adults may be related to the animal's response to stress. This issue is particularly important in as much as precautions to minimize stressful conditions were not always followed in the earlier studies. Therefore, we investigated the response characteristics of the β-endorphin system to standardized stresses.

In the first study, rats were removed from their cage and placed in a footshock box for 30 seconds. They received a shock of 0.8 mAmp to the grid floor for the last 5 seconds of the session. At the end of the 30 second session, the rat was returned to a holding cage until it was removed for decapitation in an adjoining room. Baseline controls were handled for 14 days but not placed in the footshock box. Animals were sacrificed either 3, 10, or 30 minutes after the footshock. The brains were dissected rapidly into seven regions and frozen for determination of β-endorphin by radioimmunoassay.

The results of this study are presented in Table I and Figure 3. Certain brain regions, namely, the septal region, respond to the stress with signifi-

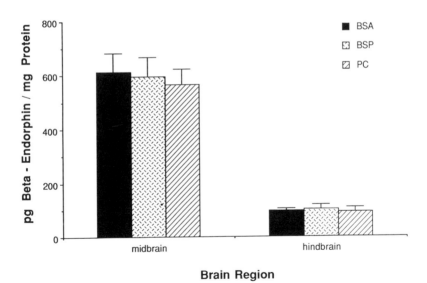

Brain Region

Fig. 2. Levels of β-endorphin in the midbrain (including the diencephalon) and hindbrain (pons and medulla) of prenatally ethanol-exposed adult rats (BSA, n = 24, black bars), their pair-fed controls (BSP, n = 6, stippled bars), and normally fed controls (PC, n = 6 lined bars). Data are expressed as described in Figure 1. Rats are of approximately the same age as those shown in Figure 1; however, in this experiment, the rats were sacrificed immediately after removal from the home cage in order to minimize stress. No difference in level of β-endorphin is evident in either brain region for any of the three experimental groups.

cantly decreased β-endorphin at 3 minutes post-stress; other regions show the same tendency for decreased β-endorphin. We interpret this decrease as resulting from secretion or release of the peptide. In rats sacrificed 10 and 30 minutes post-stress, β-endorphin had returned to levels not significantly different from baseline. Other regions (the amygdala, hypothalamus less the arcuate nucleus, and the midbrain) respond only slightly. Data from the septal region, a responsive area, and the amygdala, a non-responsive area, are plotted in curves versus time in Figure 3 to better visualize these responses. The arcuate region is a very small area at the base of the hypothalamus and contains all of the cell bodies which synthesize brain β-endorphin (i.e., the other six regions represent sites of high β-endorphin fiber or terminal density). The response in the arcuate is unlike the terminal regions in that it may reflect post-release peptide processing in the cell body coincident with the release that is occurring in many of the terminal regions.

A corollary study (Baker and Shoemaker, 1991b) examined the effect of prenatal exposure to ethanol on the post-stress release of β-endorphin. All testing was done on adults and both mild (5 second-footshock) and prolonged (30 second-footshock) acute stressors were used. The results from these studies indicate that the offspring of ethanol-fed dams did not differ from controls when tested with the mild stressor, but they were hyporesponsive in β-endorphin release for the more prolonged (30 second-footshock) stressor. That is, 3 minutes after the stress, those brain regions that normally contain decreased peptide levels in the control groups, remained unchanged in the ethanol-exposed group. This pattern of β-endorphin unresponsiveness or hyporesponsiveness in the offspring of ethanol-fed dams is parallel to the behavioral unresponsiveness described below in the 10-day-old offspring of the ethanol-fed dams.

TABLE I. Change in β-Endorphin After Footshock Stress in Different Brain Regions

Brain region	Mean unstressed level (ng peptide/mg protein)	Minutes post-stress (% of unstressed level)		
		3	10	30
Septal region	0.52 ± 0.08	47[a]	76	110
Amygdala	0.16 ± 0.01	109	112	107
Hypothalamus	2.55 ± 0.14	113	114	124
Thalamus	0.59 ± 0.08	90	96	123
Midbrain	0.30 ± 0.02	103	114	115
Medulla/pons	0.20 ± 0.03	80	96	110
Arcuate nucleus				
ng/mg protein	12.43 ± 1.83	126	165	193
ng/tissue	3.87 ± 0.58	143	191	131

[a]Significantly decreased over unstressed; see Figure 3 for methods and statistical analysis.

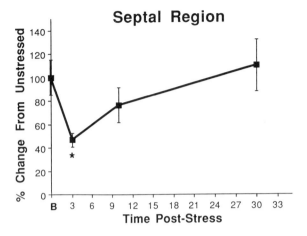

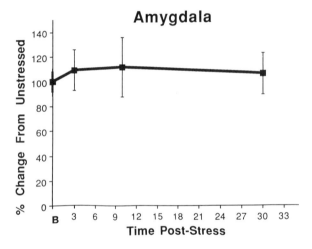

Fig. 3. Change in level of β-endorphin peptide following 5 second-footshock stress. The mean level of β-endorphin for unstressed rats, handled daily for 14 days prior to experiment, is calculated for each of the 3 consecutive days of the experiment. The percent deviation from the daily mean for individual rats tested on each experimental day is then calculated and the mean (100%) is plotted as the unstressed baseline ± the SEM, indicated by the dark line on the Y axis. On each experimental day, the percent change of each stressed rat from the daily mean is calculated, and the mean percent change with SEM is plotted. Time post-stress reflects the time between termination of the stress and sacrifice, and the baseline unstressed level (B) is equated to 100% for each of the three different experimental groups. In the septal region, at 3 minutes post-stress, the percent β-endorphin levels compared to unstressed levels is significantly different (denoted by *, $P < 0.05$ by ANOVA), while in the amygdala there is no change in the percent β-endorphin levels compared to unstressed levels at any time post-stress. This method of normalizing baseline β-endorphin levels to 100% and comparing the percent of stressed to unstressed levels was followed for all brain regions studied (see Table I).

PRENATAL ALCOHOL EFFECTS ON OPIOID-MEDIATED BEHAVIORS

Recent research has described the development of neonatal behaviors that are dependent on endogenous opioid systems for their normal expression (Kehoe, 1988; Kehoe and Harris, 1989). These opioid-mediated behavioral systems appear to play a role in adaptation to stressful situations and learnedaffectional behaviors. Moreover, children diagnosed with FAS have difficulty in learning and adjusting their behavior to specific situations (Streissguth and Randels, 1988); thus, it appeared logical to test neonates that are prenatally exposed to ethanol for behaviors that are opioid mediated. The responsiveness of prenatally ethanol exposed 10-day-old rat pups to opioid-mediated behaviors was tested by measuring isolation-induced vocalizations and subsequent morphine- and stress-induced analgesia. Morphine, an opiate that mimics the effects of the endogenous peptides, has been shown to suppress isolation-induced vocalizations and reduce pain sensitivity (Kehoe and Blass, 1986a, b, c). In addition, the effect of naltrexone, an opioid receptor antagonist that increases ultrasonic vocalizations and increases pain sensitivity of the isolate, was also examined. These opiate agonist and antagonist drugs assist us in defining the status of the endogenous opioid systems following prenatal treatments.

The behavioral studies were carried out on 10-day-old offspring of mothers that were fed either a 5.0% ethanol-containing liquid diet (BSA), pair-fed an isocaloric non-alcoholic form of the same liquid diet (BSP), or fed a diet of a control chow (PC) pellets (Kehoe and Shoemaker, 1991). All mammalian infants who are separated from their parents and siblings emit vocalizations, a quantifiable emotional behavior, in response to separation. Neonatal rats, under a variety of social and thermal conditions, vocalize in the ultrasonic range of 30–50 KHz, beyond the range of human hearing (Allin and Banks, 1972; Noirot, 1972). Therefore, 15 minutes after saline, naltrexone, or morphine injection, pups were isolated for 15 minutes in an environmental chamber with clean bedding at 32°C. During this 15 minutes the pups' ultrasonic vocalizations, made audible through a QMC Instruments Bat Detector, were counted and recorded. The rat pups were then tested for pain responsivity on a hot plate at 48°C. All tests were done by experimenters who were blind to pup's prenatal diet or postnatal drug treatment. All pups, isolated or not, were tested for responsivity to heat. Those pups not isolated were injected with saline, morphine, or naltrexone, returned to the nest for 15 minutes, and then taken directly from the nest for analgesia testing.

Prenatal exposure to ethanol significantly affects the number of vocalizations emitted by the pup (Fig. 4; Kehoe and Shoemaker, 1991). Ethanol-exposed pups that were given saline vocalized considerably less than the two control groups. The reduction in calling behavior by pups prenatally exposed to ethanol was also seen in pups pretreated with morphine. In contrast to saline and morphine pretreatments, naltrexone treatment reduced calling in both pair-fed (BSP) and ethanol (BSA) groups when compared to chow controls (PC). The vocalization results in the BSA-exposed group would appear to be a combination of the ethanol exposure and the concomitant undernutrition that accompanies it, since the pair-fed control group does display some deficiency in calling behavior, provoked by blocking opioid receptors with naltrexone.

As in adult rats, endogenous opioid systems also appear to be involved when neonates respond to pain and stress. Stress caused by isolation from mother and sibs produces an analgesia that is blocked by the opiate antagonist naltrexone (Kehoe and Blass, 1986a, b, c). The effect of prenatal exposure to ethanol on isolation-induced analgesia, with and without the opiate active drugs, can be seen in Figure 5 (Kehoe and Shoemaker, 1991). Here, PC and BSP groups present a similar profile of a doubling of paw-lift latency after isolation, as well as a return to non-isolated levels with naltrexone. The ethanol-exposed pups (BSA group), however, fail to show an isolation-induced increase in paw-lift latency. Since the change in pain threshold is naltrexone-reversible, it appears that the alcohol-exposed pups may be deficient in the opioid mediation of this analgesic response to isolation. That is, ethanol-exposed rats are hyporesponsive both neurochemically and behaviorally to an environmental stress.

COMPARISON BETWEEN BEHAVIORS IN ANIMAL MODELS AFTER PRENATAL ETHANOL AND FAS CHILDREN

Chen et al. (1982) described altered suckling behaviors in rat pups prenatally exposed to ethanol. The exposed pups displayed longer latencies to attach to the nipple, as well as failure to shift from one nipple to another

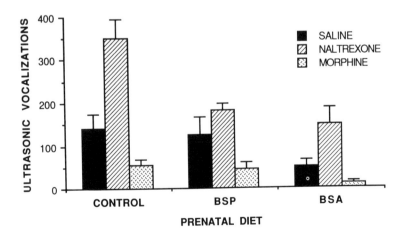

Fig. 4. Mean number of ultrasonic vocalizations for each prenatal treatment group (chow-pellet control, pair-fed BSP, and alcohol diet BSA) monitored on postnatal day 10 during 5 minutes of isolation, 15 minutes after receiving an intraperitoneal injection of saline, naltrexone (0.5 mg/kg body weight), or morphine (0.5 mg/kg body weight). (Reproduced from Kehoe and Shoemaker, 1991, with permission.)

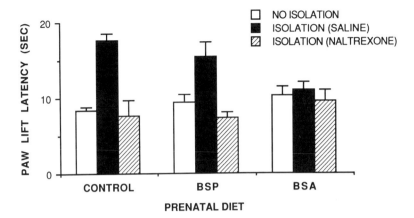

Fig. 5. Mean paw removal latency (sec) from a 48°C hot plate for each prenatal treatment group (chow-pellet control, pair-fed BSP, and alcohol diet BSA) tested either directly from the nest (no isolation) or at the end of the 5 minute isolation period prior to which an injection of saline or naltrexone (0.5 mg/kg body weight) had been administered. (Reproduced from Kehoe and Shoemaker, 1991, with permission.)

(Riley and Rockwood, 1984). These findings are analogous to the results of early developmental studies of humans which report a variety of feeding difficulties in infants of chronic alcoholics (Ouellette et al., 1977; Ulleland, 1972). Martin et al. (1979) studied a large group of children with FAS and described their suckling behavior as being delayed and displaying a weak suck. Moreover, studies with rats exposed to ethanol during gestation document hyperactivity from 12–76 days of age (Bond and DiGiusto, 1976; Branchey and Friedhoff, 1979; Shaywitz et al., 1979), increased exploratory behavior independent of general activity even up to adulthood (Riley, 1982; Riley et al., 1986), deficits in spontaneous alternation (Abel, 1982; Riley et al., 1979), passive avoidance learning (Lochry and Riley 1980), and an increased startle reaction (Anadem et al., 1980). According to Riley (1982), all of these behaviors have in common a deficit of inhibitory responsiveness. Long-term studies of FAS children indicate that these children have difficulty in learning from experience, adjusting their behavior to specific situations, and do not respond normally to punishment, even as young adults (Streissguth and Randels, 1988). Additionally, in the Ainsworth "strange-situation" procedure (Ainsworth et al., 1978), human infants exposed to moderate and high levels of alcohol prenatally show greater disorganized behavior and more insecure attachment behavior than infants not exposed to ethanol prenatally (O'Connor et al., 1987).

Another animal model of FAS that has been extensively studied utilizes pigtailed macaques, in which pregnant females receive weekly doses of ethanol during gestation. Since the developmental profile and behavioral repertoire of this non-human primate may more closely model the human situation, the behavioral and neurochemical results are particularly interesting. Furthermore, the once-a-week dosing of ethanol in this study approximates "binge" drinking, a common pattern for female drinkers. This primate model has been studied with regard to pregnancy outcome (Clarren et al., 1987), physical and behavioral development (Clarren et al., 1988), and neuroanatomical and neurochemical abnormalities of the dopamine system (Clarren et al., 1990). Of interest here is that the offspring exposed to even moderate doses (< 2.0 gm/kg once a week) exhibit developmental delays in tests of object permanence, visual recognition, and motor development (Clarren et al., 1988). Higher prenatal doses are associated with increased deviation from control means. Most of the more than 30 offspring in the study had no physical stigmata resulting from the prenatal ethanol. The picture that emerges from both the rodent and primate studies is quite similar to a description of the fundamental neurological and developmental abnormalities seen in individuals with attention deficit disorder, a condition in children characterized by poor impulse control, distractibility, and hyperactivity. Furthermore, Nanson and Hiscock (1990) demonstrated that although FAS/FAE children are more impaired intellectually, their attentional deficits and behavioral problems are similar to children with attention deficit disorder.

The question posed here is whether there is a link between the failure of animals prenatally exposed to ethanol to respond to normal environmental stimuli, as measured by opioid-mediated behaviors and β-endorphin secretion, and the attention deficits exhibited by FAS children.

RESPONSIVENESS TO ADMINISTERED OPIATES IN PRENATALLY EXPOSED ANIMALS

In our studies of prenatal ethanol exposure on opioid-mediated responses, a curious finding appeared. We observed that the administration of morphine to rats exposed to ethanol in utero elicits a response greater than that in controls (Kehoe and Shoemaker, 1991). This hyperresponsiveness to morphine occurs even though the ethanol-exposed group is deficient in the secretion of its own endogenous opioids. A good example of this phenomenon is depicted in Figure 6. Offspring from the three treatment groups were given morphine alone or with 5 minutes isolation. Notice that in the ethanol-exposed (BSA) pups, the analgesia due to morphine alone is greater than that seen in controls. At the same time, the effect of the isolation-induced analgesia (presumed to result from endogenous opioid secretion) produces a significant enhancement of morphine analgesia only in controls.

In the vocalization behaviors in which morphine quiets the pups crying, the ethanol-exposed (BSA) pups are quieted significantly more by the morphine treatment than are controls (Fig. 4). The hyperresponsiveness to administered opiates has been described by Nelson el al. (1986), who demonstrate that adult rats prenatally exposed to ethanol exhibit a greater response to morphine on analgesia tests than controls. In addition, Taylor et al. (1988), in a review of maternal alcohol consumption and neuroendo-

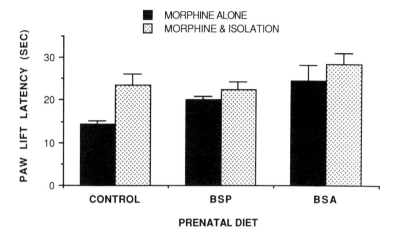

Fig. 6. Mean paw removal latency (sec) from a 48°C hot plate for each prenatal treatment group (chow-pellet control, pair-fed BSP, and alcohol diet BSA) tested after an injection of morphine (0.5 mg/kg body weight) either directly from the nest or following a 5 minute isolation period. (Reproduced from Kehoe and Shoemaker, 1991, with permission.)

crine responsiveness in offspring, summarize their results as demonstrating that prenatal ethanol ". . . leads to enhanced responsiveness of the brain-pituitary-adrenal axis in stress . . ." The combination of *hyporesponsiveness* of endogenous opioid systems to external stimuli and *hyperresponsiveness* to administered opiate is unusual, but could be related physiologically. If the normally encountered stimuli for the secretion of endogenous opioids produce little or no opioid secretion in ethanol prenatally exposed animals, the post-synaptic elements could become supersensitive, as occurs in denervated or transmission-blocked situations with other transmitter systems (Fischbach and Cohen, 1973). A common response to denervation or blocked transmission is an increase in the number of receptors by the post-synaptic cell. At present, since no one has demonstrated that any opiate receptor or binding site is "up-regulated" after prenatal alcohol exposure, the supersensitivity must be manifest by means other than receptor number.

EVIDENCE THAT SOME FAS CHILDREN MAY HAVE ABNORMAL OPIOID RESPONSIVENESS

Recent studies reveal that a subset of FAS children have autism in addition to their FAS symptomatology (Nanson, 1991). Although not commonly considered part of the behavioral profile of FAS children, Nanson reports a dual diagnosis of FAS and autism in six children. Conceivably, the numbers may be greater since the overwhelming behavioral disturbances of autism may have masked the diagnosis of FAS in other cases. The connection between FAS children with autism and the endogenous opioid systems is supported by a number of recent reports of beneficial results with naltrexone, the opiate antagonist, in the treatment of autism. Herman et al. (1987) reported that the self-injurious behavior in three severe autistic children was markedly reduced with naloxone treatment. Self-injurious behavior is one of the most damaging and difficult to treat symptoms in autism. Sandman et al. (1983) have reported that naloxone attenuates self-abusive behavior in developmentally disabled adults.

It is appealing to speculate that self-injurious behavior is an attempt by the individual to stimulate the pleasure-sensing aspects of endogenous opiate secretion. In this view, this behavior of the autistic individual may be related to an addiction to its own endogenous opioids. Three factors can be cited as fitting with our animal model derived hypothesis. First, the stimuli usually encountered by the individual in its daily activity would not produce sufficient endogenous opioid release. More potent stimuli would be needed (like head banging or other self-injurious behavior) in order to produce the normal tone of β-endorphin release. Second, in the prenatally ethanol exposed offspring, β-endorphin producing cell bodies increase the levels of the peptides following stress (Baker and Shoemaker, 1991b). The increased peptide levels in cell body regions may be related to the reduced release of β-endorphin in the terminals. In ethanol-exposed offspring of our rat study, in addition to the failure to respond by releasing from terminals at 3 minutes, increased levels of β-endorphin were noted at 30 minutes post-stress. The accumulated levels of β-endorphin in the terminals may eventually respond to very potent stimuli, thereby flooding the synapse with large amounts of β-endorphin. If such a situation occurs in FAS autistic children, it is possible that the frequent use of self-injurious behavior is an attempt to gain pleasure from their endogenous stores of opioid peptide. Naltrexone would then be an effective treatment since this drug dissociates the release of stored peptide from the pleasurable response triggered by the receptor action. Third, while naltrexone has only minimal effect on normal healthy subjects, the more profound effect in these individuals could also be due to the supersensitivity of their opioid system that results from the lack of normal tonal release.

While there is still much speculation in the interpretation of the human studies, it is hoped that additional research, both basic and clinical, would lead to more effective treatments for all of those born with FAS.

REFERENCES

Abel EL (1982): In utero alcohol exposure and developmental delay of response inhibition. Alcohol Clin Exp Res 6:369–376.

Ainsworth MDS, Blehar MC, Waters E, Wall S (1978): "Patterns of Attachment." Hillsdale, NJ: Lawrence Erlbaum Associates.

Allin JT, Banks EM (1972): Functional aspects of ultrasound production by infant albino rats (Rattus norvegicus) Anim Behav 20:175–185.

Anandam N, Feleg W, Stern JM (1980): In utero alcohol heightens juvenile reactivity. Pharmacol Biochem Behav 13:531–535.

Baker RA, Shoemaker WJ (1991a): β-endorphin immunoreactive neurons in the hypothalamus and medulla of the rat brain. Effect of prenatal ethanol. Neuroscience (submitted).

Baker RA, Shoemaker WJ (1991b): Effect of prenatal ethanol and stress on brain β-endorphin. Alcohol Clin Exp Res 15:339.

Baker RA, Shoemaker WJ (1988): β-endorphin immunoreactive cells in rats prenatally exposed to ethanol. Abst Soc Neurosci 14:543.

Bayon A, Shoemaker WJ, Bloom FE, Mauss A, Guillemin R (1979): Perinatal development of the endorphin-enkephalin-containing systems in the rat brain. Brain Res 179:93–101.

Bond NW, DiGiusto EL (1976): Effects of prenatal alcohol consumption on open-field behavior and alcohol preference in rats. Psychopharmacology 46:163–168.

Branchey L, Friedhoff AJ (1979): Response perseveration in rats exposed to alcohol prenatally. Pharmacol Biochem Behav 10:255–259.

Bronstein DM, Przewlocki R, Akil H (1990): Effects of morphine treatment on pro-opiomelanocortin systems in rat brain. Brain Res 519:102–111.

Chen JS, Driscoll CD, Riley EP (1982): Ontogeny of suckling behavior in rats exposed to alcohol prenatally. Teratology 26:145–153.

Clarren SK, Astley SJ, Bowden DM, Lai H, Milam AH, Rudeen PK, Shoemaker WJ (1990): Neuroanatomic and neurochemical abnormalities in non-human primate infants exposed to weekly doses of ethanol during gestation. Alcohol Clin Exp Res 14:674–683.

Clarren SK, Astley SJ, Bowden DM (1988): Physical anomalies and developmental delays in non-human primate infants exposed to weekly doses of ethanol during gestation. Teratology 37:561–570.

Clarren SK, Bowden DM, Astley SJ (1987): Pregnancy outcomes after weekly oral administration of ethanol during gestation in pigtailed macaques (Macaca nemestrina). Teratology 35:345–354.

Elkabes S, Peng Loh Y, Nieburgs A, Wray S (1989): Prenatal ontogenesis of proopiomelanocortin in the mouse central nervous system and pituitary gland: An in situ hybridization and immunocytochemical study. Dev Brain Res 46:85–95.

Fischbach GD, Cohen SA (1973): The distribution of acetylcholine sensitivity over uninnervated and innervated muscle fibers grown in cell culture. Dev Biol 31:147–162.

Herman BH, Hammock MK, Arthur-Smith A, Egan J, Chatoor I, Werner A, Zelnik, N (1987): Naltrexone decreases self-injurious behavior. Ann Neurol 22:550–552.

Kehoe P (1988): Opioids, behavior, and learning in mammalian development. In Blass EM (ed): "Developmental Psychobiology and Behavioral Ecology (9th ed.)." New York: Plenum Press, (pp 309–340).

Kehoe P, Blass EM (1986a): Behaviorally functional opioid systems in infant rats: II. Evidence for pharmacological, physiological, and psychological mediation of pain and stress. Behav Neurosci 5:624–630.

Kehoe P, Blass EM (1986b): Central nervous system mediation of positive and negative reinforcement in neonatal albino rats. Dev Brain Res 27:69–75.

Kehoe P, Blass EM (1986c): Opioid-mediation of separation distress in 10-day-old rats: Reversal of stress with maternal stimuli. Dev Psychobiol 19:385–398.

Kehoe P, Harris JC (1989): Ontogeny of noradrenergic effects on ultrasonic vocalizations in rat pups. Behav Neurosci 5:1099–1107.

Kehoe P, Shoemaker WJ (1991): Opioid-dependent behaviors in infant rats: Effects of prenatal exposure to ethanol. Physiol Biochem Behav 39:389–394.

Khachaturian H, Alessi NE, Munfakh N, Watson SJ (1983): Ontogeny of opioid and related peptides in the rat CNS and pituitary: An immunocytochemical study. Life Sci 33(supplement):61–64.

Khachaturian H, Lewis ME, Alessi NE, Watson SJ (1985): Time of origin of opioid peptide-containing neurons in the rat hypothalamus. J Comp Neurol 236:538–546.

Lochry EA, Riley EP (1980): Retension of passive avoidance and T-maze escape in rats exposed to alcohol prenatally. Neurobehav Toxicol 2:107–115.

Martin DC, Martin JC, Streissguth AP, Lund CA (1979): Sucking frequency and amplitude in newborns as a function of maternal drinking and smoking. In Gallanter M (ed): "Currents in Alcoholism (Vol. 5)." New York: Grune and Stratton, pp 359–366.

McGivern RF, Clancy AN, Mousa S, Couri D, Noble EP (1983): Prenatal alcohol exposure alters enkephalin levels without affecting ethanol preference. Life Sci 34:585–590.

Millan MJ, Przewlocki R, Jerlicz M, Gramsch Ch, Hollt V, Herz A (1981): Stress-induced release of brain and pituitary β-endorphin: Major role of endorphins in generation of hyperthermia, not analgesia. Brain Res 208:325–338.

Miller MW (1988): Effect of prenatal exposure to ethanol on the development of cerebral cortex: I. neuronal generation. Alcohol Clin Exp Res 12:440–449.

Nanson JL (1991): Autism in fetal alcohol syndrome: A report of six cases. Alcohol Clin Exp Res (in press).

Nanson JL, Hiscock M (1990): Attention deficits in children exposed to alcohol prenatally. Alcohol Clin Exp Res 14:656–661.

Nelson BK, Brightwell WS, MacKenzie-Taylor DR, Burg JR, Massari VJ (1988): Neurochemical, but not behavioral, deviations in the offspring of rats following prenatal or paternal inhalation exposure to ethanol. Neurotoxicol Teratol 10:15–22.

Nelson LR, Taylor AN, Lewis JW, Branch BJ, Liebeskind JC (1986): Morphine analgesia potentiated in adult rats prenatally exposed to ethanol. Brain Res 372:234–240.

Noirot E (1972): Ultrasound and maternal behavior in small rodents. Dev Psychobiol 5:371–387.

O'Connor MJ, Sigman M, Brill N (1987): Disorganization of attachment in relation to maternal alcohol consumption. Consult Clin Psychol 55:831–836.

Ouellette EM, Rosett HL, Rosman NP, Weiner L (1977): Adverse effects on offspring of maternal alcohol abuse during pregnancy. N Eng J Med 297:528–530.

Perry MLS, Carrasco MA, Dias RD, Izquierdo I (1984): β-endorphin-like immunoreactivity of brain, pituitary gland and plasma of rats submitted to postnatal protein malnutrition: Effect of behavioral training. Peptides 5:15–20.

Riley EP (1982): Ethanol as a behavioral teratogen: Animal models. In NIAAA Monograph Series 2: Biomedical Processes and Consequences of Alcohol Use, DHHS Pub. #83-1191:311–334.

Riley EP, Barron S, Hannigan JH (1986): Response inhibition deficits following prenatal alcohol exposure: A comparison to the effects of hippocampal lesions in rats. In West JW (ed): Alcohol and Brain Development." New York: Oxford University Press, pp 71–102.

Riley EP, Lochry EA, Shapiro NR, Baldwin J (1979): Response perseveration in rats exposed to alcohol prenatally. Pharmacol Biochem Behav 1:255–259.

Riley EP, Rockwood GA (1984): Alterations in suckling behavior in preweanling rats exposed to alcohol prenatally. Nutr Behav 1:289–299.

Rosett HL, Weiner L (1984): "Alcohol and the Fetus." New York: Oxford University Press.

Rossier J, French ED, Rivier C, Ling N, Guillemin R, Bloom FE (1977): Foot-shock induced stress increases β-endorphin levels in blood but not brain. Nature 270:618–620.

Sandman CA, Datta PC, Barron J (1983): Naloxone attenuates self-abusive behavior in developmentally disabled clients. Appl Res Ment Retard 4:5–11.

Shaywitz BA, Griffieth GG, Warshaw JB (1979): Hyperactivity and cognitive deficits in developing rat pups born to alcoholic mothers: An experimental model of the expanded fetal alcohol syndrome (EFAS). Neurobehav Toxicol 1:113–122.

Shoemaker WJ, Baetge G, Azad R, Sapin V, Bloom FE (1983): Effects of prenatal alcohol exposure on amine and peptide neurotransmitter systems. Monog Neural Sci 9:130–139.

Streissguth AP, Randels S (1988): Long term effects of fetal alcohol syndrome. In Robinson GC, Armstrong RW (eds): "Alcohol and Child/Family Health." Vancouver, BC: University of British Columbia, pp 135–151.

Swaab DF, Visser M, Tilders FJH (1976): Stimulation of intra-uterine growth in rat by α-melanocyte-stimulating hormone. J Endocrinol 70:445–455.

Taylor AN, Branch BJ, Van Zuylen JE, Redci E (1988): Maternal alcohol consumption and stress responsiveness in offspring. In Chrousos G, Loriaux DL, Gold PW (eds): "Mechanisms of Physical and Emotional Stress." New York: Plenum Press, pp 311–317.

Ulleland CN (1972): The offspring of alcoholic mothers. Ann NY Acad Sci 197:167–169.

van Ree JM, Bohus B, Csontos KM, Gispen WH, Greven HM, Nijkamp FP, Opmeer FA, de Rotte GA, van Wimersma Greidanus TB, Witter A, de Wied D (1981): In Ciba Foundation Symposium 81, Peptides of the pars intermedia, 263–276.

Vavrousek-Jakuba E, Baker RA, Shoemaker WJ (1991): Effect of ethanol on maternal and offspring characteristics: Comparison of three liquid diet formulations fed during gestation. Alcohol Clin Exp Res 15:129–135.

Vendite D, Wofchuk S, Souza DO (1985): Effects of undernutrition during suckling on footshock escape behavior and on related neurochemical parameters in rats. J Nutr 115:1418–1424.

Weinberg J, Nelson L, Taylor AN (1986): Hormonal effects of fetal alcohol exposure. In West JR (ed): "Alcohol and Brain Development." New York: Oxford University Press, pp 343–372.

West JR (1986): Alcohol and brain development. New York: Oxford University Press.

Index